T0155813

Evolutionary Anatomy of the Primate Cerebral Cortex

Studies of brain evolution have moved rapidly in recent years, building on the pioneering research of Harry J. Jerison. This book provides state-of-the-art reviews of primate (including human) brain evolution. The book is divided into two sections: the first gives new perspectives on the developmental, physiological, dietary and behavioral correlates of brain enlargement. It has long been recognized however, that brains do not merely enlarge globally as they evolve, but that their cortical and internal organization also changes in a process known as reorganization. Species-specific adaptations therefore have neurological substrates that depend on more than just overall brain size. The second section explores these neurological underpinnings for the senses, adaptations and cognitive abilities that are important for primates. With a prologue by Stephen J. Gould and an epilogue by Harry J. Jerison, this is an important new reference work for all those working on brain evolution in primates.

DEAN FALK is Professor of Anthropology and Adjunct Professor of Psychology at the University at Albany, and an Honorary Professor of Anthropology at the University of Vienna. Her research focuses on early hominids, primate brain evolution, comparative neuroanatomy and the evolution of cognition, language and intelligence. Her previous books include *Braindance: New Discoveries about Human Origins and Brain Evolution* (1992) and *Primate Diversity* (2000).

KATHLEEN R. GIBSON is Professor and Chair of Basic Sciences at the University of Texas, Houston, and Adjunct Professor of Anthropology at Rice University. She is a member of the Executive Board of the American Anthropological Association. She has also co-edited *Language and 'Intelligence' in Monkeys and Apes* (1990), *Tools, Language and Cognition in Human Evolution* (1993), *Mammalian Social Learning* (1999), *Brain Maturation and Cognitive Development: Comparative and Cross-Cultural Perspectives* (1991), and *Modelling the Early Human Mind* (1996).

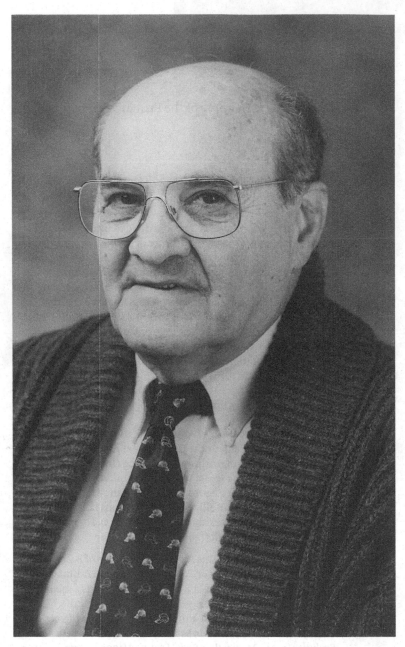

Harry J. Jerison

Evolutionary Anatomy of the Primate Cerebral Cortex

Edited by
DEAN FALK & KATHLEEN R. GIBSON

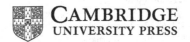

CAMBRIDGE UNIVERSITY PRESS
Cambridge, New York, Melbourne, Madrid, Cape Town, Singapore, São Paulo, Delhi

Cambridge University Press
The Edinburgh Building, Cambridge CB2 8RU, UK

Published in the United States of America by Cambridge University Press, New York

www.cambridge.org
Information on this title: www.cambridge.org/9780521642712

© Cambridge University Press 2001

First published 2001
This digitally printed version 2008

A catalogue record for this publication is available from the British Library

Library of Congress Cataloguing in Publication data
Evolutionary anatomy of the primate cerebral cortex / edited by Dean Falk & Kathleen Gibson.
    p.   cm.
  ISBN 0 521 64271 X
  1. Cerebral cortex – Anatomy. 2. Cerebral cortex – Evolution. I. Falk, Dean. II. Gibson, Kathleen.
  QM455 ·E95 2001
  611′.81–dc21   00-063067

ISBN 978-0-521-64271-2 hardback
ISBN 978-0-521-08995-1 paperback

For Harry and Irene Jerison,
with love, respect, and admiration

Contents

List of contributors

LESLIE C. AIELLO
Department of Anthropology, University College London, Gower Street, London WC1E 6BT, England

NICOLA BATES
Department of Anthropology, University College London, Gower Street, London WC1E 6BT, England

MICHAEL BERAN
3401 Pantherville Road, Decatur, Georgia 30034, USA

FRED L. BOOKSTEIN
Center for Human Growth and Development, University of Michigan, Ann Arbor, Michigan 48109, USA

DOUGLAS C. BROADFIELD
Department of Anthropology, City University of New York, New York, New York 10029, USA

BRUNETTO CHIARELLI
Institute and Museum of Anthropology and Ethnology, University of Florence, Via del Proconsolo 112, 501122 Florence, Italy

GLEN CONROY
Department of Anatomy and Neurobiology, Washington University School of Medicine, St. Louis, Missouri 63110, USA

DEAN FALK
Department of Anthropology, The University at Albany, Albany, New York 12222, USA

BARBARA L. FINLAY
Department of Psychology, Cornell University, Ithaca, New York 14853, USA

PATRICK J. GANNON
Department of Otolaryngology, Mount Sinai School of Medicine, New York, New York 10029, USA

KATHLEEN R. GIBSON
Department of Basic Sciences, University of Texas Houston Health Science Center – Dental Branch, P.O. Box 20068, Houston, Texas 77035, USA

EMMANUEL GILISSEN
Department of Anatomical Sciences, University of the Witwatersrand, Medical School, Wits 2050, 7 York Road, Parktown 2193 Johannesburg, South Africa

STEPHEN J. GOULD
Museum of Comparative Zoology, Harvard University, Cambridge, Massachusetts 02138, USA

PATRICK R. HOF
Fishberg Research Center for Neurobiology & Kastor Neurobiology of Aging Laboratory, Mount Sinai School of Medicine, New York, New York 10029, USA

MICHEL A. HOFMAN
Netherlands Institute for Brain Research, Meibergdreef 33, 1105 AZ Amsterdam, The Netherlands

RALPH L. HOLLOWAY
Department of Anthropology, Columbia University, New York, New York 10029, USA

HARRY J. JERISON
Department of Psychiatry and Biobehavioral Sciences, UCLA Health Sciences Center, 760 Westwood Plaza, Los Angeles, CA 90024, USA

TRACEY JOFFE
Department of Anthropology, University College London, Gower Street, London WC1E 6BT, England

PETER M. KASKAN
Department of Psychology, Cornell University, Ithaca, New York 14853, USA

NANCY M. KHECK
Department of Otolaryngology, Mount Sinai School of Medicine, New York, New York 10029, USA

DAVID R. KORNACK
Section of Neurobiology, Yale University School of Medicine, New Haven, CT 06510, USA

TODD M. PREUSS
Institute of Cognitive Science, Cognitive Evolution Group, University of Louisiana at Lafayette, 4401 West Admiral Doyle Drive, New Iberia, Louisiana 70560, USA

HERMANN PROSSINGER
Institute for Anthropology, University of Vienna, Althanstrasse 14, 1090 Wien, Austria

PASKO RAKIC
Section of Neurobiology, Yale University School of Medicine, New Haven, CT 06510, USA

DUANE RUMBAUGH
Department of Psychology, Georgia State University, Atlanta, Georgia 30303, USA

KATRIN SCHÄFER
Institute for Anthropology, University of Vienna, Althanstrasse 14, 1090 Wien, Austria

HORST SEIDLER
Human Biology Institute, University of Vienna, Althanstrasse 14, 1090 Wien, Austria

KATERINA SEMENDEFERI
Department of Anthropology, University of California, San Diego, La Jolla, California 92093, USA

PHILLIP V. TOBIAS
Department of Anatomical Sciences, University of the Witwatersrand, Johannesburg, South Africa

MICHAEL S. YUAN
Department of Anthropology, Columbia University, New York, New York 10029, USA

Preface

Beginning with the 1973 publication of his classic monograph, *Evolution of the Brain and Intelligence*, Harry Jerison's ongoing research has had a profound impact on the questions, methods, and theoretical framework that continue to shape the field of brain evolution. On April 2, 1998, researchers from Europe, Africa, and the United States gathered in Salt Lake City at the sixty-seventh annual meeting of the American Association of Physical Anthropologists to take part in a symposium that recognized and celebrated Harry Jerison's intellectual influence on the development of our discipline. The session, entitled 'Current findings on mammalian, primate, and human brain evolution: A symposium in honor of Harry J. Jerison', was the impetus for the present volume. In addition to contributions from participants at that symposium, several prominent investigators who could not be present have also contributed chapters. Although the fourteen chapters that comprise the bulk of this volume were intended to be 'state-of-the-art' reviews of the different sub-areas of brain evolution, many authors have gone much further by contributing new results of original research that would normally appear in peer-reviewed journals, and by providing glimpses of where they think the field is headed as we enter the twenty-first century. That they have chosen to do so is a reflection of their admiration, respect, and fondness for Harry Jerison.

Dean Falk   *Albany, New York*
Kathleen R. Gibson   *Houston, Texas*
April 2000

Prologue

Size matters and function counts

Standard proverbs often give us no guidance because they come in contradictory pairs, as in the relevant contrast for this preface: 'Fools rush in where angels fear to tread' vs. 'Nothing ventured, nothing gained' or 'In for a penny, in for a pound.' The best scientists try to balance these extremes by not wasting precious time on the truly undoable and unanswerable, while remaining open (indeed eager) to try the 'crazy' experiment that just might work. Science would become stodgy and stymied if practitioners did not often risk the second part of this pairing. (In one of the saddest 'science stories' I have ever heard, developmental biologist Eddy de Robertis told me that, when he proposed his utterly nutty, and brilliantly successful, experiment to search for homologs of *Drosophila* homeobox genes in vertebrates, only two members of his lab refused to participate for fear of being branded as fools – both graduate students. I do understand that pressures for conformity may fall more strongly upon beginners than upon established seniors. But if people won't think big and take risks at the outset of their careers, how will they ever develop this most essential of all habits among truly accomplished scientists?)

I met Harry Jerison in the early 1960s, when I was an undergraduate at Antioch College, and he a scientist at a local research lab, and a professor. We were both working – at the maximally disparate levels of undergraduate research projects vs. professional papers – on the application of allometric equations (power functions) to problems of growth and evolutionary size increase: I on the domed shapes of land snail shells, he on the history of vertebrate brain sizes.

I thought, in all the arrogance of youth, that his bold project could never work (whereas my petty, little contained study could at least be brought to rigorous completion, albeit without earthshaking results).

I had two major objections, both recording the timidity of a tyro, to Jerison's procedures. First, why should something so coarse and general as overall brain volume measure anything of biological significance? Second, how (especially in fossils) could one hope to get reliable measures in any case, especially for the independent variable of body size required by the allometric analysis? I expressed my doubts to Harry, and he had the courtesy, and professorial skill, to respond with bemusement, but not derision or condescension – and to warn me about the dangers of stifling prejudgment (a lesson I never forgot).

The results embodied Mark Twain's famous comment about his changing perceptions of his father's mental capacities: that Twain, when in his late teens, had considered his father a fool, but then, ten years later, became amazed as at how much the old man had learned during the intervening decade. My snail studies proceeded nicely and rightly; perhaps half a dozen people read the published results. Harry's work culminated in one of the most influential books of the late twentieth century organismal biology: *Evolution of the Brain and Intelligence*, published in 1973 and still inspiring new thoughts and researches, as this volume so directly and amply testifies.

Harry's work succeeded so brilliantly for two basic reasons (that I, as an undergraduate, had been too inexperienced and generally sophomoric to understand). First, Harry's methodology had been right and sophisticated for the circumstances. Yes, size may seem too coarse to yield anything meaningful, but how can you know until you try? And what else do you have to work with you, at least for the fossil record, in any case? Science, as my favorite biologist and essayist Peter Medawar wrote in a book title, is 'the art of the soluble.' Better to try with something measurable and operational, however crude, than to grouse at nature's recalcitrance and do nothing. Moreover, even if a measure of volume does not record the desired mental property directly *in se*, size may still serve us as well as an operational surrogate (and perhaps the only accessible one at that) through its predictable correlation with the attribute we seek to assess.

Second, Harry delivered the goods in a series of simple, robust and elegant results. Two stand out in my memory. (1) Throughout the Tertiary, and within broad taxa at a similar level of habitus and heritage, the log–log 'mouse to elephant' interspecific curve of brain size vs. body size for mammalian species maintains the same slope, but increases in y-intercept – thus yielding the same proportional increase of brain size at any body size between two successive curves through time. (2) Within this general pattern, sensible finer divisions can be discerned. For example, the brain–body curve for carnivores lies higher than that of their potential herbivorous prey at any common time, as does the primate curve vs. the general curve for all mammals – also yielding the result of a constant proportional advantage in brain size at any body size for carnivores vs. herbivores and primates vs. averages for all other mammals.

As a student of the history of science, I must also confess my partisanship towards Harry's formulation, and wry naming, of the 'encephalization quotient' – or EQ in an obviously sardonic reference to the dubious IQ of our traditions for assessing our own species – as the proper and best single number for expressing brain size in an allometric world. Ever since Aristotle, scientists have known that absolute brain size would not suffice, due to the correlation with body size. Ever since Cuvier, scientists have understood that the simple brain/body ratio wouldn't work either, due to negative allometry (and our resulting unwillingness to declare shrews smarter than us). Ever since Dubois, scientist have recognized that simple power functions could provide a good first approximation for the allometric relationship. Thus, Jerison's EQ, or the ratio of a particular creature's brain size to the expected brain size for its group at its body size (as given by the allometric curve), embodies all these refinements of more than two millennia of study.

As with any pathbreaking work based upon such an audacious methodology, Jerison's results and procedures quickly became enmeshed in controversy – the best of all criteria for recognizing fruitful scientific endeavors. I only regret that our all-to-human propensity for dichotomization made the dispute more acrimonious (and perhaps less productive, or at least less quickly productive) than necessary – as too many participants parsed the issue as a controversy between two extremes of evolution by pure size increase (based on a view of the brain as a basically non-modular instrument acting as a coherent entity despite any measured specializations of subregions), and evolution by reorganization among constituent parts (based on the concept of a modular brain with effectively independent regions of distinctly different function). I don't think that any major participant ever held, or could hold, anything close to either of these obviously extreme positions – but we do tend to so caricature our adversaries in the heat of battle.

Perhaps Jerison did overemphasize Lashley's principle of mass action. (After all, once one has decided to use a general measure – brain volume in this case – even if only as a surrogate for estimating particulars of greater specificity and localization, one may be excused for also citing, and perhaps even exaggerating the importance or reliability, of the only coherent theoretical defense ever offered for considering the general measure as a meaningful biological property in itself as well.) But Jerison also, and consistently, argued that he used general size measures as operational criteria, and as estimators for desired properties, and not as direct assessments of mental mights and powers. Moreover, he has always recognized that subparts of the brain do not grow in isometry as the general mass increases. He has, for example, emphasized, as a prominent theme and finding, the lack of correlation between the size of the olfactory bulbs and that of other brain structures.

In any case, as Shakespeare noted, what's past is prologue. I think that this controversy has been resolved at an appropriate golden mean, with devotees of volume allowing a greater role for subtle reshuffling of sizes and spaces, and especially for dramatic changes at the cellular level; and with devotees of special qualities allowing that sizes, both absolute and relative, and of both parts and wholes, yield important insights not obtainable by other means.

This remarkable book, appearing nearly 30 years after Jerison's pioneering volume, proves the continuing vitality of the subject, and the importance of Jerison's focus and prod. Moreover, the commingling of cellular with biometric studies, and of growths and sizes of parts and wholes with research on microarchitectural and cellular reorganization, testifies to the healing of past controversies, and to a coordinated approach using the most fruitful themes of both sides in a falsely perceived dichotomy.

As just one interesting and emblematic example of the need for such joint approaches, and of complexities in interpretation, consider the finding of Gannon et al., reported in this volume, that the differential enlargement of the left planum temporale, an asymmetry once viewed as distinctively human and related to our unique capacity for language, also exists in apes, and perhaps in Old World monkeys as well. The authors then inquire about the meaning of these extended results: should we now claim that 'the markedly asymmetric planum temporale is involved with ape "language" or other species specific, interindividual communication modalities'? But the authors then realize that the morphological similarity (and presumed homology) need not imply functional identity. Perhaps this area operates differently in apes and humans? Perhaps we have been wrong in assuming that the human asymmetry is 'involved with high-level receptive language processing, but may simply represent an early stage relay station' – in which case, we could more easily argue for functional similarity in apes and humans, while revising our traditional hypothesis about the actual function. In any case, we needed Jerisonian size date to make the discovery itself, and we will need histological data on cellular reorganization and experimental data on neurological operation to resolve the key issues about function and evolutionary meaning.

In further examples of fruitful extensions from Jerison's methods and approaches, Kaskan & Finlay proceed beyond Jerison's traditional bivariate approach to apply multivariate factor analysis to volumes of neural structures among species in several mammalian orders. In affirmation of Jerison's conclusion about the relative independence of olfactory bulbs, they identify two primary and orthogonal factors, with overall brain size (unsurprisingly) as the focus of the much larger first factor (with most brain parts loading strongly on this factor), but with a second factor dominated by olfactory and limbic structures. Interestingly, whereas diurnal mammals tend to plot with high values on the first factor, many nocturnal mammals may be distinguished by high projections on the second factor, thus supporting a functional separation that often transcends genealogical boundaries.

Further integration of metric and cellular or developmental approaches also leads to insights about evolutionary mechanisms. Kaskan & Finlay find a correlation between length of cytogenesis in embryonic development and areas of the brain with largest relative increases as the entire structure grows. Following this theme, Rakic & Kornack suggest that the cortical neuronal precursor cells of the human brain may undergo three or four extra mitotic divisions, in comparison with macaques. Both results suggest that the evolutionary process of heterochrony, or changes in developmental timing for structures already present in ancestors, may play a major role in restructuring the brain by superintending changes in the relative sizes of parts as consequences of differential rates of growth and cell division – yet another example of interesting evolutionary hypotheses (large and meaningful outcomes from potentially small and simple genetic imputs in this case) exemplified by a combination of metric and cellular approaches.

Harry Jerison, dear professor of my formative years, you are truly a work in progress – as young as the new millennium, and as full of promise.

The evolution of brain size

Introduction to Part I

Jerison's now classic volume, *Evolution of the Brain and Intelligence* (1973), drew inspiration from the words of Karl Lashley

> The only neurological character for which a correlation with behavioral capacity in different animals is supported by significant evidence is the total mass of tissue, or rather, the index of cephalization, measured by the ratio of brain to body weight, which seems to represent the amount of brain tissue in excess of that required for transmitting impulses to and from the integrative centers. (Lashley, 1949, p. 33, cited Jerison, 1973, p. 3.)

Jerison expanded Lashley's views in key respects. First, he postulated that brain size is a *natural biological statistic* that can be readily used to estimate other anatomical characteristics of the brain including the size of other neural structures, the degree of fissurization, and neuronal density. He recognized, however, one major exception to this rule – the size of the olfactory bulbs appears to have little relationship to that of other brain structures. Second, Jerison articulated the principle of proper mass – 'the mass of neural tissue controlling a particular function is appropriate to the amount of information processing involved in performing the function.' (Jerison, 1973, p. 8). Third, Jerison recognized that brain mass varies with body mass, and he developed a model of brain/body size relationships according to which, with increasing body size, brain size expands in a mathematically predictable way in each vertebrate class. In Jerison's framework, mammals were the most intelligent vertebrates, and those mammals whose brain sizes exceeded the predicted brain sizes of other mammals of similar body size were the most intelligent mammals. Relatively, large-brained mammals were assumed to have extra neurons above and beyond those needed to handle their basic sensorimotor and body functions.

Jerison also presented a model of the evolution of mental processes (Jerison, 1973). He speculated that the nervous systems of mammals and birds construct minds and systems of consciousness to handle the overwhelming amounts of information that reach them. In his view, the evolution of these mental constructional processes began with the invasion of nocturnal niches by early mammals. Many modern reptiles rely heavily upon the visual sense, and they appear to be capable of primarily detecting and responding to visual stimuli in a stereotyped way. In contrast, early nocturnal mammals depended heavily upon the olfactory and auditory senses and used auditory input to construct spatial concepts. This meant that, for the first time, nervous systems met the challenge of constructing complex perceptions from temporal sequences of sensory information. When mammals reinvaded diurnal niches, they again relied heavily upon the visual modality. Jerison (1973) notes, however, that mammalian visual systems are more complex than those of reptiles, in that they are modeled on mammalian auditory systems and, hence, use sequential perceptions to construct spatial relationships.

In Jerison's model, later mammals also developed enhanced capacities to integrate information from varied sensory modalities. As mammals, including primates and humans, grew larger brains they expanded on the basic characteristics of temporal/sequential analysis and cross-model integration, and these abilities served as the foundation for higher levels of intelligence. The capacity to note temporal contingencies is, for example, the essence of the ability to detect causality. According to Jerison (1973), this ability may also be a key component to our understandings of ourselves as continuing self-contained beings. Otherwise, we would simply note each sensory input or experience as it comes, rather than construct mental models of ourselves as individuals with changing perceptual and experiential worlds.

The editors and contributors to this volume have often drawn inspiration from Jerison's writings. Hence, the chapters that follow repeatedly return to issues that he addressed. The six chapters in Part 1, in particular, explore the brain size issues that served as the central focus of Jerison's research and provide new perspectives on the developmental, physiological, dietary and behavioral correlates of brain enlargement.

Kaskan & Finlay (Chapter 1) reinforce key aspects of Jerison's work. They demonstrate that in insectivores, bats, and primates, absolute brain size correlates very strongly ($r^2 > 0.96$) with the size of all neural structures except for the main olfactory bulb. The correlation between olfactory bulb size and absolute brain size is, nonetheless, strong -0.696. Factor analysis indicates that two primary factors account for most brain size variation in these groups: an overall brain size factor accounts for 96% of the variation in brain size and an olfactory–limbic factor accounts for 3% of the variance (Finlay & Darlington, 1995). Diurnal mammals have the greatest overall brain enlargement and, hence, the greatest weighting on the first factor. Nocturnal mammals exhibit the largest olfactory and limbic structures, and, hence, the greatest weighting on the second factor. These findings support Jerison's views that absolute brain size serves as a natural biological statistic for the sizes of other neural structures, that olfactory systems may be subject to somewhat different selective pressures than are other portions of the brain, and that the brains of nocturnal and diurnal mammals may exhibit differential adaptations.

Adult brain size depends, in part, on the numbers of neurons produced and retained during ontogeny. Kaskan & Finlay focus on the first of these issues – the production of neurons and neuronal precursors. They find that neural areas differ in the length of the embryonic period of cytogenesis of neuronal precursor cells. Portions of the brain that exhibit the greatest enlargement with increasing brain size, such as the neocortex, experience the longest periods of cytogenesis, whereas those which enlarge proportionately less, such as the medulla, have shorter cytogenetic periods. It follows that heterochrony (changes in developmental timing) could account for species variations in absolute brain size and in the relative size of individual neural structures. Kaskan & Finlay postulate that the relatively smaller size of limbic structures in monkeys as compared to rats may, in fact, reflect species differences in the relative duration of cytogenesis of limbic and isocortical structures in these animals.

That two major factors account for most of the variation in brain size in bats, insectivores, and primates implies that two major genes or gene complexes may be responsible for much of this size variation: one gene or gene complex affecting overall brain growth and another affecting the growth of the limbic system. Although such genes have not yet been delineated, a protein has been identified that is differentially associated with the limbic system in rat brains (Levitt, 1984). When antibodies to the limbic associated membrane protein (LAMP) are injected into developing rat brains, the result is reduced size of the hippocampus. Kaskan & Finlay note that the percentage of LAMP expressing cells can be altered by the introduction of growth factors into cell populations. Further studies of

LAMP and similar antigens may ultimately help us delineate the genetic and developmental factors responsible for species variations in brain size and proportions.

Rakic & Kornack (Chapter 2, this volume) extend these developmental and genetic themes by presenting their radial unit hypothesis of the development and evolution of the neocortex. Cortical neurons are formed from precursor cells that line the cerebral ventricles. These neurons migrate radially along glial fascicles until they reach their ultimate cortical destination. The neurons that are generated earliest join the deepest cortical layers. As later neurons are formed, they join progressively more superficial cortical layers with the result that the most superficial cortical layer is the last to receive its neuronal complement. Cells derived from the same regions of the ventricular zone remain together in the same radial columns. The numbers of columns generated determines the cortical surface area, while the numbers of cells incorporated within each column determines cortical thickness.

The neocortical surface area of the human brain is approximately 10 times as large as that of the macaque, but humans and macaques differ minimally in cortical thickness. This suggests that the human neocortical expansion primarily reflects the generation of increased numbers of radial units (Rakic & Kornack, Chapter 2, this volume). One factor that could account for this is an increase in the numbers of mitotic cell divisions involved in the production of neurons prior to or during the early stages of the initial formation of radial units. For example, macaque cortical neuronal precursor cells experience 28 mitotic cell divisions in the ventricular zone prior to neuronal migration, whereas, in mice, the neuronal precursors experience only 11 mitotic cycles prior to migration. Rakic & Kornack hypothesize that the enlargement of the human brain, in comparison to the macaque brain, requires approximately three or four extra mitotic divisions or a few extra days of mitosis prior to neuronal migration. A second factor that could contribute to increased brain size is decreased rates of apoptosis – programmed death of neurons and neuronal precursor cells. These findings of Rakic & Kornack complement those of Kaskan & Finlay in confirming that minor changes in developmental processes, potentially controlled by only a few genes that affect cell division and cell death, may account for species variations in brain size.

All neocortical areas share similar anatomical features in that all are organized into columns and layers. They differ from each other, however, in the relative development of specific layers and columns, in neurochemistry, and in functional connectivity (Preuss, Chapter 7, this volume). Two distinct hypotheses have been proposed to account for such differences. According to the first, each neocortical area begins as a *tabula rosa*. Cytoarchitectonic differences develop secondarily to the receipt of cortical input from afferent fibers. Alternately, cytoarchitectonic differences may be genetically preprogrammed. Developmental evidence provided by Rakic & Kornack indicates that the second view is more likely to be correct. In monkeys and rats, cytoarchitectonic differences are apparent in the embryonic period prior to cell migration and prior to afferent inputs reaching their final cortical destinations.

Jerison (1973) found that, in mammals, on average, each unit increase in mean species body size results in a 0.67 increment in mean species brain size. He interpreted this to mean that brain size scales in relationship to body surface area. Later work indicated that mammalian species variations in brain size actually scale at a 0.75 rate with body size (Martin, 1996). As basal metabolic rate also scales at a 0.75 rate with body size, these findings suggest that metabolic factors place limits on brain size. In Martin's view, fetal and neonatal brain size are constrained by maternal metabolism. Aiello, Bates & Joffe (Chapter 3, this volume) explore the possibility of a relationship between metabolism and brain size in adults. They note that animals with large brains do not have higher basal metabolic rates than similarly sized animals with smaller brains. They interpret this to mean that, in relatively large-brained mammals, excess neural metabolic requirements are mitigated by decreased metabolic demands of other body systems. Specifically, they evaluate the expensive tissue hypothesis. This postulates an inverse relationship between brain size and the size of another metabolically expensive organ system – the gut. Humans, for example, have a small gut in comparison to many similarly sized mammals, and the authors find an inverse correlation between gut size and brain size ($r^2 = 0.47$) in a sample of 18 Anthropoidea. They find no significant correlation, however, between brain size and gut size in a larger series of mammals or in birds. Moreover, it appears that the nature of the sample and of the data used strongly affects the statistical results. Thus, it remains impossible to conclusively test the expensive tissue hypothesis at the present time. Nonetheless, these preliminary findings are extremely important because they are helping to initiate a new area of study – ecophysiology.

Fetal and infantile brains have even greater energy requirements than adult brains, and neural demand for lipids, amino acids, and other nutrients is extremely high during periods of rapid brain growth. In hunting and gathering societies, human children nurse for three to four years, and their brain growth continues for several years beyond the weaning period. Human children, however, have smaller guts than adults and ingest less food. As a consequence, in order to foster appropriate brain growth, children require an easily digestible, nutrient-rich diet (see, for example, Tobias, Chapter 12, this volume). Most nutrient-rich human foods, such as meat, fish, tubers, and grains can be obtained and processed only by means of tool-using techniques that humans do not master until late childhood or adolescence. Hence, human adults must provision human children for some years subsequent to weaning. These long nursing periods and needs for long-term, post-weaning food provisioning place huge demands upon human mothers. These demands may be responsible for major differences between human and great ape social structures. Human males, in most human societies, for instance, routinely provision or financially support their female partners, and, in many societies, grandmothers provide food for their grandchildren (Hawkes et al., 1997). Aiello et al. (Chapter 3, this volume) provide additional arguments in favor of the hypothesis that provisioning of grandchildren may have been a major factor that selected for menopause and grandmothering.

Aiello et al. assume that humans adopted a high-energy diet as a result of decreased gut size – in other words, dietary change was secondary to brain enlargement and gut reduction. Other information suggests that the opposite might be true – dietary change may have precipitated gut reduction and selection for brain enlargement. Primate gut size, for example, is plastic in response to dietary change (Milton, 1995), and it has been suggested that the sensorimotor and cognitive requirements for finding and processing embedded, high-energy, foods may have demanded enhanced sensorimotor skills, cognition, and brain size in human and non-human primates (Clutton-Brock & Harvey, 1980; Gibson, 1986; Milton, 1988; Parker & Gibson, 1977, 1979).

Irrespective of the exact selection pressures that may have produced enhanced brain size, it is clear that the human brain must mediate behaviors that provide powerful survival or reproductive advantages. Otherwise, the heavy metabolic, nutritive, and social demands of the human brain would have selected for reduced brain size. A critical issue, however, is what aspect of brain size provides behavioral advantages:

absolute size of the brain, absolute size of specific components of the brain, or brain size measures that take body size into account. Jerison defined two key parameters of potential significance for intelligence, the encephalization quotient (EQ) and extra neurons (Jerison, 1973). Encephalization quotients represent the degree to which brain size in a particular mammalian species exceeds or falls below the brain size of typical mammals of similar body size. Extra neurons are the additional neurons that highly encephalized mammals are thought to possess above and beyond those needed to handle the needs of a larger body. Bauchot & Stephan (1969) defined a very similar parameter to Jerison's encephalization quotient, the index of progression (IP), which represents the extent to which brain size in a given mammalian species exceeds or falls below that expected for an insectivore of similar body size.

Most authors have assumed that EQs and IPs are better measures of intelligence than absolute brain size. At the time these parameters were defined, however, little was known about the cognitive and learning capacities of non-human primates. Gibson, Rumbaugh & Beran (Chapter 4, this volume) examine EQs, IPs, extra neurons, and absolute brain size and body size measures from the standpoint of current knowledge of non-human primate cognitive capacities. They find that absolute brain size, extra neurons and body size all correlate very strongly with performance on a test of mental flexibility, the transfer index test. EQ does not correlate with performance on this test.

Much modern behavioral evidence indicates that great apes exceed monkeys in their performance on varied human-like cognitive tasks related to tool behaviors, self-awareness, language, and social intelligence (Gibson & Jessee, 1999; Parker, 1996; Parker & Gibson, 1979, Parker & McKinney, 1999). Absolute brain size, extra neurons, and the absolute size of various neural structures including the neocortex, cerebellum, corpus striatum, and hippocampus distinguish apes from monkeys, but EQs and IPs do not. Hence, extra neurons, absolute size of the brain and absolute size of several brain structures predict the cognitive differences that distinguish apes from monkeys. Measures of encephalization do not. Absolute brain size strongly correlates with extra neurons (Rumbaugh et al., 1996) and with the size of most brain structures (Finlay & Darlington, 1995; Gibson & Jessee, 1999). Hence, absolute brain size not only predicts some aspects of cognitive capacity in non-human primates, it also predicts other quantitative neural factors that relate to cognitive capacity.

Although encephalization measures do not correlate with cognitive capacities in non-human primates, they do correlate with dietary strategies. Specifically, primates and bats that eat high energy diets have higher EQs and IPs than do herbivores (Clutton-Brock & Harvey, 1980; Gibson, 1986; Milton, 1988). Hence, Gibson *et al.* suggest that, in non-human primates, encephalization measures reflect metabolic relationships between brain and body size rather than cognitive capacities. As noted by Aiello *et al.* (Chapter 3, this volume) animals that eat nutrient dense foods have short guts. They also tend to have relatively smaller bodies than herbivores. Hence, they would be expected to have large encephalization quotients irrespective of their actual levels of intelligence.

Although interspecies variations in brain size have been the focus of most work on brain evolution, intraspecies brain size variations also occur. Among humans and several non-human primate species, some of the most pronounced intraspecies brain size variations occur between males and females. The nature and meaning of these variations is the focus of Falk's paper (Chapter 5, this volume). At any given stature or body mass, human males have approximately 100 extra grams of neural tissue, and similar sex differences are found in rhesus monkeys. In absolute terms, human male brains have greater amounts of gray matter, white matter, and cerebrospinal fluid. Female brains, however, have a higher percentage of gray matter than do male brains. Hence, much of the male brain expansion may relate to increases in the length, thickness or number of myelinated fibers that transmit information over long distances, rather than to increases in neuronal processing capacity.

Falk suggests that sex differences in brain structure relate to the differential performance of males and females on spatial versus verbal tasks. Spatial abilities, including the mental rotation of objects, the use of projectiles, and geographical navigation, may demand more integration between distantly separated neural processing areas than do language functions. Male superiority on tests of spatial ability may reflect the greater amounts of white matter, hence, connectivity in male brains.

Recent work indicates that genomal imprinting impacts brain development (Keverne *et al.*, 1996). In mice, duplicated paternal genomes result in enhanced body size and enhanced development of the hypothalamus and septum. In contrast, duplicated maternal genomes result in enhanced overall brain growth and enhanced growth of the neocortex, striatum, and hippocampus. Falk suggests that differential male and female reproductive strategies have selected for these effects on brain enlargement. Females of all mammalian species nurture young. Males in most mammalian species do not. Thus, enhanced development of those brain regions that mediate long term planning and vocal communication skills is in the best reproductive interests of females. Male reproductive interests, in contrast, are best served by enhancement of those capacities that provide increased access to mates such as enhanced body size, sexual promiscuity, competitiveness, and spatial navigation skills.

Why isn't the human brain even larger? Is there an optimum brain size? Hofmann (Chapter 6, this volume) notes that energetic, metabolic, and neural processing constraints all place upper limits on brain size. For example, the human brain generates 15 watts of energy. A progressive energy build up could readily lead to brain overheating and 'cooking'. Human brain expansion was rendered possible, in part, by changes in venous drainage that permitted the more efficient removal of excess heat (Falk, 1990). The increased metabolic demands of enlarged brains also require enhanced neural arterial blood flow for the delivery of oxygen and nutrients. In Hofman's view, however, each of these demands are readily met, and neither is likely to pose insurmountable obstacles to increased brain size.

Greater challenges are posed by neural processing constraints: the larger the brain, the greater the distance between neural processing units and the greater the difficulty integrating and comparing information. Hence, enlarged brains demand more rapid neural transmission and, if information is to be widely shared among neural processing units, they demand greater amounts of long distance axonal communication. This accounts for Hofman's finding that, with brain expansion in the primate order, axonal mass has increased proportionately more than gray matter. Even so, it is likely that individual neurons in large brained animals communicate with a smaller fraction of the total brain neurons than is the case in smaller brained species. Other problems could result from the disproportionate increase in size of the neocortex with increasing primate brain size. With ever increasing brain size, the neocortex would theoretically enlarge to the point that it crowded other neural structures and forced them to reduce in size, thereby reducing their neural processing capacities.

These considerations imply that brains built on the primate *bauplan* would become inefficient information processors if they reached excessive size. Hofman suggests that the human brain could approximately double in size and continue to function effectively, but that it could not increase beyond that point. In essence, the human brain is almost as large as it can be. Further increases in information processing capacities will continue to require the external computational devices that our brain-sized mediated neural processing capacities have allowed us to invent.

References

Bauchot, R. & Stephan, H. (1969). Encephalisation et niveau evolutif chez les Simiens. *Mammalia*, **33**, 225–275.

Clutton-Brock, T. H. & Harvey, P. H. (1980). Primates, brains and ecology. *Journal of Zoology*, **190**, 309–323.

Finlay, B. L. & Darlington, R. B. (1995). Linked regularities in the development and evolution of mammalian brains. *Science*, **268**, 1578–1584.

Falk, D. (1990). Brain evolution in *Homo*: The 'radiator' theory. *Behavioral and Brain Sciences*, **13**, 333–381.

Gibson, K. R. (1986). Cognition, brain size and the extraction of embedded food resources. In *Primate Ontogeny, Cognition, and Social Behaviour*, eds. J. G. Else & P.C. Lee, pp. 93–103. Cambridge: Cambridge University Press.

Gibson, K. R. & Jessee, S. (1999). Language evolution and the expansion of multiple neurological processing areas. In *The Origins of Language: What Nonhuman Primates Can Tell Us*, ed. B. J. King, pp. 189–227. Santa Fe: SAR Press.

Hawkes, K., O'Connell, J. F. & Blurton-Jones, N. G. (1997). Hadza women's time allocation, offspring provisioning, and the evolution of post-menopausal lifespans. *Current Anthropology*, **38**, 551–577.

Jerison, H. J. (1973). *Evolution of the Brain and Intelligence*. New York: Academic Press.

Keverne, E. B., Fundele, R., Narasimha, M., Barton, Sc. D. & Surani, M. A. (1996). Genomic imprinting and the differential roles of parental genomes in brain development. *Developmental Brain Research*, **92**, 91–100.

Lashley, K. S. (1949). Persistent problems in the evolution of mind. *Quarterly Review of Biology*, **24**, 28–42.

Levitt, P. (1984). A monoclonal antibody to limbic system neurons. *Science*, **223**, 299–301.

Martin, R. (1996). Scaling of the mammalian brain: the maternal energy hypothesis. *News in the Physiological Sciences*, **11**, 149–156.

Milton, K. (1988). Foraging behaviour and the evolution of primate intelligence. In *Machiavellian Intelligence*, eds. R. Byrne & A. Whiten, pp. 285–305. Oxford: Clarendon Press.

Milton, K. (1995). Reply to Aiello and Wheeler. *Current Anthropology*, **36**, 214–216.

Parker, S. T. (1996). Apprenticeship in tool-mediated extractive foraging: the origins of imitation, teaching, and self-awareness in apes. In *Reaching into Thought:The Minds of the Great Apes*, eds. A. E. Russon, K. Bard & S. T. Parker, pp. 348–370. Cambridge: Cambridge University Press.

Parker, S. T. & Gibson, K. R. (1977). Object manipulation, tool use, and sensorimotor intelligence as feeding adaptations in cebus monkeys and great apes. *Journal of Human Evolution*, **6**, 623–641.

Parker, S. T. & Gibson, K. R. (1979). A developmental model for the evolution of language, intelligence and the brain. *Behavioral and Brain Sciences*, **2**, 367–408.

Parker, S. T. & McKinney, M. L. (1999). *Origins of Intelligence: the Evolution of Cognitive*

Development in Monkeys, Apes, and Humans. Cambridge: Cambridge University Press.

Rumbaugh, D., Savage-Rumbaugh, E.S. & Washburn, D. (1996). Toward a new outlook on primate learning and behavior: Complex learning and emergent processes in comparative perspective. *Japanese Psychological Research*, **38**, 113–125.

1
_____

Encephalization and its developmental structure: how many ways can a brain get big?

Harry Jerison argued in his *Evolution of the Brain and Intelligence* that the initial enlargement of the brain of ancestral mammals resulted from refinement of the sensory processes of audition and olfaction, improving adaptation to life in nocturnal niches (Jerison, 1973). Every relationship and transition hypothesized in this statement is an intriguing subject for investigation. Twenty-five years later, challenged by Jerison's vision, we (and he) have learned a great deal about the variation in the structure of the brains of extant mammals and of those mammals represented in the fossil record (Jerison, 1991). Concurrently, the explosion of knowledge in neuroscience has profoundly changed our view of the organization, localization and development of functional systems in the brain. We can now make much better sense of variation in neural structure in terms of behavioral function. In particular, appreciation of how functions can be distributed over multiple brain components is coming to replace our initial single structure-single function models. Furthermore, we can now extend Jerison's initial evolutionary question to ask how brain changes come about developmentally.

In this review, we first examine the extent to which specific structures in the brain may be the targets of selection, or whether change occurs at the level of interconnected functional systems, other organizational units, or at the most global level of brain size. After we have described where variation occurs in the brains of extant mammals, and at which level or levels this variation occurs, our job as developmental neurobiologists is to describe how development produces these differences. Our most basic and important assumption is that evolution proceeds through the selection of individuals with advantageous adult phenotypes, which are in turn the result of robust and flexible developmental programs. The causal explanations in this account are distinctly bidirectional and perhaps multidirectional. There are limitations to the morphologies produced, and though particular selective pressures are the ultimate cause of changes in brains, some morphologies may truly be impossible given the embedded developmental constraints all evolving animals carry with them.

A wonderful view of developmental mechanism, adult phenotype and evolutionary change has been synthesized (Gerhart & Kirschner, 1997; Kirschner & Gerhart, 1998). Their view reconciles the notions of phenotypic variability and conserved molecular and cellular developmental processes. It has been claimed that the basic molecular and cellular processes, or core processes, such as signalling pathways, the cell cycle, or metabolic pathways have been constrained because of their deep integration within other mechanisms. If this were the case, Gerhart & Kirschner argue, variation and change would be detrimental and possibly lethal. Their main point is that the conservation of these core processes is due not to their inherent advantage or deep embedment within other processes, but to the fact that they confer flexibility and interdependence upon other processes. In light of this, as developmental neurobiologists, we want to know what aspects of the nervous system are constrained and why, and what features of these nervous systems, if any, might confer flexibility in behavior. A good developmental account of brain change should integrate what is known of specific selection pressures, developmental constraint, and the evolution of flexibility.

Neurogenesis and the structure of encephalization

We will briefly review some general trends in brain size and their corresponding developmental mechanisms, which have been published previously (Finlay & Darlington, 1995; Finlay et al., 1998). There are two complementary research traditions in brain evolution, which might be generically termed the allometric, as exemplified in the work of Jerison, and the neuroethological. The allometric approach looks at size changes in the entire brain or generous subdivisions in light of the phylogenetic or niche relationships of animals (for example, brain size changes in Carnivora (Gittleman, 1995); differences in the size of brain components for nocturnal versus diurnal animals (Jolicoeur et al., 1984)). The neuroethological approach maps specific behaviors to specific structures (for example, song repertoire size to the number of neurons in song control

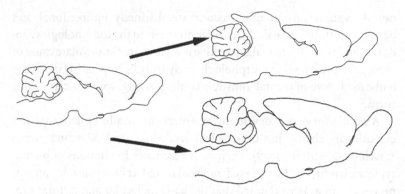

Fig. 1.1. Top, an example of local increase in one structural subdivision of the brain, the midbrain tectum. Bottom, coordinated enlargement of the entire brain. The statistical analyses reported are designed to discriminate these contrasting patterns.

nuclei (DeVoogd *et al.*, 1993); size of home range to the volume of the hippocampus (Jacobs & Spencer, 1994)). These traditions involve both an analysis of some aspect of behavior and a mapping onto brain size, but have very different assumptions about the nature of that mapping. While integrating these is beyond the scope of this review, explication of the developmental mechanisms related to these different classes of change is a good place to begin the integration.

Overall changes in brain size and associated developmental mechanisms

In line with the allometric/neuroethological contrast, we attempted to see how much variation in the brains of extant mammals could be accounted for by variation in individual structures versus coordinated variation of the entire brain (Finlay & Darlington, 1995). In Fig. 1.1 we show an example of the sort of variation we attempted to distinguish, in this case, isolated enlargement of the midbrain tectum (top) versus enlargement of the whole brain. We attempted to distinguish these competing possibilities by deriving a general rule of the allometric variety; residual variation not accounted for by allometry could then be further partitioned into individual species variation (the possible target of directed selection), sex and individual differences. Using the Stephan data set of size of brain structures in 137 simians, prosimians, bats and insectivores (Stephan *et al.*, 1981; Frahm *et al.*, 1982; Stephan *et al.*, 1982;

Baron *et al.*, 1983; Frahm *et al.*, 1984a; Baron *et al.*, 1988; Baron *et al.*, 1987; Stephan *et al.*, 1987; Stephan *et al.*, 1988; Baron *et al.*, 1990) we found that the sizes of all structures correlated 0.960 or higher with total brain size, except for the main olfactory bulb, for which the correlation was only 0.696 (Fig. 1.2; Finlay & Darlington, 1995).

Shown in Fig. 1.2 are sample graphs to show scaling of the olfactory bulb, 'paleocortex,' and isocortex on brain size ('paleocortex' in the Stephan nomenclature includes the lateral olfactory tract, the nucleus of the lateral olfactory tract, the anterior olfactory nucleus, the prepyriform cortex, olfactory tubercle and substantia innominata, but not the entorhinal cortex (Baron *et al.*, 1987)). These three graphs demonstrate two principles. First, the predictability of brain component variation varies, with olfactory bulb clearly variable in both slope and intercept, 'paleocortex' intermediate, and isocortex most predictable – note that for each taxa, the slopes of the olfactory bulb and 'paleocortex' are related. Second, averaging across the represented taxa, the three structures have different overall mean slopes, with isocortex steepest, the 'paleocortex' lower, and the olfactory bulb variable. What should be noted here, on the whole, is the disproportionate and predictable enlargement of some structures as brain size increases. For example, the isocortex increases faster in size than the entorhinal cortex as the whole brain enlarges. We are interested in what developmental mechanisms might produce these overall relationships.

The sizes of brain structures composed of gray matter, such as the isocortex or 'paleocortex,' are due to the number of neurons or supporting cells. An increase in the number of cells in a structure can be caused by an increase in the rate at which precursors are produced or by an increase in the duration of precursor production. These precursor cells, early in the expanding ventricular zone of the premature nervous system, divide and produce two daughter cells, each of which can further divide. These symmetric divisions produce an exponentially growing number of precursors. The birthday of a neuron is said to occur when a precursor cell divides 'asymmetrically' and the resulting cell migrates from its initial position in the ventricular zone of the neural tube to a distant position, where it differentiates into a neuron.

The time from conception to the peak of neuronal birthdays in a structure is a measure of the duration of cytogenesis for that particular structure. The longer peak birthdays are delayed, the more precursor cells are produced, which will increase the size of the particular structure. We

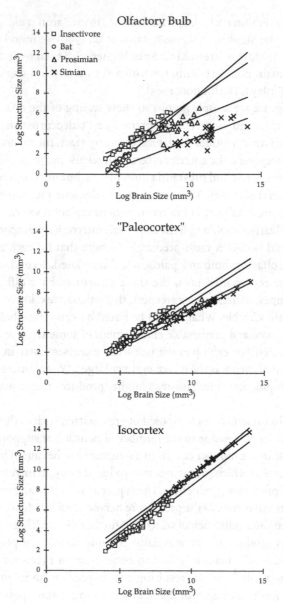

Fig. 1.2. The scaling of the olfactory bulb, 'paleocortex' and isocortex on brain size is shown here for 137 mammalian species. The term 'paleocortex' includes the lateral olfactory tract, the nucleus of the lateral olfactory, the anterior olfactory nucleus, the prepyriform cortex, olfactory tubercle and the substantia innominata (Baron *et al.*, 1987). Both the predictability and the slope of scaling of each of these brain components varies. The isocortex increases in size more rapidly than either 'paleocortex' or olfactory bulb, with respect to brain size.

found that structures which enlarged rapidly with increasing brain size, such as the isocortex or cerebellum, had characteristically late birthdays, whereas those which enlarged to a lesser extent, such as the medulla or basal forebrain, had earlier birthdays (Finlay & Darlington, 1995). A diagram of the underlying increases in the number of brain precursor cells, and the consequences for the relative sizes of structures that are born early or late is shown in Fig. 1.3. Any change in development that increases the number of cell divisions, and consequently the number of cells, will produce these increasing disparities in structure size (Finlay *et al.*, 1998).

How might the birth dates of neural cells along the neuraxis be organized? Is this related to which structures become disproportionately large? The location of brain structures with late birth dates can be understood in terms of basic brain segmentation. The duration of cytogenesis can be predicted in part by location in the primordial neural tube, using the prosomeric segmentation model of Rubenstein (Rubenstein *et al.*, 1994) – alar and anterior components produce cells for a longer amount of time. Thus, the basic pattern by which vertebrate nervous systems will tend to differentiate and enlarge can be found in the segmentation of the most primitive vertebrate brain.

Two component structure in brain enlargement

A number of previous investigators have noted how poorly the main olfactory bulb scales with brain size (Baron *et al.*, 1983; Stephan *et al.*, 1988; Barton *et al.*, 1995). This trend was again shown to exist by carrying out a principal components analysis of the Stephan data (Fig. 1.2). It was found that a two component model could account for 99.19% of the variance in structure size. The first of these two components, which is essentially brain size, accounted for 96.29% of the variance, and loaded most heavily on the isocortex, cerebellum, and diencephalon. The second component, or limbic component, accounted for 3.00% of the total variance, and loaded most heavily on the olfactory bulb, paleocortex, and hippocampus, as well as other limbic structures (Fig. 1.2; Finlay & Darlington, 1995; previously noted in general form by Gould, 1975; Jolicoeur *et al.*, 1984; Barton et al., 1995). Thus, slightly more than 99 % of the variance in these brain structure sizes can be accounted for by (1) overall brain size and (2) the 'limbic component.' These two factors map neatly onto two features of brain evolution that Jerison pointed out as critical in *Evolution of the Brain and Intelligence* (1973) – the predictability of encephalization, and the

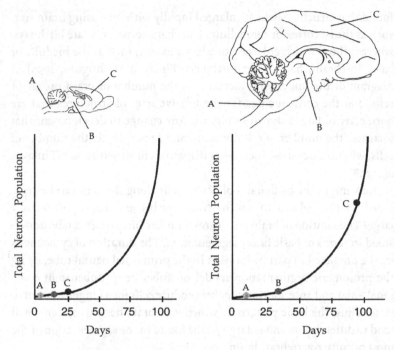

Fig. 1.3. Multiplying populations of precursors to neurons follow an exponential growth curve. In mammals, the basic order of events is preserved across species, but the fact that this order is superimposed on a nonlinear curve produces brains with different sized components. In this example, the sizes of structures A, B, and C in the rodent are similar. In the primate, structure C becomes relatively much, much larger than A or B because it lies much further along the growth curve with its precursors proliferating for a longer amount of time.

importance of the movement back and forth between nocturnal and diurnal niches in driving brain evolution.

As different as night and day

The rising and the setting of the sun is one of the most predictable features of life on earth – so much so that virtually every species examined encodes in its genome a version of the circadian clock. Even the intricate features of photoreceptor and eye design are conserved across invertebrate and vertebrate species (see review in Fernald, 1997). Though there are rather few mammals that could be viewed as exclusively nocturnal or diurnal, most have become specialists in some period of the day or night.

The nocturnal/diurnal distinction is built wholesale into our nervous system, in every sense – dynamic, developmental and evolutionary. For example, most vertebrate retinas dynamically switch between cone-based daylight vision and rod-based night vision, using many of the same cellular elements of the retina to switch between one type of visual analysis and another. During development, the eyes use experience to assess whether the nocturnal (large, even cell distribution) or diurnal (size constrained by the development of an area centralis or fovea) eye is the more appropriate conformation (Finlay & Snow, 1998). Since any extant mammal derives from an evolutionary history of ancestors specialized for both niches, it seems unusually likely that naturally-occurring genetic variation in the developmental programs of vertebrates might reflect those constellations of brain structures and sensory systems best adapted for either the nocturnal or diurnal niche. Diurnal prosimians would benefit most from a visual system adapted to foraging in the daylight, while nocturnal prosimians derive greater benefit from acute olfaction (though neither becomes anosmic or blind!). Here we argue that the 'limbic component' we see in the structure of brain size variation could reflect an evolutionarily derived nocturnal/diurnal distinction.

There is good empirical support for this position in the pattern of natural variation in brain component size. Baron and colleagues have detailed the variation in the volumes of the main olfactory bulb for primates, with respect to nocturnal or diurnal niches (Baron et al., 1983). Prosimians with larger bulbs tend to be nocturnal whereas prosimians with smaller bulbs tend to be diurnal. In simians, most of which are diurnal, main olfactory bulb size indices were smaller than in the prosimians. The nocturnal simian Aotus had the largest main olfactory bulb size index, whereas Pan and Homo had some of the smaller indices (Baron et al., 1983).

More recently, Barton and colleagues have looked at correlations between the sizes of visual and olfactory structures after removing the effect of overall brain size (Barton et al., 1995). These authors have shown that for primates, bats, and insectivores, the relationships within each sensory modality are positive. For the primates, correlations between visual and olfactory structures are negative. They have also shown that nocturnal lineages tend to have larger olfactory structures than diurnal or partially diurnal lineages. Among primate species, those within diurnal niches have larger primary visual cortices. We find evidence of a persistent trade-off between olfaction and vision during primate evolution – the same feature Jerison had pointed out with respect to primitive mammals.

There is a deeper division of the nervous system, going back to the first differentiation of vertebrates, that is not fully isomorphic with the limbic/non-limbic distinction, but has enough overlap to be tantalizing. Chordate nervous systems contain somatic sensory cells and motor neurons, but chordates have no gut musculature or the sensory or motor neurons to innervate it. In vertebrates, additional ectodermal tissue, the neural crest, is committed to a neural fate, and gives rise to the sympathetic and parasympathetic nervous systems. The components of the spinal cord innervating and innervated by the sympathetic and parasympathetic nervous systems have quite a different intrinsic organization than the pre-existing somatic sensory and motor neurons, characterized principally by short-axoned pathways – the 'visceral core' of the nervous system that extends to and includes the hypothalamus (Fig. 1.4). At the same time, the entire forebrain elaborates with its special sense organs and various neural divisions, some of which are limbic, and some not. There is a fair degree of commonality of the limbic system with the visceral core, the hypothalamus and its connections. We speculate that these ancient divisions may later be partially 'exapted' to fit the requirements of new contingencies, such as the diurnal/nocturnal distinction.

Developmental mechanisms of coordinated reduction in limbic system size

Limbic system neurogenesis is shortened in the monkey

In accord with our previous hypothesis that a reduction in the relative amount of time of precursor neurogenesis will reduce the relative size of the structures directly affected, we examined our original data set on neurogenesis to determine if terminal neurogenesis in the limbic system was advanced in the rhesus monkey compared with the rat. We compressed the duration of monkey neurogenesis to the time scale of rat neurogenesis, and plotted these durations next to one another. The limbic system structures of the monkey undergo an early and synchronous birth compared to those of the rat (Finlay & Darlington, 1995). Fig. 1.5 shows this relatively early onset of neuron production in the primate limbic system and the relatively delayed onset of neuronal production in the isocortex. We propose this accounts for the smaller relative size of the limbic system in the monkey.

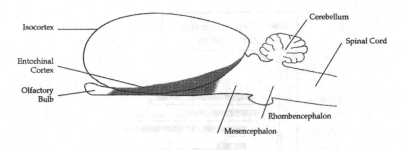

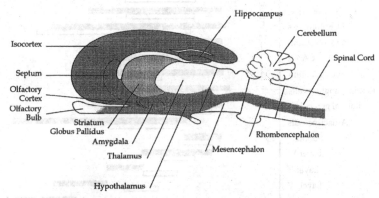

Fig. 1.4. This diagram represents the locations of the limbic system associated membrane protein, in a lateral and midline view, plotted from the distribution of LAMP-positive areas described in Levitt (1984). Areas shaded in dark gray represent a strong LAMP-positive signal, those in light gray represent a less strong LAMP-positive signal.

This observation, however, is only the beginning of a developmental inquiry into mechanism. Just what directs the entire limbic system into premature neurogenesis? If we knew the answer to this question, at the level of cell biology, we could then begin to look for such effects at a less wholesale level, forming a basis for an integration of allometric and neuroethological approaches to comparative brain structure. In the following section, we go into this question in some detail, as a model for such an approach.

The various components of the limbic system come from different regions on the neural tube, and while these disparate areas are richly connected with each other, they are not uniformly connected with each other – the cells of the limbic system are not in direct contact with each other during development. What cellular mechanism could coordinate neurogenesis in these spatially distributed structures?

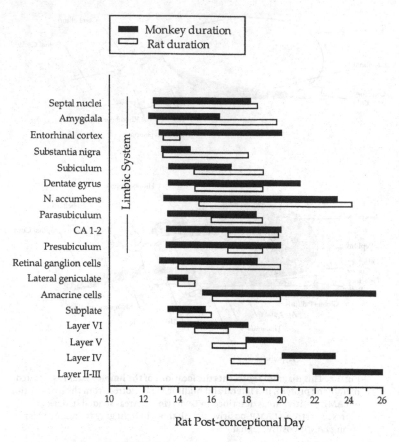

Fig. 1.5. Neurogenesis in the monkey has been compressed in this example to the time scale of neurogenesis in the rat, so that the relative times of neurogenesis onset and offset can be compared for limbic and isocortical structures in the two species. We propose that the smaller relative size of limbic structures in the primate are due to a synchronous and early birth of the neurons in those structures relative to those in the rodent.

Limbic-associated membrane protein and clues to the coordination of cell proliferation

In 1984, Levitt reported that an antibody to rat hippocampal cell membranes labeled a whole series of brain structures, all primarily associated with the limbic system. Levitt suggested that this molecule might play a role in the assembly of the limbic system (Levitt, 1984). Levitt *et al.* (1986) later reported that the limbic system associated membrane protein (LAMP) was distributed in the developing brain in the same patterns as in the adult brain. When an antibody to LAMP was introduced into the developing rat brain, hippocampal volumes were significantly reduced, suggesting the molecule did play an organizing developmental role (Levitt *et al.*, 1986). Within the brain, the presence of 'recognition molecules' or marker proteins sets particular areas apart from others, but none so markedly as the limbic system-associated membrane protein. As a unifying developmental feature of the limbic system, this may allow the distributed limbic system to be a single 'object' of selection. Is it possible that the LAMP protein itself allows cells to be selectively receptive to a systemic signal regulating neurogenesis?

The LAMP protein is not expressed in the areas of ventricular zone giving rise to the limbic system, however, ruling out this first guess. Horton & Levitt (1988) reported that LAMP was first expressed on the surfaces of axons and soma in the developing rat brain at embryonic day 15, 24 to 36 hours after neuronal precursors underwent their final mitosis. This occurred in the intermediate zone, superficial to the precursor population. Further research revealed that there is a period when cortical precursor cells and early differentiating neurons remain uncommitted to a particular cortical phenotype. The commitment of cortical cells to a limbic fate, via whatever mechanism, was reported to occur between final cell division and the first part of settling in their terminal region (Barbe & Levitt, 1991).

The LAMP protein itself serves in cell–cell interactions. For example, when tissue from perirhinal cortical areas on embryonic day 14 was transplanted to a sensorimotor host area it was innervated by fibers from both limbic and somatosensory thalamic nuclei – no limbic fibers would normally go to this area (Barbe & Levitt, 1992). LAMP-transfected cells facilitate neurite outgrowth of primary limbic neurons. In culture, LAMP facilitates the binding of limbic system neurons to one another (Zhukareva & Levitt, 1995). The administration of anti-LAMP *in vivo* resulted in abnormal growth of the mossy fiber projection from the developing granule neurons of the hippocampal dentate gyrus. Overall, LAMP functions most clearly as a short-range recognition molecule rather than a general guidance signal (Pimenta *et al.*, 1995).

We must therefore go back one step and ask what causes all the various distributed limbic areas to express LAMP, and how that event could be coordinated in a systemic way. Local signals can influence the differentiation of cortical progenitors (Ferri & Levitt, 1995). In culture, approximately 80% of E12 limbic cells express LAMP, whereas only 20% of presumptive (E12) sensorimotor cells do. Growth factors introduced into the presumptive sensorimotor population, such as transforming growth factor alpha, TGF-α, when cells are grown on collagen type VI, can alter the percentage of LAMP expressing cells, depending upon where in the cell-cycle manipulations are made. Embryonic day 12 sensorimotor cells, grown in culture upon collagen type VI, and exposed to TGF-α after 48 hours did not alter their expression of LAMP – thus only cells actively proliferating are responsive to this signal. Significant alteration of LAMP expression occurred only after 20 hours of TGF-α exposure, beginning at the start of culture (Levitt *et al.*, 1997).

These growth factor receptors are expressed rather generally in the telencephalon, and have not yet yielded any substantial clues to what differentiates the early limbic system proliferative areas from the rest. Both collagen type IV and the epidermal growth factor receptor (TGF-α being one of its ligands) have been mapped in the embryonic rat telencephalon. Both proteins are coexpressed throughout the ventricular zone throughout corticogenesis. The majority of immunoreactivity within the subventricular zone is due to the presence of the EGF receptor, with little staining due to collagen type IV. Postmitotic cells migrating from the generative zones are negative for the receptor, but upon settling in the cortical plate once again express it. By the end of corticogenesis, both proteins are coexpressed only within the pathway leading to the olfactory bulb (Eagleson *et al.*, 1997).

While the cell biology of the developing limbic system cannot yet tell us the precise mechanism by which cells are specified as limbic, developmental neurobiologists are closing in on the location and the few hours in development when this occurs, and some candidate molecules that can at least indicate what cellular mechanisms are brought into play in the specification process have been identified. This might be a case where comparative, evolutionary neurobiology could provide clues to inform developmental neurobiology; by identifying the differences in the sequence of events of cytogenesis in the primate compared to the rodent that leads to the relatively early production of the primate limbic system. The next fifteen years spent studying the evolution of the brain should put us solidly into a mechanistic account, at the level of cell biology, of how different developmental trajectories are selected to produce particular neurobiological adaptations in different species.

Summary

Developmental neurobiology can now confirm in large part the findings Harry Jerison based on allometric analyses – the developing brain is not a patchwork of uncoordinated proliferative zones, but in many ways acts as a single organ, enlarging in different species in a nonlinear manner through a statable and stable set of developmental rules. In addition to coordinated enlargement of the entire brain, there is a second way brains show structure in change – the distributed limbic system can appear to act as a single, selectable entity. This mechanism may have its original roots in the separate evolution of the somatic and visceral brains at the beginning of the vertebrate ancestry, and it may be engaged as vertebrates go from nocturnal to diurnal niches and back again.

Casual inspection still tells us, however, that the products of vertebrate evolution are not just variously sized tree shrews, but a range of animals differing profoundly in sensory specializations, motor abilities and cognitive capacities. We still have not answered the neuroethological challenge of how to produce behavioral diversity with a brain so conservative in its structure. By stating what does not change, however, the mechanisms of diversification will show in best relief.

References

Barbe, M. F. & Levitt, P. (1991). The early commitment of fetal neurons to the limbic cortex. *Journal of Neuroscience*, **11**, 519 –533.

Barbe, M. F. & Levitt, P. (1992). Attraction of specific thalamic input by cerebral grafts depends on the molecular identity of the implant. *Proceedings of the National Academy of Sciences USA*, **89**, 3706–3815.

Baron, G., Frahm, H. D., Bhatnagar, K. P. & Stephan, H. (1983). Comparison of brain structure volumes in insectivora and primates. III. Main olfactory bulb (MOB). *Journal für Hirnforschung*, **24**, 551–558.

Baron, G., Stephan, H. & Frahm, H. D. (1987). Comparison of brain structure volumes in insectivora and primates. VI. Paleocortical components. *Journal für Hirnforschung*, **28**, 463–477.

Baron, G., Frahm, H. D. & Stephan, H. (1988). Comparison of brain structure volumes in Insectivora and Primates. VIII. Vestibular Complex. *Journal für Hirnforschung*, **29**, 509–523.

Baron, G., Stephan, H. & Frahm, H. D. (1990). Comparison of brain structure volumes in Insectivora and Primates. IX. Trigeminal complex. *Journal für Hirnforschung*, **31**, 193–200.

Barton, R. A., Purvis, A. & Harvey, P. H. (1995). Evolutionary radiation of visual and olfactory brain systems in primates, bats, and insectivores. *Philosophical Transactions of the Royal Society of London, B* **348**, 381–392.

DeVoogd, T., Krebs, J.R., Healy, S.D. & Purvis, A. (1993). Relations between song repertoire size and the volume of brain nuclei related to song: comparative evolutionary analyses among oscine birds. *Proceedings of the Royal Society of London, B* **254**, 75–82.

Eagleson, K.L., Ferri, R.T. & Levitt, P. (1997). Complementary distribution of collagen type IV and the epidermal growth factor receptor in the rat telencephalon. *Cerebral Cortex*, **6**, 540–548.

Fernald, R.D. (1997). The evolution of eyes. *Brain, Behavior and Evolution*, **50**, 253–259.

Ferri, R.T. & Levitt, P. (1995). Regulation of regional differences in the differentiation of cerebral cortical neurons by EGF family-matrix interactions. *Development*, **121**, 1151–1160.

Finlay, B.L. & Darlington, R.B. (1995). Linked regularities in the development and evolution of mammalian brains. *Science*, **268**, 1578–1584.

Finlay, B.L., Hersman, M. & Darlington, R.B. (1998). Patterns of vertebrate neurogenesis and paths of vertebrate evolution. *Brain, Behavior and Evolution*, **52**, 232–242.

Finlay, B.L. & Snow, R.L. (1998). Scaling the retina, micro and macro. In *Development and Organization of the Retina: From Molecules to Function*, eds. L.M. Chalupa & B.L. Finlay, pp. 245–258. New York: Plenum Press.

Frahm, H.D., Stephan, H. & Stephan, M. (1982). Comparison of brain structure volumes in Insectivora and Primates. I. Neocortex. *Journal für Hirnforschung*, **23**, 375–389.

Frahm, H.K., Stephan, H. & Baron, G. (1984a). Comparisons of brain structure volumes in Insectivora and Primates. V. Area striata. *Journal für Hirnforschung*, **25**, 537–557.

Frahm, H.K., Stephan, H. & Baron, G. (1984b). Comparisons of accessory olfactory bulb volumes in the common tree shrew (*Tupaia glis*). *Acta Anatomica*, **119**, 129–135.

Gerhart, J. & Kirschner, M. (1997). *Cells, Embryos and Evolution*. Malden, Massachusetts: Blackwell Science.

Gittleman, J.L. (1995). Carnivore brain size, behavioral ecology and phylogeny. *Journal of Mammology*, **67**, 23–36.

Gould, S.J. (1975). Allometry in primates with emphasis on scaling and the evolution of the brain. *Contributions to Primatology*, **5**, 244–292.

Horton, H.L. & Levitt, P. (1988). A unique membrane protein is expressed on early developing limbic system axons and cortical targets. *Journal of Neuroscience*, **8**, 4653.

Jacobs, L.F. & Spencer, W.D. (1994). Natural space-use patterns and hippocampal size in kangaroo rats. *Brain, Behavior and Evolution*, **44**, 125–132.

Jerison, H.J. (1973). *Evolution of the Brain and Intelligence*. New York: Academic Press.

Jerison, H.J. (1991). Fossil brains and the evolution of the neocortex. In *The Neocortex: Ontogeny and Phylogeny*, eds. B.L. Finlay, G. Innocenti & H. Scheich, pp. 5–20. New York: Plenum Press.

Jolicoeur, P., Pirlot, P., Baron, G. & Stephan, H. (1984). Brain structure and correlation patterns in insectivora, chiroptera and primates. *Systematic Zoology*, **33**, 14–29.

Kirschner, M. & Gerhart, J. (1998). Evolvability. *Proceedings of the National Academy of Sciences USA*, **95**, 8420–8427.

Levitt, P. (1984). A monoclonal antibody to limbic system neurons. *Science*, **223**, 299–301.

Levitt, P., Pawlak-Byczkowska, E., Horton, H.L. & Cooper, V. (1986). Assembly of functional systems in the brain: molecular and anatomical studies of the limbic system. In *Neurobiology of Down Syndrome*, ed. C.J. Epstein, pp. 195–210. New York: Raven Press.

Levitt, P., Eagleson, K.L., Chan, A.V., Ferri, R.T. & Lillien, L. (1997). Signaling pathways that regulate specification of neurons in the developing cerebral cortex. *Developmental Neuroscience*, **19**, 6–8.

Pimenta, A.F., Zhukareva, V., Barbe, M.F., Reinoso, B.S., Grimly, C., Henzel, W., Fischer, I. & Levitt, P. (1995). The limbic system-associated membrane protein is an Ig superfamily member that mediates selective neuronal growth and axon targeting. *Neuron*, **15**, 287–297.

Rubenstein, J.L.R., Martinez, S., Shimamura, K. & Puelles, L. (1994). The embryonic vertebrate forebrain: the prosomeric model. *Science*, **266**, 578–579.

Stephan, H., Baron, G. & Frahm, H.D. (1982). Comparison of brain structure volumes in insectivora and primates. II. Accessory olfactory bulb. *Journal für Hirnforschung*, **23**, 571–595.

Stephan, H., Baron, G. & Frahm, H.D. (1988). Comparative size of brain and brain components. *Comparative Primate Biology*, **4**, 1–38.

Stephan, H., Frahm, H. & Baron, G. (1981). New and revised data on volumes of brain structures in insectivores and primates. *Folia Primatologica*, **35**, 1–29.

Stephan, H., Frahm, H.D. & Baron, G. (1987). Comparison of brain structure volumes in insectivora and primates. VII. Amygdaloid components. *Journal für Hirnforschung*, **28**, 571–584.

Zhukareva, V. & Levitt, P. (1995). The limbic system-associated membrane protein (LAMP) selectively mediates interactions with specific central neuron populations. *Development*, **121**, 1161.

2

Neocortical expansion and elaboration during primate evolution: a view from neuroembryology

The neocortex is a hallmark of mammalian brain evolution and is the structure that provides the basis of human mental capacity and uniqueness. Since the time of its emergence in a mammalian ancestor perhaps 250 million years ago, the neocortex has expanded in both relative and absolute size independently in several mammalian lineages. This expansion is particularly apparent in anthropoid primates, in which the neocortex comprises up to 80% of the brain mass. The expansion occurs primarily in the surface area rather than in thickness. Further, the neocortex is parcellated into different cytoarchitectonic areas, which increased in number, size and complexity during the cortical evolution.

Traditionally, our insights into the evolution of the neocortex have come from physical anthropology and comparative anatomy (e.g. Ariëns Kappers et al., 1936; Armstrong & Falk, 1982; Butler, 1994; Herrick, 1948; Jerison, 1991; Kaas, 1988; Nauta & Karten, 1970; Northcutt & Kaas, 1995; Preuss, 1993). In contrast, genetic, molecular and cellular mechanisms by which the cerebral cortex might have evolved are only beginning to be scientifically explored (e.g. Simeone, 1998; Smith Fernandez et al., 1998). The present review is an attempt to interpret some of the recent advances in neuroembryology within the context of neocortical evolution. That the embryonic development of living species can provide clues about possible mechanisms underlying evolution is a well-established approach in evolutionary biology that has been used extensively (e.g. Gerhart & Kirschner, 1997; Gould, 1977; Haeckel, 1879; Richardson et al., 1997; Striedter, 1997, 1998). However, recent advances in developmental neurobiology provide new insights into possible genetic and cellular mechanisms at a level of analysis that was not possible in the past.

One of the most prominent features of the cerebral cortex in all species, particularly in primates, is its parcellation into distinct laminar, radial, and areal domains (Mountcastle, 1997; Rakic & Singer, 1988). The neocortex consists of six basic cellular layers, each having distinct neuronal organization and connections: layers 5 and 6 contain neurons that project to subcortical structures, layer 4 contains local circuit neurons, and layers 2 and 3 are composed mostly of neurons that project to other cortical areas, both ipsilaterally and contralaterally. The neocortex is also organized into radial groups of neurons that are linked synaptically in the vertical dimension (Mountcastle, 1997; Rakic & Singer, 1988). Furthermore, the neocortex is parcellated into structurally and functionally distinct cytoarchitectonic areas, which increased in number, size and proportions during the evolution of bigger brains (Brodmann, 1909). Recent reexamination of cortical parcellation by modern hodological, cytochemical and physiological methods indicates that the definition as well as the border assignments of areas in the cortex may be more complex than previously thought by Brodmann and others. Nonetheless the principle of functional localization remains the same (Felleman & Van Essen, 1991).

Understanding the evolution of the cerebral cortex can be approached from the standpoint of (i) its origin from phylogenetically older structures, (ii) the expansion of its size once it has been established, and (iii) the parcellation and elaboration of the neocortex into functionally and structurally specialized domains, or 'cytoarchitectonic maps.' We will interpret various aspects of cortical development in the embryo within the context of cortical evolution. In particular we will focus on the cellular events that must have changed to build a larger and more parcellated cortex.

Origin of the neocortex

The phylogenetic origin of the neocortex in vertebrate evolution has been a focus of interest to evolutionary biologists for more than a century (Darwin, 1871). Although the neocortex is recognized as a neural structure unique to mammals, its possible evolutionary antecedents and its homologues in the brains of other vertebrates are still not universally agreed upon (see reviews by Butler, 1994; Karten, 1997; Northcutt, 1981; Northcutt & Kaas, 1995; Smith Fernandez et al., 1998; Striedter, 1997). Perhaps the most frequently stated hypothesis is that the mammalian neocortex developed as an enlargement of the reptilian dorsal pallium

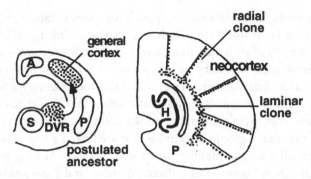

Fig. 2.1. Comparative studies suggest that during evolution the general cortex of a mammalian ancestor expanded and propelled the archicortex (A; hippocampus, H) and the paleocortex (P; pyriform cortex, P) toward the medial wall of the telencephalon. It has also been postulated that neuroblasts of the dorsal ventricular ridge (DVR) located in the dorsal striatum (S) migrated and incorporated into the general cortex in ancestral mammals to result in the modern six-layered isocortex (Nauta & Karten, 1970). One possible explanation of the coexistence of radial and laminar clones in the mouse cerebral cortex is that these two phylogenetically distinct populations of cells remain ontogenetically segregated and are allocated differently. (From Kuan *et al.*, 1997, modified after Nauta & Karten, 1970.)

(e.g. Herrick, 1948; Northcutt, 1981). Another frequently mentioned concept, although no longer tenable, is that the neocortex is an elaboration of the olfactory system (Ariëns Kappers *et al.*, 1936). One attractive hypothesis, proposed in the early 1970s, was based on the comparative anatomy of neuronal organization, and suggested that the neocortex may have originated from two sources of cells from lower parts of the neuraxis (Karten, 1997; Nauta & Karten, 1970). The basic idea is based on comparative anatomical studies that suggest that the lateral 'pallium,' or general cortex, of amphibians, birds and reptiles may be homologous to the six-layered mammalian neocortex (reviewed in Northcutt, 1981). The basic tenet of this 'dual origin' hypothesis is that during evolution, the expansion of the lateral pallium was associated with displacement of the archicortex (hippocampal formation) and the paleocortex (pyriform cortex) toward the medial wall of the telencephalon (Fig. 2.1). Furthermore, it was suggested that the lateral pallium was simultaneously transformed from a simple neural structure into a more complex six-layered mammalian cortex.

The cellular events underlying these complex cytoarchitectonic changes are unknown. In particular, it is not clear how the predecessors of the neurons that eventually form the neocortex arose during evolution.

One possibility is that during evolution, the neuroblasts of the dorsal ventricular ridge (DVR) of ancient reptiles shifted into the lateral pallium and provided additional cells for the six-layered neocortex (Nauta & Karten, 1970). Not everyone is convinced that the DVR has a homologue in the mammalian telencephalon or that the isocortex originates in topographically different pallial compartments (e.g., Aboitiz, 1999). Nevertheless, according to Nauta & Karten's hypothesis, the mammalian neocortex is formed by contributions from two distinct populations of founder cells. However, supporting developmental evidence for this concept was lacking.

Recent results from studies of chimeric mice give implicit support for the dual origin hypothesis, and in addition indicate that the two phylogenetically discrete populations remain segregated during ontogeny as the separate laminar and radial clones within the mammalian cerebral cortex (Kuan *et al.*, 1997). This is an example how new methods in developmental biology may provide new insights into evolutionary questions. As elaborated below, neuroembryology provides not only new evidence to evaluate existing hypotheses, but can also generate new ideas of how the cortex may have evolved. An instructive example is the radial unit hypothesis of cortical expansion (see below).

Critical developmental events

Because our view of cortical evolution depends on data and ideas obtained from neuroembryology, we will first briefly review major developmental events that lead to the formation of the cerebral cortex. We will describe primarily the timing and sequence of cellular events that occur in the macaque monkey, since the focus of this review is on cortical evolution in primates.

During the fifth week of gestation in rhesus monkeys and humans, the process of differential cell proliferation causes the anterior-most end of the embryonic neural tube to 'balloon' outwards, forming a pair of telencephalic vesicles, which will become the cerebral hemispheres (Sidman & Rakic, 1982). It is within the dorsal walls of these vesicles that the neocortex forms. It was initially suspected from observations in human embryos, by using classical methods, and later confirmed by the tritiated thymidine autoradiographic technique, that the neurons of the mammalian neocortex are generated only during a restricted period of early development, the period of neurogenesis. Unlike most species that have been examined, in which cortical neurogenesis lasts until birth or shortly thereafter, primates including humans acquire their full complement of cortical neurons before the last trimester (Rakic, 1974, 1988b; Rakic & Sidman, 1968; Sidman & Rakic, 1973).

The use of the autoradiographic method also revealed that cortical neurons are not generated within the cortex itself, but rather, are generated near the surface of the cerebral ventricle (reviewed in Rakic, 1974, 1982, 1988b; Sidman & Rakic, 1973) (Fig. 2.2). The progenitors of cortical neurons are confined to the narrow ventricular zone, where they form a transient pseudostratified epithelium (Rakic, 1972). Dividing cells in the ventricular zone are attached to each other at the ventricular surface by their endfeet and have radial processes that protrude towards the pial surface and into the outer cell-free marginal zone (Fig. 2.2c).

Besides harboring progenitors, the ventricular and subventricular zones contain a population of elongated radial glial cells that span the entire embryonic cerebral wall, from the ventricular to the pial surface (Levitt et al., 1981; Rakic, 1972; Schmechel & Rakic, 1979a). This class of non-neuronal cells is present transiently in all mammals, but is particularly prominent in the large primate telencephalon (Schmechel & Rakic, 1979b). These cells do not divide during the phase of neuronal migration, and their fibers, which connect ventricular and pial surfaces, elongate as the cerebral wall widens (Schmechel & Rakic, 1979a). Postmitotic neurons produced in succession within the proliferative zones migrate outwards along radial glial fascicles and traverse the intermediate and subplate zones before entering the developing cortical plate (Fig. 2.2c). Upon entering the cortical plate, they settle in an orderly inside-out temporospatial gradient, such that the earliest-born neurons form the deepest layer and successively later-born cells make progressively more superficial layers (Rakic, 1974). Although some postmitotic cells do not obey radial constraints (Misson et al., 1991; Rakic et al., 1974; Rubenstein et al., 1994; Schmechel & Rakic, 1979b; Ware et al., 1999) and a selective population may exhibit tangential, neurophilic modes of movement (O'Rourke et al., 1992; Rakic, 1990; Ware et al., 1999), the majority of neurons in a given column of the cortex are generated in the underlying sectors of the ventricular zone and migrate radially by gliophilic interactions (Luskin et al., 1988; Nakatsuji et al., 1991; Rakic, 1978, 1995a; Tan & Breen, 1993; Tan et al., 1998). The use of the retroviral-gene transfer method to trace cell lineages in the fetal monkey shows that even in the large convoluted primate cerebrum, clones of neurons in the cortex remain in strict radial alignment (Kornack

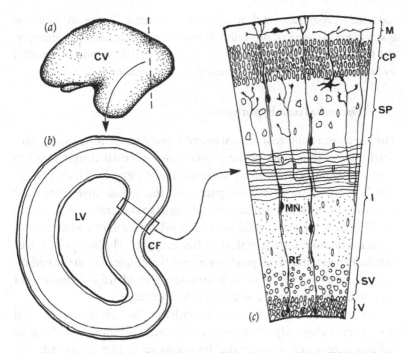

Fig. 2.2. The cytological organization of the primate cerebral wall during the first half of gestation. (*a*) The cerebral vesicle (CV) of a 60–65 day old monkey fetus is still smooth and lacks the characteristic convolutions that will emerge in the second half of gestation. (*b*) A coronal section across the occipital lobe at the level indicated by a vertical dashed line in (*a*). The lateral ventricle (LV) at this age is still relatively large and only the identification of the incipient calcarine fissure (CF) marks the position of the prospective visual cortex. (*c*) A block of the tissue dissected from the upper bank of calcarine fissure. At this early stage one can recognize six embryonic layers from the ventricular surface (bottom) to the pial surface (top): ventricular zone (V); subventricular zone (SV); intermediate zone (I); subplate zone (SP); cortical plate (CP); and marginal zone (M). Note the presence of migrating neurons (MN) moving along radial glial fibers (RF) which span the full thickness of the cortex. The early afferents from the brain stem, thalamus and other cortical areas invade the cerebral wall and accumulate in the subplate zone, where they make transient synapses before entering the cortical plate. (From Rakic, 1990.)

& Rakic, 1995). Postmitotic neurons that are confined to a radial pathway exhibit a strong affinity for the radial glial cells (Gadisseux *et al.*, 1990; Rakic, 1972, 1978, 1988a). The class of migrating cells that use a glial substrate are termed 'gliophilic,' in contrast to 'neurophilic' cells, which move preferentially along axonal pathways (Rakic, 1990). The identity of surface molecules that provide differential adhesion between migrating neurons and glial fibers is being actively investigated (reviewed in Hatten & Mason,

1990; Rakic, 1997; Rakic *et al.*, 1994). In the context of the present article, it is sufficient to state that this cellular system may be an essential prerequisite for building a cerebral cortex as a sheet of radial columns intersected by horizontal layers of isochronously generated neurons.

The radial unit hypothesis

The increase in number of cortical neurons precedes the formation of connections and thus must be the primary and essential change that has occurred during evolution. In addition, the manner by which a larger number of postmitotic cells migrate from the proliferative ventricular zone to become deployed in the cortical plate as a sheet rather than a lump (as they do, for example, in the neostriatum) is crucial for understanding cortical expansion during evolution (Rakic, 1995b). The interpretation of the data on kinetics of cell production and their allocation in the embryonic telencephalon has led to the postulate of the radial unit hypothesis of cortical development and evolution (Rakic, 1988b).

According to the radial unit hypothesis, the developing cortical plate consists basically of arrays of ontogenetic columns. The dynamic cellular events that underlie the development of this organization in the embryonic cerebral wall are presented schematically in Fig. 2.3. Autoradiographic studies of neuronal origin indicate that neurons within a given radial column originate from several clones (polyclones) that share the same birthplace, migrate along a common pathway, and settle on top of each other within the same ontogenetic column (Rakic, 1988b). This has been confirmed by retroviral lineage tracing experiments in primates (Kornack & Rakic, 1995) and rodents (Reid *et al.*, 1995) and in chimeric and transgenic animals (Nakatsuji *et al.*, 1991; Soriano *et al.*, 1995; Tan & Breen, 1993). Progenitor cells within the individual radial units that generate neurons destined for the cortical plate are coupled by specialized junctions that allow for intercellular communication (Bittman *et al.*, 1997). These radial units may form the developmental basis of functional columns or modules that are observed in the adult cerebral cortex (Eccles, 1984; Mountcastle, 1997; Szenthágothai, 1978). However, the relation of ontogenetic columns to functional columns of the adult cortex remains to be defined.

According to the radial unit hypothesis, tangential (horizontal) coordinates of cortical neurons are determined by the relative position of their precursor cells in the ventricular zone, while their radial (vertical) position is determined by the time of their origin (Rakic, 1988b). Moreover, the number of the ontogenetic columns determines the size of the cortical surface, whereas the number of cells within the columns determines the thickness. Therefore questions about the evolution of cortical size and thickness become translated into questions about developmental regulation of total cell number, and how this regulation was modified during evolution.

Cortical expansion

Even cursory examination of cerebral hemispheres in a series of living adult mammals reveals a dramatic difference in the number of cortical neurons and overall size of cortical surface. For example, the surface area of the neocortex in mouse, macaque monkey and human has an approximate ratio of 1: 100: 1000 respectively, while the thickness barely varies by a factor of two (Blinkov & Glezer, 1968). The difference in the size of the neocortex between human and macaque monkey is particularly instructive as their basic cytoarchitectonic and hodological organization are rather similar (Polyak, 1957; Shkol'nik-Yarros, 1971). Thus, it appears that in the 23 million years since the macaque monkey and human have diverged from a common ancestor (Fleagle, 1988), the cerebral cortex of these two Old World primate species has undergone different rates of expansion in cell number and cortical surface without a significant increase in the thickness of the cortical mantle. According to the radial unit hypothesis, the increase in the cortical surface without a comparable increase in its thickness during mammalian evolution can be accounted for by changes in the proliferation kinetics of founder cells in the ventricular zone that increase the number of radial units without significantly changing the number of neurons within each unit (Rakic, 1995b). How was this expansion initiated and, once established, how was it preserved? What is the explanation that about 15-fold more postmitotic cells in humans (compared to macaques) become generated and deployed to a form of a thin, regular sheet? This question can be further extended to the approximately 100-fold difference between the surface of the mouse and monkey neocortex.

Control of cortical number

In principle, total neuronal number in the cortex is determined by five basic parameters: (i) the number of founder cells; (ii) the duration of the

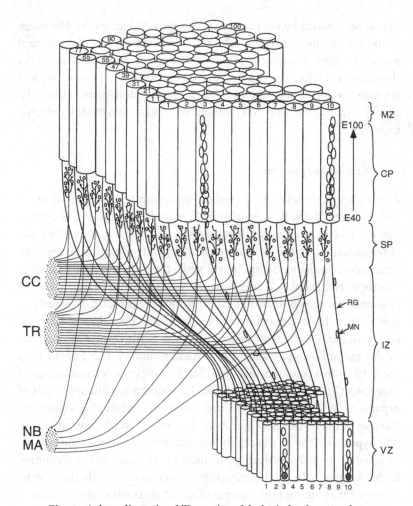

Fig. 2.3. A three-dimensional illustration of the basic developmental events
and types of cell–cell interactions occurring during early stages of
corticogenesis, before formation of the final pattern of cortical connections.
(From Rakic, 1988.) This cartoon emphasizes radial migration, a predominant
mode of neuronal movement that, in primates, underlies the elaborate
columnar organization of the neocortex. After their last division, cohorts of
migrating neurons first traverse the intermediate zone (IZ) and then the
subplate zone (SP) where they have an opportunity to interact with 'waiting'
afferents arriving sequentially from the nucleus basalis and monoamine
subcortical centers (NB, MA), from the thalamic radiation (TR), and from
several ipsilateral and contralateral cortico-cortical bundles (CC). After newly
generated neurons bypass the earlier generated ones, situated in the deep
cortical layers, they settle at the interface between the developing cortical plate
(CP) and marginal zone (MZ) and eventually form a radial stack of cells that

cell-division cycle; (iii) the number of successive cell cycles during the period of neurogenesis; (iv) the modes of cell division; and (v) selective cell death. Recent progress in understanding the relevance of these parameters and their genetic control to cortical expansion is described below.

Kinetics of cell division

The length of the cell cycle is a major determinant of the number of cells produced because it determines the total number of successive cell divisions that elapse over the entire period of neurogenesis. Accordingly, to gain insight into which parameters were modified during the evolution of larger cortices, we measured the length of the cell cycle of progenitor cells that generate neurons of the primary visual cortex in fetal macaque monkeys and compared it to cell cycle measurements in the smaller-brained mouse. Surprisingly, we found that the duration of the cell-cycle in monkeys is as much as five times longer than that in the mouse neocortex (Kornack & Rakic, 1998). Nevertheless, owing to the greatly extended duration of cortical neurogenesis in primates (60 days in monkeys compared to 6 days in mice), substantially more successive rounds of cell division elapse during neurogenesis in monkeys than in mice. Specifically, the generation of cortical cells in monkeys requires at least 28 successive rounds of cell division in the ventricular zone, in contrast to the much smaller cortex of mice which is produced by only 11 mitotic cycles. Moreover, in contrast to the progressive slowing of the cycle described in rodents (Caviness et al., 1995), the rate of cell division accelerated during neurogenesis of the enlarged cortical layers in monkeys (Kornack & Rakic, 1998). This evolutionary amplification in the number of successive cell-division cycles that generate cortical cells could account for the expansion of the monkey cortical surface and the hypercellularity of upper layers in the monkey visual cortex. Thus, evolutionary modification of the duration and number of progenitor cell divisions has contributed to both the

share a common site of origin but are generated at different times. For example, neurons produced between embryonic day E40 and E100 in radial unit No. 3 follow the same radial glial fascicle and form ontogenetic column No. 3. Although some cells, presumably neurophilic, may detach from the cohort and move laterally, guided by an axonal bundle, most are gliophilic, i.e. have an affinity for the glial surface, and strictly obey constraints imposed by transient radial glial cell scaffolding. This cellular arrangement preserves relationships between the proliferative mosaic of the ventricular zone (VZ) and the corresponding protomap within the SP and CP, even though the cortical surface in primates shifts considerably during the massive cerebral growth during mid-gestation. (For details see Rakic, 1972, 1988a, b.)

expansion and laminar elaboration of the primate neocortex. Uncovering the genes and cellular signals that control the length of cell cycle and duration of neurogenesis in ontogeny may provide clues to how these changes have occurred during evolution. Already progress has been made in identifying particular genes and signaling molecules that influence proliferation during cortical development in the mouse. For example, deleting the gene for the winged helix transcription factor, BF-1, decreases the proliferation of progenitor cells in the forebrain and results in greatly reduced cerebral hemispheres (Xuan et al., 1995).

Modes of cell division
In addition to the length of the cell cycle and the total duration of neurogenesis, the mode of cell division that produces (i) two equal progenitors (symmetric, non-terminal mode); (ii) one progenitor and one postmitotic cell (stem or asymmetrical mode); or (iii) two postmitotic cells (symmetric, terminal mode) can also significantly influence the total output of the proliferative ventricular zone (Kornack & Rakic, 1995; Rakic, 1995b). Since, as reviewed above, the entire cortical plate is created by neurons generated in the ventricular zone, the way they are generated may have profound consequences on their allocation in the cortex. In the macaque monkey, which has a 165-day gestation, before the 40th embryonic day (E40), all cells in the ventricular zone are dividing symmetrically: each progenitor produces two additional progenitor cells during each mitotic cycle (Rakic, 1988b). With each extra round of symmetric divisions the number of founder cells in this phase doubles the number of progenitor cells, resulting in an exponential increase in the size of the ventricular zone (Fig. 2.5a). Conceivably, a slight prolongation of this phase of telencephalic development of proliferation could be indirectly responsible for the large surface enlargement of the cerebral cortex (Rakic, 1995b).

After E40 in macaque monkeys and humans, some progenitor cells begin to produce postmitotic neurons that leave the ventricular zone, differentiate into neurons and will never divide again (Rakic, 1974, 1985). Autoradiographic and retroviral analyses of the patterns of cell division indicate that, after E40, many precursors begin to divide asymmetrically (Kornack & Rakic, 1995; Rakic, 1988b) (Figs. 2.4a, 2.5b). This mode of division, also known as 'stem cell' division, produces one daughter cell that is permanently postmitotic, and the other, which continues to divide or dies. The postmitotic cell that will become a neuron detaches from the ventricular surface and begins to migrate toward the pial surface, eventually settling in the cortical plate (Figs. 2.4a, 2.5b). The other daughter cell

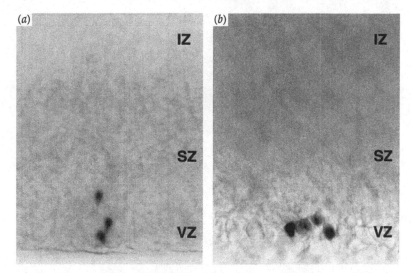

Fig. 2.4. The distribution of retrovirally labeled cell clones in the inner
cerebral wall of a fetal monkey near the end of corticogenesis, three weeks after
an intraventricular injection of retroviral vectors carrying the histological
marker gene, *lac z*. These distribution patterns of labeled cells provide evidence
for the coexistence of two distinct modes of cell division in the proliferative
ventricular zone (VZ), i.e. asymmetric and symmetric. (*a*) The radial alignment
of these three clonally related cells suggests that they are the offspring of an
asymmetrically dividing progenitor. The innermost cell, near the ventricular
surface, is most likely the progenitor that produced, in sequence, the outer two
'sibling' cells, which are migrating outward toward the developing cortical
plate. (*b*) Clonally related cell clusters that remain in the VZ are most likely
progenitor cell 'cousins' that are the offspring of a symmetrically dividing
progenitor. Note the lateral displacement of the resultant progenitors (SZ,
subventricular zone; IZ, intermediate zone). (Modified from Kornack & Rakic,
1995.)

remains attached to the ventricular surface by the endfoot and usually
continues to divide, producing an additional pair of unequal cells: one
progenitor and one postmitotic neuron that departs for the cortical plate.
This pattern of cell division in the monkey fetus proceeds during the next
30–60 days depending on the cortical area (Rakic, 1974, 1976, 1982). The
number of cells contributing to each column depends on the duration of
the period of corticogenesis and length of the cell cycle.

In primates (Kornack & Rakic, 1995) and other mammals (Caviness
et al., 1995; Chenn & McConnell, 1995; Mione *et al.*, 1997) many precursors
continue to divide symmetrically into the second phase (i.e. after the
onset of neurogenesis) (Fig. 2.4*b*). During the course of neurogenesis, this
mode appears to be gradually supplanted by the asymmetric mode until

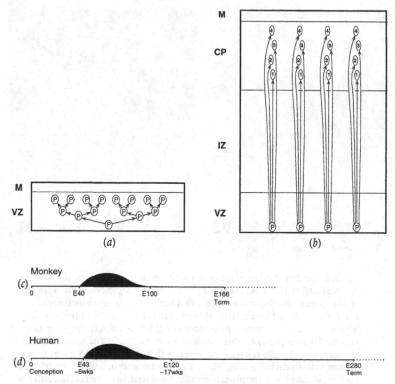

Fig. 2.5. (a) A schematic model of symmetric cell divisions, which predominate before the 40th embryonic day (E40). At this early embryonic age the cerebral wall consists of only the ventricular zone (VZ), where all cells proliferate and the marginal zone (M), where some of them extend their radial processes. Symmetric division produces two progenitors (P) during each cycle and causes rapid horizontal lateral spread. (b) A model of asymmetric or stem division, which becomes predominant in the monkey embryo after E40. During each asymmetric division a progenitor (P) produces one postmitotic neuron which leaves the ventricular zone and another progenitor which remains within the proliferative zone and continues to divide. Postmitotic neurons migrate rapidly across the intermediate zone (IZ) and become arranged vertically in the cortical plate (CP) in reverse order of their arrival (1, 2, 3, 4). (c) A diagrammatic representation of the time of neuron origin in macaque monkey. The data are obtained from the 3H-thymidine autoradiographic analyses (Rakic, 1974). (d) An estimate of the time of neuron origin in the human neocortex based on the number of mitotic figures within the ventricular zone, supravital DNA synthesis in slice preparations of fetal tissue and the presence of migrating neurons in the intermediate zone of the human fetal cerebrum. (Based on Rakic, 1978, and Rakic & Sidman, 1968.)

the ventricular zone becomes exhausted as a source of cortical neurons and neurogenesis ceases (Caviness *et al.*, 1995; Kornack & Rakic, 1998; Rakic, 1988b, 1995b). However, the retrovirus gene transfer method of labeling clonally related cells in both rodent and primate embryos supports the hypothesis that neurons produced by a single asymmetrically dividing stem cell migrate radially and settle in the same ontogenetic column (Kornack & Rakic, 1995; Luskin *et al.*, 1988; Misson *et al.*, 1991; Reid *et al.*, 1995). It should be emphasized that even neurons produced from symmetrical division that become distributed over several columns, after their terminal division, nevertheless appear to migrate radially and settle within the same layer (Kornack & Rakic, 1995; Rakic, 1995a). The elimination of the isochronously dividing cells by low doses of ionizing radiation in monkey embryos at different stages of development supports this concept (Algan & Rakic, 1997). Specifically, irradiation of monkey embryos before E40 results in a decrease in cortical surface with little effect on its thickness, whereas irradiation after E40 deletes individual layers, and reduces cortical thickness without overall decrease in total surface.

In summary, the kinetics of mitotic activity in the macaque ventricular zone can be divided into two broad phases: (1) the phase before E40, when most of the founder cells of the prospective cerebral cortex are formed; and (2) the phase of ontogenetic column formation, which proceeds mainly by asymmetric and terminal symmetric divisions that begin after E40 and continue until the completion of corticogenesis in a given region (Rakic, 1988b). The duration of the first phase, and of the cell cycle, determines the number of radial units and indirectly, the size of the cortical areas. The duration of the second phase regulates the number of neurons within each ontogenetic column. It is also during this second phase that the laminar phenotype of generated neurons is determined (reviewed in McConnell, 1995). It was proposed that the switch between the two phases of cortical development may be triggered by the activation of putative regulatory genes that control the mode of mitotic division in the ventricular zone (Rakic, 1995b). This activation is initiated within the telencephalon prior to the arrival input from the periphery.

Several lines of evidence from experimental manipulation as well as the pathogenesis of particular cortical malformations in humans suggest that these two phases can be separately affected: a deficit occurring during the first phase produces a cortex with a small surface area but normal or enlarged thickness (lissencephaly), whereas a defect during the phase of ontogenetic column formation produces a thin cortex with a relatively normal or larger surface size (polymicrogyria) (reviewed in Rakic, 1988b).

Programmed cell death

An additional mechanism that may be involved in the control of cell production in the ventricular zone is the extent of apoptosis, or programmed cell death (PCD). Several lines of evidence support the notion that PCD is an active, inherently regulated phenomenon of selective cell elimination that is clearly distinct from cell necrosis, which occurs in response to harmful mechanical or chemical injuries (Kerr et al., 1972). Although PCD has been considered a major factor contributing to the formation of the vertebrate brain (Glucksman, 1951), current research has focused on histogenetic cell death occurring at late developmental stages where it is primarily involved in eliminating 'incorrect' axonal connections (Cowan et al., 1984; Oppenheim, 1991; Rakic, 1986). Relatively little attention has been paid to the reports documenting sporadic cell death in the ventricular zone (e.g. Rakic, 1972) or more massive elimination of cells that fail to migrate away from the proliferative centers, prior to formation of any connections (Rakic & Sidman, 1973). Recently, the use of methods that identify dying cells by labeling the exposed ends of their fragmented nuclear DNA suggests that early apoptosis may be much more widespread than generally assumed (Blaschke et al., 1996). The possibility of studying this issue in mammals at the cellular/molecular level has dramatically increased in the past few years with the identification of regulatory genes that regulate PCD (Ellis & Horvitz, 1986). Because biologically important molecules tend to be conserved during evolution, we can use the same genes that were identified, for example, in Drosophila or the nematode, C. elegans, and examine their function in mice. We can, for example, delete, over-express, under-express, or differentially express genes as nerve cells are produced or allocated. This can be illustrated by our recent work on genes controlling apoptosis in the mouse (Kuida et al., 1996, 1998). We have reduced apoptosis by inactivating genes for casapase 3 and casapase 9, which must be expressed for a cell to die. In mice lacking both copies of the gene, apoptosis is reduced in the cerebral ventricular zone at early stages, during production of the founder progenitor cells.

The main finding, relevant to the subject of this article, is that in accord with the radial unit hypothesis, a larger-than-normal number of founder cells resulted in a cortex with an increased surface area and the formation of convolutions. By this single gene mutation, a lyssencephalic mouse cortex was transformed into a gyrencephalic cerebrum, which is usually a hallmark of larger brains, as if there was a recapitulation of evolution. In this instance, the mutation resulting in more cortical neurons was not good for the homozygous mice; most of the mice died before birth. However, during evolution over millions of years, numerous mutations that increase the number of founder cells by either changes in the kinetics of proliferation or cell death could occur, and at some point supernumerary cells may have formed functionally useful connections that have helped in the survival of the species. Although the developmental mechanisms underlying the natural occurrence and patterning of cortical gyri in other species remain largely unknown, several theories have been proposed, which are beyond the scope of this review (Armstrong *et al.*, 1995; Van Essen, 1997; Welker, 1990). This experiment with apoptotic genes addresses this issue and illustrates the remarkable power of molecular and developmental neurobiology: here we used a gene identified in a roundworm that may help the understanding of principles of cortical development that could be extrapolated to primate evolution. In summary, the size of the cortex results from interactions of genes involved in progenitor proliferation and genes that cause the death of some of those progenitors.

Relevance of the radial unit hypothesis to cortical expansion

The radial unit hypothesis of cortical development provides a useful framework for understanding cortical expansion during evolution: the larger the number of radial units in a given species, the larger the surface of the neocortex (e.g. Fig. 2.3). The radial unit hypothesis predicts that the difference in cortical surface area between two species depends on the difference in the number of founder cells generated during the first phase of unit formation (Rakic, 1995b). As evident from Fig. 2.5, during this phase, each round of symmetric cell divisions could double the number of founder cells whereas, during the second phase, when asymmetrical divisions begin to predominate, each additional mitotic cycle adds only a single neuron to a given ontogenetic column. Indeed, in the monkey the second phase begins 4 weeks later than it does in the mouse (E40 and E11, respectively). Thus although the length of cell cycle at the onset of neuron production is about twice as long in primates as that in mice (Kornack &

Rakic, 1998), the size of the proliferative pool at the comparable embryonic stages is much larger in monkey than in mouse. However, it takes
only a few days to account for the difference of an order of magnitude of
cortical expansion between monkey and human (Fig. 2.5c, d). If the length
of cell cycle in these two Old World primates is comparable, a delay in the
onset of the second phase of a few days that allows three to four extra
rounds of mitosis would result in a 2^3-fold to 2^4-fold increase in founder
cells, which would generate an 8- to 16-times larger number of columns
and therefore the proportionally larger cortical surface (Fig. 2.5c, d). In
contrast, a 20-day longer duration of the second phase in human compared to monkey (E100 and E120) would add only about 10 more cells per
ontogenetic column. Assuming that each column consists of about 100
neurons (Rakic, 1988b) such an addition would increase cortical thickness
by only 10%. These numbers, as well as the descriptions of developmental
events, are oversimplifications of more complex cellular processes that
occur during this developmental period. For example, this model does
not take into account the possible changes in the proportion of symmetrical cell divisions during the second phase, the growth in size of individual
neurons, the contribution of glial cells and myelin, or the rate of cell
death, all of which may also influence surface expansion to different
extents in each species. However, these developmental and structural differences are relatively minor between the two Old World primate species
that we selected for comparison. The enlargement of the number of radial
units must be the most prominent and decisive evolutionary factor.

The developmental events described here indicate that the evolutionary expansion of the neocortex in primates could be attributed, to a large
extent, to a change in genetic mechanisms that control the onset, cessa-
tion, rate, and/or mode of cell division (Rakic, 1995b). According to the
proposed model, the species-specific size of the cortex is determined at
early stages by the pool of founder cells before corticogenesis starts, and
before there is any input from the periphery. Although the evolutionary
construction of the mammalian brain may require as many genes as were
needed for all morphogenetic and metabolic functions in phyletic history
(John & Gabor Miklos, 1988), a small modification of a regulatory gene(s)
may have played a significant role in the evolutionary expansion of the
neocortex, as has presumably occurred in other bodily systems (Medawar,
1953). Therefore, the explanation for cortical expansion between mammalian species rests predominantly upon the process of heterochrony
whereby changes in the timing of developmental events increase the

number of founder cells and consequently the surface of the cortical plate (Kornack & Rakic, 1998; Rakic, 1995b).

The protomap hypothesis of cortical expansion

In addition to expanding more than 1000 times in surface area during evolution, the neocortex also became divided into more complex and more distinct cytoarchitectonic maps by both the differential growth of existing areas, as well as the introduction of novel ones. For example, compared to small-brained mammals (e.g. insectivores, rodents), large-brained primates, including macaque monkeys and humans, display a larger number as well as more pronounced differences between cytoar-chitectonic features, distribution of neurotransmitter receptor complements and neuronal circuitry (Rakic & Singer, 1988). How might such differences emerge? Again, to get some insight into how this could have occurred during evolution, we have devised scenarios based on advances in understanding ontogenetic development.

As reviewed above, the initial number of radial units in a given species is likely to be set up early in embryogenesis by a few regulatory genes that control cell production. However, the final pattern and relative size of cytoarchitectonic subdivisions of the neocortex are probably regulated by a different set of genes and, in addition, they must be coordinated through reciprocal cell–cell interactions with various afferent systems.

Ten years ago, one of us proposed a protomap hypothesis of cortical parcellation (Rakic, 1988b). This hypothesis postulates that intersecting gradients of molecules might be expressed across the embryonic cerebral cortex that guide and attract specific afferent systems to appropriate cortical regions where they can interact with the responsive set of cells. The prefix 'proto' indicates the malleable character of this primordial map, as opposed to the generally accepted 'tabula rosa' hypothesis, which considers the cortical plate as an undifferentiated primordium that is shaped and subdivided entirely by afferents, as advocated effectively by Otto Creutzfeldt in the mid-1970s (Creutzfeldt, 1977). However, in the past decade, there has been increasing evidence of differential gene expression across the embryonic cerebral wall that indicates prospective subdivisions of the neocortex. Some of these molecules may be expressed in a region-specific manner before and/or independently of the input (Arimatsu et al., 1992; Barbe & Levitt, 1991; Cohen-Tannoudji et al., 1994; Donoghue & Rakic, 1999a,b; Ferri & Levitt, 1993; Gitton et al., 1999a,b;

Kuljis & Rakic, 1990; Levitt *et al.*, 1997; Rubenstein & Rakic, 1999). This independence is supported by finding that animals devoid of input from the periphery (as in experimentally induced and congenital anophthalmia) nevertheless develop region-specific cytoarchitecture and appropriate local and topographic connections (Bourgeois & Rakic, 1996; Kaiserman-Abramof *et al.*, 1989; Kennedy & Dehay, 1993; Kuljis & Rakic, 1990; Rakic & Lidow, 1995; Miyashita-Lin *et al.*, 1999). In addition, there is an emerging body of evidence for the existence of areal differences in the duration and rate of cell production in the macaque ventricular zone that can be detected prior to overt cell differentiation (Dehay *et al.*, 1993; Rakic, 1976). Finally, regional differences in the embryonic cerebral wall (either in the subplate or cortical plate) seem to be capable of attracting axons that originate from distinct diencephalic nuclei (Agmon *et al.*, 1995; De Carlos & O'Leary, 1992; Kostovic & Rakic, 1990; Letang *et al.*, 1998). This selective attraction may be due a gradient of recognition molecules distributed across the cerebral wall (Boncinelli *et al.*, 1993; Bulfone *et al.*, 1995; Donoghue & Rakic, 1999a,b; O'Leary & Koester, 1993; Simeone, 1998).

It should be emphasized that these hypothetical primordial protomaps merely provide an oriented blueprint and a biological potential that, in turn, is translated into a species-specific archetype of neural connections through reciprocal interactions between interconnected levels. Numerous studies have shown that perturbation of afferent connections and local circuitry result in changes within these regions (e.g. Algan & Rakic, 1997; O'Leary & Stanfield, 1989; Rakic, 1981, 1988b; Rakic *et al.*, 1991), implicating cellular connectivity as a necessary but not sufficient determinant of regional specification. These interactions begin before birth (Rakic, 1981) and therefore may be influenced by spontaneous electrical activity (Shatz, 1996). However, numerous experimental studies in the developing brain indicate that basic species-specific topology develops autonomously and that neural activity may play more of a permissive rather than an instructive role (reviewed in Crair, 1999). However, input from sensory receptors at the periphery may not be essential for the establishment of basic species-specific connections (Crair, 1999; Kuljis & Rakic, 1990; Rakic, 1995b).

In the primate visual system, such interactions continue until the time of puberty (Bourgeois & Rakic, 1993), when most structural and biochemical properties become stabilized through visual stimulation from the environment. Such interactions are bidirectional, i.e. from photoreceptors at the periphery toward the central structures in the cortex, and back from the cortex toward the retina. Disruption, or even a short delay in a single communication step in either direction may cause a cascade of reactions affecting heterogeneous cell classes, leading to an abnormal organization of the entire system and, consequently, to abnormal function (Bourgeois & Rakic, 1996; Hubel *et al.*, 1977; Rakic, 1983; Shatz, 1996). Thus, once connected with the appropriate input, neurons at each visual center may have a species-specific response, depending on the complement of genes that become differentially expressed.

The enlargement of cortical surface area or even the differential expansion of the individual areas in themselves is not sufficient to account entirely for the elaboration of cortical connectivity that occurred during evolution (Rakic, 1995b). The increase of cortical surface by the introduction of new radial units, as well as the expansion and elaboration of areas, provides only an opportunity for creating novel input/target/output relationships with other structures that, if heritable, may be subject to natural selection. The new synaptic relationships resulting from these neuronal interactions may be adverse, neutral, or may enhance the capacity for behavioral adaptation. As pointed out by Jacob (Jacob, 1977), a new structural feature does not have to be optimal, but must be 'good enough' to provide a survival advantage for the species. For example, reducing mortality by advantages of increased cognitive capacity, and thereby prolonging the sexually active period of individuals with a larger cortex might improve their lifetime reproductive success and propagate this trait. Although the introduction of novelty in evolution by the process of heterochrony has been proposed to explain morphological changes of non-neural organs of the body (Alberch *et al.*, 1979), understanding the role of heterochrony in the phylogenetic development of the brain presents special problems because of the complex interplay among multiple epigenetic factors that regulate gene expression during development (Changeux & Chavaillon, 1995; Edelman, 1988; Purves, 1988; Rakic, 1995b). During the genesis of the cerebral cortex, such cellular interactions probably play a more significant role than in any other organ, and this, as well as the paucity of crucial comparative developmental studies, is perhaps why progress in this field has been slow. Modern methods in molecular and developmental neurobiology – employed within a comparative context that includes primate models – may speed up this pace and provide new insights into the biological basis of our ascent.

References

Aboitiz, F. (1999). Comparative development of the mammalian isocortex and the reptilian dorsal ventricular ridge. Evolutionary considerations. *Cerebral Cortex*, 9, 783–791.

Agmon, A.A, Yang, L.T., Jones, G.E. & Dowd, D.K. (1995). Topological precision in the thalamic projection to the neonatal mouse. *Journal of Neuroscience*, 15, 549–561.

Alberch, P., Gould, S.J., Oster, G.F. & Wake, D.B. (1979). Size and shape in ontogeny and phylogeny. *Paleobiology*, 5, 296–317.

Algan, O. & Rakic, P. (1997). Radiation-induced, lamina-specific deletion of neurons in the primate visual cortex. *Journal of Comparative Neurology*, 381, 335–352.

Ariëns Kappers, C.U., Huber, G.C. & Crosby, E.C. (1936). *The Comparative Anatomy of the Nervous System of Vertebrates, Including Man*. Reprinted 1960. New York: Hafner.

Arimatsu, Y., Miyamoto, M., Nihonmatsu, I., Uratani, Y., Hatanaka, Y. & Takiguchi-Hoyashi, K. (1992). Early regional specification for a molecular neuronal phenotype in the rat neocortex. *Proceedings of the National Academy of Sciences USA*, 89, 8879–8883.

Armstrong, E. & Falk, D. (1982). *Primate Brain Evolution. Methods and Concepts*. New York: Plenum.

Armstrong, E., Schleicher, A., Omram, H., Curtis, M. & Zilles, K. (1995). The ontogeny of human gyrification. *Cerebral Cortex*, 1, 56–63.

Barbe, M.F. & Levitt, P. (1991). The early commitment of fetal neurons to the limbic cortex. *Journal of Neuroscience*, 11, 519–533.

Bittman, K., Owens, D.F. & Kriegstein, A.R. (1997). Cell coupling and uncoupling in the ventricular zone of developing neocortex. *Journal of Neuroscience*, 17, 7037–7044.

Blaschke, A.J., Staley, K. & Chun, J. (1996). Widespread programmed cell death in proliferative and postmitotic regions of the fetal cerebral cortex. *Development*, 122, 1165–1174.

Blinkov, S.M. & Glezer, I.I. (1968). *The Human Brain in Figures and Tables: a Quantitative Handbook*. New York: Plenum Press.

Boncinelli, E., Gulisano, M. & Broccoli, V. (1993). Emx and Otx homeobox genes in the developing mouse brain. *Journal of Neurobiology*, 24, 1356–1366.

Bourgeois, J.-P. & Rakic, P. (1993). Changes of synaptic density in the primary visual cortex of rhesus monkey from fetal to adult stages. *Journal of Neuroscience*, 13, 2801–2820.

Bourgeois, J.-P. & Rakic, P. (1996). Synaptoarchitecture of the occipital cortex in macaque monkey devoid of retinal input from early embryonic stages. *European Journal of Neuroscience*, 8, 942–950.

Brodmann, K. (1909). *Vergleichende Lokalisationslehre der Grosshirnrinde in ihren Prinzipien dargestellt auf Grund des Zeelinbaues*. Liepzig: Barth.

Bulfone, A., Smiga, S.M., Shimamura, K., Peterson, A., Puelles, L. & Rubenstein, J.L.R. (1995). T-brain-1: a homolog of *Brachyury* whose expression defines molecularly distinct domains within the cerebral cortex. *Neuron*, 15, 63–78.

Butler, A.B. (1994). The evolution of the dorsal pallium in the telencephalon of amniotes: cladistic analysis and a new hypothesis. *Brain Research Reviews*, 19, 66–101.

Caviness, V.S. Jr., Takahashi, T. & Nowakowski, R.S. (1995). Numbers, time and neocortical neuronogenesis: a general developmental and evolutionary model. *Trends in Neurosciences*, 18, 379–383.

Changeux, J.-P. & Chavaillon, J. (eds.) (1995). *Origins of the Human Brain*. New York: Oxford University Press.

Chenn, A. & McConnell, S.K. (1995). Cleavage orientation and the asymmetric inheritance of Notch1 immunoreactivity in mammalian neurogenesis. *Cell*, **82**, 631–641.

Cohen-Tannoudji, M., Babinet, C. & Wassef, M. (1994). Early determination of a mouse somatosensory cortex marker. *Nature*, **368**, 460–463.

Cowan, W.M., Fawcett, J.W., O'Leary, D.D.M. & Stanfield, B.B. (1984). Regressive events in neurogenesis. *Science*, **225**, 1258–1265.

Crair, M.C. (1999). Neuronal activity during development: permissive or instructive? *Current Opinion in Neurobiology*, **9**, 88–93.

Creutzfeldt, O.D. (1977). Generality of the functional structure of the neocortex. *Naturwissenschaften*, **64**, 507–517.

Darwin, C. (1871). *The Descent of Man and Selection in Relation to Sex (2nd edn, 1889)*. London: Murray.

De Carlos, J.A. & O'Leary, D.D.M. (1992). Growth and targeting of subplate axons and establishment of major cortical pathways. *Journal of Neuroscience*, **12**, 1194–1211.

Dehay, C., Giroud, P., Berland, M., Smart, I. & Kennedy, H. (1993). Modulation of the cell cycle contributes to the parcellation of the primate visual cortex. *Nature*, **366**, 464–466.

Donoghue, M.J. & Rakic, P. (1999a). Molecular evidence for early specification of presumptive functional domains in the embryonic primate cerebral cortex. *Journal of Neuroscience*, **19**, 5967–5979.

Donoghue, M.J. & Rakic, P. (1999b). Molecular gradients and compartments in the embryonic primate cerebral cortex. *Cerebral Cortex*, **9**, 586–600.

Eccles, J.C. (1984). The cerebral neocortex. A theory of its operation. In *Cerebral Cortex, Vol. 2*, eds. E.G. Jones & A. Peters, pp. 1–36. New York: Plenum.

Edelman, G.M. (1988). *Topobiology. An Introduction to Molecular Embryology*. Basic Books.

Ellis, H.M. & Horvitz, H.R. (1986). Genetic control of programmed cell death in the nematode *C. elegans*. *Cell*, **44**, 817–829.

Felleman, D.D. & Van Essen, D.C. (1991). Distributed hierarchical processing in the primate cerebral cortex. *Cerebral Cortex*, **1**, 1–47.

Ferri, R.T. & Levitt, P. (1993). Cerebral cortical progenitors are fated to produce region-specific neuronal populations. *Cerebral Cortex*, **3**, 187–198.

Fleagle, J.G. (1988). *Primate Adaptation and Evolution*. New York: Academic Press.

Gadisseux, J.-F., Kadhim, H.J., van den Bosch de Aguilar, P., Caviness, V.S. & Evrard, P. (1990). Neuron migration within the radial glial fiber system of the developing murine cerebrum: an electron microscopic autoradiographic analysis. *Developmental Brain Research*, **52**, 39–56.

Gerhart, J. & Kirschner, M. (1997). *Cells, Embryos, and Evolution*. Malden, MA: Blackwell Science.

Gitton, Y., Cohen-Tannoudji, M. & Wassef, M. (1999a). Role of thalamic axons in the expression of H-2Z1, a mouse somatosensory cortex specific marker. *Cerebral Cortex*, **9**, 611–620.

Gitton, Y., Cohen-Tannoudji, M. & Wassef, M. (1999b). Specification of somatosensory area identity in cortical explants. *Journal of Neuroscience*, **19**, 4889–4898.

Glucksman, A. (1951). Cell deaths in normal vertebrate ontogeny. *Biological Reviews*, **26**, 59–86.

Gould, S. J. (1977). *Ontogeny and Phylogeny*. Cambridge, MA: Harvard University Press (Belknap Press).

Haeckel, E. (1879). *The Evolution of Man: A Popular Exposition of the Principle Points of Human Ontogeny and Phylogeny*. New York: D. Appleton and Company.

Hatten, M. E. & Mason, C. A. (1990). Mechanism of glial-guided neuronal migration *in vitro* and *in vivo*. *Experientia*, **46**, 907–916.

Herrick, C. J. (1948). *The Brain of the Tiger Salamander*. Chicago: University of Chicago Press.

Hubel, D. H., Wiesel, T. N. & LeVay, S. (1977). Plasticity of ocular dominance columns in monkey striate cortex. *Philosophical Transactions of the Royal Society of London* B**278**, 377–409.

Jacob, F. (1977). Evolution and Tinkering. *Science*, **196**, 1161–1166.

Jerison, H. J. (1991). *Brain Size and the Evolution of Mind*. New York: American Museum of Natural History.

John, B. & Gabor Miklos, G. L. (1988). *The Eukaryote Genome in Development and Evolution*. Boston: Allen & Unwin.

Kaas, J. H. (1988). Development of cortical sensory maps. In *Neurobiology of Neocortex*, eds. P. Rakic & W. Singer, pp. 101–113. New York: John Wiley & Sons.

Kaiserman-Abramof, I. R., Graybiel, A. M. & Nauta, W. J. H. (1989). The thalamic projection to cortical area 17 in congenitally anophthalmic mouse strain. *Neuroscience*, **5**, 41–52.

Karten, H. J. (1997). Evolutionary developmental biology meets the brain: The origins of mammalian cortex. *Proceedings of the National Academy of Sciences USA*, **94**, 2800–2804.

Kennedy, H. & Dehay, C. (1993). Cortical specification of mice and men. *Cerebral Cortex*, **3**, 171–186.

Kerr, J. F., Wyllie, A. H. & Currie, A. R. (1972). Apoptosis: a basic biological phenomenon with wide ranging implications in tissue kinetics. *British Journal of Cancer*, **26**, 239–257.

Kornack, D. R. & Rakic, P. (1995). Radial and horizontal deployment of clonally related cells in the primate neocortex: relationship to distinct mitotic lineages. *Neuron*, **15**, 311–321.

Kornack, D. R. & Rakic, P. (1998). Changes in cell-cycle kinetics during the development and evolution of primate neocortex. *Proceedings of the National Academy of Sciences USA*, **95**, 1242–1246.

Kostovic, I. & Rakic, P. (1990). Developmental history of the transient subplate zone in the visual and somatosensory cortex of the macaque monkey and human brain. *Journal of Comparative Neurology*, **297**, 441–470.

Kuan, C., Elliott, E. A., Flavell, R. A. & Rakic, P. (1997). Restrictive clonal allocation in the chimeric mouse brain. *Proceedings of the National Academy of Sciences USA*, **94**, 3374–3379.

Kuida, K., Haydar, T. F., Kuan, C., Gu, Y., Taya, C., Karasuyama, H., Su, M. S.-S., Rakic, P. & Flavell, R. A. (1998). Reduced apoptosis and cytochrome c-mediated caspase activation in mice lacking caspase 9. *Cell*, **94**, 325–337.

Kuida, K., Zheng, T. S., Na, S., Kuan, C., Yang, D., Karasuyama, H., Rakic, P. & Flavell, R. A. (1996). Decreased apoptosis in the brain and premature lethality in CPP32-deficient mice. *Nature*, **384**, 368–372.

Kuljis, R. O. & Rakic, P. (1990). Hypercolumns in the primate visual cortex develop in the absence of cues from photoreceptors. *Proceedings of the National Academy of Sciences USA*, **87**, 5303–5306.

Letang, J., Gaillard, A. & Roger, M. (1998). Specific invasion of occipital-to-frontal grafts by axons from the lateral posterior thalamic nucleus consecutive to neuronal lesion of the rat occipital cortex. *Experimental Neurology*, **152**, 64–73.

Levitt, P., Barbe, M.F. & Eagleson, K.L. (1997). Patterning and specification of the cerebral cortex. *Annual Reviews Neuroscience*, **20**, 1–24.

Levitt, P., Cooper, M.L. & Rakic, P. (1981). Coexistence of neuronal and glial precursor cells in the cerebral ventricular zone of the fetal monkey: An ultrastructural immunoperoxidase analysis. *Journal of Neuroscience*, **1**, 27–39.

Luskin, M.B., Pearlman, A.L. & Sanes, J.R. (1988). Cell lineage in the cerebral cortex of the mouse studied *in vivo* and *in vitro* with a recombinant retrovirus. *Neuron*, **1**, 635–647.

McConnell, S.K. (1995). Constructing the cerebral cortex: neurogenesis and fate determination. *Neuron*, **15**, 761–768.

Medawar, P.B. (1953). Some immunological and endocrinological problems raised by the evolution of viviparity in vertebrates. *Symposium Society of Experimental Biology*, **7**, 320–338.

Mione, M.C., Cavanagh, J.F.R., Harris, B. & Parnavelas, J.G. (1997). Cell fate specification and symmetrical/asymmetrical divisions in the developing cerebral cortex. *Journal of Neuroscience*, **17**, 2018–2029.

Misson, J.-P., Austin, C.P., Takahashi, T., Cepko, C.L. & Caviness, V.S. Jr. (1991). The alignment of migrating neural cells in relation to the murine neopallial radial glial fiber system. *Cerebral Cortex*, **1**, 221–229.

Miyashita-Lin, E.M., Hevner, R., Montzka Wasserman, K., Martinez, S. & Rubenstein, J.L.R. (1999). Early neocortical regionalization in the absence of thalamic innervation. *Science*, **285**, 906–909.

Mountcastle, V.B. (1997). The columnar organization of the neocortex. *Brain*, **120**, 701–722.

Nakatsuji, M., Kadokawa, Y. & Hirofumi, S. (1991). Radial columnar patches in the chimeric cerebral cortex visualized by use of mouse embryonic stem cells expressing ß-galactosidase. *Developmental Growth Differentiation*, **33**, 571–578.

Nauta, W.J.H. & Karten, H.J. (1970). A general profile of the vertebrate brain, with sidelights on the ancestry of cerebral cortex. In *The Neurosciences. Second Study Program*, ed. F.D. Schmitt, pp. 6–27. New York: Rockefeller University Press.

Northcutt, R.G. (1981). Evolution of the telencephalon in nonmammals. *Annual Reviews Neuroscience*, **4**, 301–350.

Northcutt, R.G. & Kaas, J.H. (1995). The emergence and evolution of the mammalian neocortex. *Trends in Neurosciences*, **18**, 373–379.

O'Leary, D.D.M. & Koester, S.E. (1993). Development of axon pathways and patterned connections of the mammalian cortex. *Neuron*, **10**, 991–1006.

O'Leary, D.D.M. & Stanfield, B.B. (1989). Selective elimination of axons extended by developing cortical neurons is dependent on regional locale: experiments utilizing fetal cortical transplants. *Journal of Neuroscience*, **9**, 2230–2246.

O'Rourke, N.A., Dailey, M.E., Smith, S.J. & McConnell, S.K. (1992). Diverse migratory pathways in the developing cerebral cortex. *Science*, **258**, 299–302.

Oppenheim, R.W. (1991). Cell death during development of the nervous system. *Annual Reviews Neuroscience*, **14**, 453–501.

Polyak, S.L. (1957). *The Vertebrate Visual System*. Chicago: University of Chicago Press.

Preuss, T.M. (1993). The role of the neurosciences in primate evolutionary biology: Historical commentary and prospectus. In *Primates and Their Relatives in Phylogenetic Perspective*, ed. R.D.E. MacPhae, pp. 333–362. New York: Plenum Press.

Purves, D. (1988). *Body and Brain. A Trophic Theory of Neural Connections.* Cambridge, Mass.: Harvard University Press.

Rakic, P. (1972). Mode of cell migration to the superficial layers of fetal monkey neocortex. *Journal of Comparative Neurology*, **145**, 61–84.

Rakic, P. (1974). Neurons in rhesus monkey visual cortex: Systematic relation between time of origin and eventual disposition. *Science*, **183**, 425–427.

Rakic, P. (1976). Differences in the time of origin and in eventual distribution of neurons in areas 17 and 18 of visual cortex in rhesus monkey. *Experimental Brain Research Supplement*, **1**, 244–248.

Rakic, P. (1978). Neuronal migration and contact guidance in the primate telencephalon. *Postgraduate Medical Journal*, **54** Suppl. 1, 25–40.

Rakic, P. (1981). Development of visual centers in the primate brain depends on binocular competition before birth. *Science*, **214**, 928–931.

Rakic, P. (1982). Early developmental events: cell lineages, acquisition of neuronal positions, and areal and laminar development. *Neuroscience Research Program Bulletin*, **20**, 439–451.

Rakic, P. (1983). Geniculo-cortical connections in primates: normal and experimentally altered development. *Progress in Brain Research*, **58**, 393–404.

Rakic, P. (1985). Limits of neurogenesis in primates. *Science*, **227**, 1054–1056.

Rakic, P. (1986). Mechanism of ocular dominance segregation in the lateral geniculate nucleus: competitive elimination hypothesis. *Trends in Neurosciences*, **9**, 11–15.

Rakic, P. (1988a). Defects of neuronal migration and the pathogenesis of cortical malformations. [Review.] *Progress in Brain Research*, **73**, 15–37.

Rakic, P. (1988b). Specification of cerebral cortical areas. *Science*, **241**, 170–176.

Rakic, P. (1990). Principles of neural cell migration. *Experientia*, **46**, 882–891.

Rakic, P. (1995a). Radial versus tangential migration of neuronal clones in the developing cerebral cortex. *Proceedings of the National Academy of Sciences USA*, **92**, 11 323–11 327.

Rakic, P. (1995b). A small step for the cell, a giant leap for mankind: a hypothesis of neocortical expansion during evolution. *Trends in Neurosciences*, **18**, 383–388.

Rakic, P. (1997). Intra and extracellular control of neuronal migration: relevance to cortical malformations. In *Normal and Abnormal Development of Cortex*, eds. A.M. Galaburda & Y. Christen, pp. 81–89. Berlin: Springer.

Rakic, P., Cameron, R.S. & Komuro, H. (1994). Recognition, adhesion, transmembrane signaling and cell motility in guided neuronal migration. *Current Opinions in Neurobiology*, **4**, 63–69.

Rakic, P. & Lidow, M.S. (1995). Distribution and density of neurotransmitter receptors in the visual cortex devoid of retinal input from early embryonic stages. *Journal of Neuroscience*, **15**, 2561–2574.

Rakic, P. & Sidman, R.L. (1968). Supravital DNA synthesis in the developing human and mouse brain. *Journal of Neuropathology and Experimental Neurology*, **27**, 246–276.

Rakic, P. & Sidman, R.L. (1973). Sequence of developmental abnormalities leading to granule cell deficit in cerebellar cortex of weaver mutant mice. *Journal of Comparative Neurology*, **152**, 103–132.

Rakic, P. & Singer, W. (1988). *Neurobiology of Neocortex.* New York: John Wiley & Sons.

Rakic, P., Stensaas, L. J., Sayre, E. P. & Sidman, R. L. (1974). Computer-aided three-dimensional reconstruction and quantitative analysis of cells from serial electron microscopic montages of foetal monkey brain. *Nature*, **250**, 31–34.

Rakic, P., Suñer, I. & Williams, R. W. (1991). A novel cytoarchitectonic area induced experimentally within the primate visual cortex. *Proceedings of the National Academy of Sciences USA*, **88**, 2083–2087.

Reid, C. B., Liang, I. & Walsh, C. (1995). Systematic widespread clonal organization in cerebral cortex. *Neuron*, **15**, 299–310.

Richardson, M. K., Hanken, J., Gooneratne, M. L., Pieau, C., Raynaud, A., Selwood, L. & Write, G. M. (1997). There is no highly conserved embryonic stage in the vertebrates: implications for current theories of evolution and development. *Anatomy and Embryology*, **196**, 91–106.

Rubenstein, J. L. R., Martinez, S., Shimamura, K. & Puelles, L. (1994). The embryonic vertebrate forebrain: The prosomeric model. *Science*, **266**, 578–580.

Rubenstein, J. L. R. & Rakic, P. (1999). Genetic control of cerebral cortical development. *Cerebral Cortex*, **9**, 521–524.

Schmechel, D. E. & Rakic, P. (1979a). Arrested proliferation of radial glial cells during midgestation in rhesus monkey. *Nature*, **227**, 303–305.

Schmechel, D. E. & Rakic, P. (1979b). A Golgi study of radial glial cells in developing monkey telencephalon. *Anatomy and Embryology*, **156**, 115-152.

Shatz, C. J. (1996). Emergence of order in visual system development. *Proceedings of the National Academy of Sciences USA*, **93**, 602–608.

Shkol'nik-Yarros, E. G. (1971). *Neurons and Interneuronal Connections of the Central Visual System*. New York: Plenum Press.

Sidman, R. L. & Rakic, P. (1973). Neuronal migration, with special reference to developing human brain: a review. *Brain Research*, **62**, 1–35.

Sidman, R. L. & Rakic, P. (1982). Development of the human central nervous system. In *Histology and Histopathology of the Nervous System*, eds. W. Haymaker & R. D. Adams, pp. 3–145. Springfield: C.C. Thomas.

Simeone, A. (1998). Otx1 and Otx2 in the development and evolution of the mammalian brain. *EMBO*, **23**, 6790–6798.

Smith Fernandez, A., Pieau, C., Repérant, Boncinelli, E. & Wassef, M. (1998). Expression of the Emx-1 and Dlx-1 homeobox genes define three molecularly distinct domains in the telencephalon of mouse, chick, turtle and frog embryos: implications for the evolution of telencephalic subdivisions in amniotes. *Development*, **125**, 2099–2111.

Soriano, E., Dumesnil, N., Auladell, C., Cohen-Tannoudji, M. & Sotelo, C. (1995). Molecular heterogeneity of progenitors and radial migration in the developing cerebral cortex revealed by transgene expression. *Proceedings of the National Academy of Sciences USA*, **92**, 11 676–11 680.

Striedter, G. F. (1997). The telencephalon of tetrapods in evolution. *Brain Behavior and Evolution*, **49**, 179–213.

Striedter, G. F. (1998). Progress in the study of brain evolution: from speculative theories to testable hypotheses. *Anatomical Record (New Anatomist)*, pp. 105–112.

Szenthágothai, J. (1978). The neuron network of the cerebral cortex: a functional interpretation. *Proceedings of the Royal Society of London*, B**201**, 219–248.

Tan, S.-S. & Breen, S. (1993). Radial mosaicism and tangential cell dispersion both contribute to mouse neocortical development. *Nature*, **362**, 638–640.

Tan, S.-S., Kalloniatis, M., Sturm, K., Tam, P.P.L., Reese, B.E. & Faulkner-Jones, B. (1998). Separate progenitors for radial and tangential cell dispersion during development of the cerebral neocortex. *Neuron*, **21**, 295–304.

Van Essen, D. (1997). A tension-based theory of morphogenesis and compact wiring in the central nervous system. *Nature*, **385**, 313–318.

Ware, M.L., Travazoie, S.F., Reid, C.B. & Walsh, C.A. (1999). Coexistence of widespread clones and large radial clones in early embryonic ferret cortex. *Cerebral Cortex*, **9**, 636–645.

Welker, W. (1990). Why does the cerebral cortex fissure and fold? A review of determinants of gyri and sulci. In *Cerebral Cortex, Vol. 8B*, eds. E.G. Jones & A. Peters, pp. 3–136. New York: Plenum Press.

Xuan, S., Baptista, C.A., Balas, G., Tao, W., Soares, V.C. & Lai, E. (1995). Winged helix transcription factor BF-1 is essential for the development of the cerebral hemispheres. *Neuron*, **14**, 1141–1152.

LESLIE C. AIELLO, NICOLA BATES & TRACEY JOFFE

3
_____

In defense of the Expensive Tissue Hypothesis

Modern humans have brains that are between three and five times the size that would be expected for average mammals of human body mass (Aiello & Wheeler, 1995, 1996; Aiello, 1997). Because brain tissue per unit mass has a basal metabolism that is over 22 times higher than the same amount of muscle tissue, a relatively large brain would be expected to have a significant effect on human energy budgets. In the recent literature on human evolution there has been considerable interest in the ways in which the metabolic costs of the large human brain may have either constrained or influenced adaptation and behavior. Focus has centered on how it is possible to grow such a large brain (Martin, 1996), on how adult humans might adjust their energy budgets to maintain their large brains (Aiello & Wheeler, 1995, 1996; Aiello, 1997), and on the implications of the metabolic aspects of brain growth and maintenance for human dietary evolution (Leonard & Robertson, 1992, 1994, 1997), life history evolution (Foley & Lee, 1991), social evolution (Key & Aiello, 1999, 2000), and symbolic evolution (Power & Aiello, 1997). One recent hypothesis has also suggested that the increase in relative brain size during the course of human evolution might be better explained by the metabolic resources available to mothers during gestation and lactation rather than by any specific behavioral feature (for example feeding ecology or complexity of social organization) that might be postulated to exert a selective pressure for a relative increase in brain size (Martin, 1996).

In analyzing the implications of the metabolic aspects of brain growth and maintenance in human evolution, a major problem is that there does not appear to be a simple and direct relationship between brain size and basal metabolism. For example, the human brain is a full kilogram heavier than would be expected in a mammal of human body size but the human basal metabolic rate (BMR) is virtually identical to that of the average mammal. In other words, there is no evidence of the extra energy required by the unusually large human brain (Aiello & Wheeler, 1995, 1996; Aiello, 1997). Furthermore, across mammals when brain size is corrected for body size it is much more variable than is BMR when it is corrected for body size. This means that there is no simple one-to-one relationship between relative brain size and relative metabolism in mammals (Martin, 1996). This is consistent with MacNab & Eisenberg's (1989) earlier demonstration that there is no significant correlation between relative brain size and relative BMR.

There have been at least two solutions offered to this apparent paradox. The Maternal Energy Hypothesis (Martin, 1996) simply accepts the lack of correlation between size-corrected adult brain size and size-corrected adult basal metabolic rate as relatively trivial. Rather it argues that the fundamental metabolic relationship in brain evolution is between the basal metabolic rate of the mother (as an indicator of her energy turnover in gestation and lactation) and the brain size of her developing offspring. The second solution, the Expensive Tissue Hypothesis, offers a clear explanation for the paradox and suggests that this explanation provides fundamental clues to our understanding of human evolution and adaptation (Aiello, 1996a,b, 1998a,b). The major point to be argued in this contribution is that both hypotheses, the Maternal Energy Hypothesis and the Expensive Tissue Hypothesis, are important to the understanding of the evolution of the human brain. The Maternal Energy Hypothesis is important in explaining patterns of growth and development during gestation and lactation when the infant is dependent on maternal resources. After weaning, however, the energy balance of the individual becomes important. It is at this stage in human growth and development that the Expensive Tissue Hypothesis can provide insight into factors that can best be described as 'prime releasers' during the course of human evolution.

The Expensive Tissue Hypothesis

The Expensive Tissue Hypothesis argues that there is a fundamental one-to-one relationship between adult relative brain size and relative basal metabolism in humans as well as in other animals, but this relationship is masked by the relative sizes and basal metabolic rates of other 'expensive' tissues in the body. One of the mistakes made in prior studies of the rela-

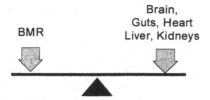

Fig. 3.1. The balance between basal metabolic rate (BMR) and the size and energetic cost of the five 'expensive' organs in the body. Other things being equal, any increase in the combined size and energetic cost of the expensive organs would be expected to require an increase in total body BMR and, conversely, any combined decrease would be mirrored in a reduced BMR. If one of the expensive organs, such as the brain, was disproportionately large this would have to be compensated by a corresponding reduction in size of another expensive organ if the BMR was to remain the same.

tionship between brain size and BMR was the assumption that the brain is the only organ in the body that might have an effect on BMR and that the relationship between brain size and basal metabolism could be understood in isolation. Even in humans the brain only accounts for about 20% of the total basal metabolic rate. Any direct relationship between brain size and total basal metabolic rate in the adult is confounded by the relative sizes and metabolic costs of the other organs in the body that account for the remaining basal metabolism. In humans four other 'expensive' organs are particularly important. These are the heart, kidneys, liver and gastrointestinal tract. The brain, together with these four other organs, accounts for about 70% of total basal metabolism in adult humans and this leaves only 30% for all of the remaining tissues of the body.

These expensive organs are the metabolic 'machinery' of the body (Daan *et al.*, 1990; Piersma & Lindström, 1997) and their sizes and energetic costs directly influence basal metabolism in the adult. If the combined mass of all of these organs is more than would be expected for an average mammal of a given size then the BMR would also be expected to be greater than that of the average mammal. Conversely, if the combined mass of these organs is less than would be expected the BMR would also be expected to be less (Fig. 3.1).

The Expensive Tissue Hypothesis posits that one way to support a relatively very large brain with an average BMR is to significantly reduce the size of one or more of the other 'expensive tissues' of the body (Aiello & Wheeler, 1995; Aiello, 1997). Allometric analyses which predict the expected organ mass for average anthropoid primates of human body

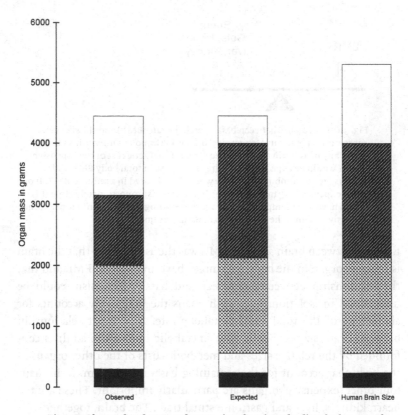

Fig. 3.2. Observed and expected organ sizes for a 'standard' 65-kg human. If this individual had the expected size of kidneys, heart, liver and gut for an average primate of his body mass but had the observed human brain size, his BMR would increase by 9.52 W, which would represent a 10.5% increase in total body BMR. Equations for the prediction of expected organ mass are from Aiello & Wheeler (1995). The observed BMR for a 65-kg human male is 90.6 W (Aschoff *et al.*, 1971).

mass show that the relatively large human brain is balanced by a corresponding reduction in the size of the gut and the metabolic costs of this reduced gut almost perfectly balance the high metabolic cost of the large brain (Aiello & Wheeler, 1995) (Fig. 3.2). The other energetically expensive organs in the human body (the heart, kidneys and liver) are all about the size expected in a mammal of human body size. If humans had the size of gut that would be expected in an average primate of human body size our basal metabolism would be over 10% higher than it is and this would have consequent feeding and fitness consequences.

If during the course of human evolution an increase in BMR was either impossible or undesirable these data imply that the metabolic costs of the evolving human brain could have been balanced, or compensated for, by a corresponding reduction in the size of the gut. Because gut size is directly related to dietary quality, the adoption of a high quality, easy to digest diet, would be necessary in order to have a relatively small gut (Aiello & Wheeler, 1995). The logical conclusion is that dietary change was a fundamental, but indirect, aspect in the evolution of the large human brain.

Testing the Expensive Tissue Hypothesis

One question in relation to the Expensive Tissue Hypothesis is whether other encephalized animals also compensate for their enlarged brains with reduced guts? Alternatively they might adopt other strategies such as, for example, elevated BMRs or alterations in the size, or metabolic cost, of any of their other expensive organs. Non-human anthropoid primates (monkeys and apes) are similar to modern humans in having a basal metabolism that would be expected for an average mammal of their body masses (Armstrong, 1985). They are also, on average, encephalized in relation to other mammals and as a result might also balance the costs of their encephalized brains by reducing the sizes of their guts (Aiello & Wheeler, 1995).

This hypothesis is more difficult to test than might be expected. There are two reasons for this. First, in order to determine whether the brain is relatively large and/or the gut is relatively small it is necessary to determine the expected brain mass and gut mass in relation to body mass. This is done by fitting 'best-fit' lines to the relationships between brain mass and body mass and gut mass and body mass. The relative size of the brain and gut are then determined in relation to these best-fit lines. If the observed size of the brain or gut lies above its appropriate line it is relatively large in relation to that line and to its expected mass based on that line. If it falls below the appropriate line it is relatively small.

The problem lies in the fact that the best-fit lines vary with the taxonomic level at which the relationship is being studied. If the best-fit line for the relationship between brain mass and body mass is fit to a sample of anthropoid primates only the slope of the line will be significantly different than if it is fit to a larger sample of primates as well as other mammals (Table 3.1). The same is true for the relationship between gut mass and body mass. For example, if relative brain mass and relative gut mass are determined in relation to the best-fit lines computed on the basis of

Table 3.1. *Anthropoid and mammalian best-fit equations for brain mass vs. body mass and gut mass vs. body mass*

	Anthropoid equations			Mammalian equations		
	Slope	Intercept	r	Slope	Intercept	r
Brain mass	0.72	1.35	0.98	0.76	1.77	0.96
Gut mass	0.85	−0.83	0.96	0.98	−1.33	0.98

Notes:
All equations are for log transformed (base 10) data and all except the mammalian brain equation are reduced major axis equations of the form: *organ mass* (g) = *slope* * *body mass* (g) + *intercept*. The anthropoid brain equation is based on data published by Stephan *et al.*, 1981, and the anthropoid and mammalian gut equations are based on data published by Chivers & Hladik, 1980, corrected for typographical errors and supplemented by additional unpublished gut weights supplied by D. Chivers and A. MacLarnon. In all cases body masses and either brain masses or gut masses come from the same individual. The mammalian brain equation is a major axis equation of the form *brain mass* (mg) = *body mass* (g) + *intercept* and is taken from Martin, 1983. In this case, body masses and brain masses are species averages.

anthropoid primates alone there is a significant negative correlation between relative gut mass and relative brain mass ($r^2 = 0.47$, $p = 0.002$ including humans, $r^2 = 0.39$, $p = 0.007$, without humans) (Fig. 3.3*a*). Those species with relatively large brains in relation to their body masses have significantly small guts relative to their body masses. This inverse relationship would appear to support the hypothesis that anthropoid primates balance the costs of their encephalized brains with relatively small guts (Aiello & Wheeler, 1995). However, if relative brain mass and relative gut mass are determined in relation to the best-fit lines computed on the basis of a larger mammalian sample, the negative correlation between relative brain mass and relative gut mass is weaker and is non-significant when humans are excluded from the relationship (Fig. 3.3*b*; $r^2 = 0.33$, $p = 0.012$ with humans, $r^2 = 0.16$, $p = 0.119$ without humans).

The second problem in testing the inverse relationship between brain size and gut size is the quality of the data available. Reliable total body composition data are not available for significant numbers of anthropoid primates. This means that it is not possible at the present time to study the relationship between relative brain mass and relative gut mass in single individuals. This is unfortunate because the brain mass data may come from a particularly large individual while the gut mass may come from a particularly small individual, confounding assessments of the

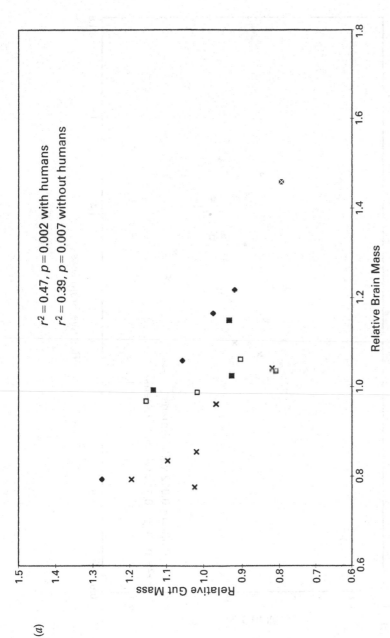

Fig. 3.3. Bivariate plots of relative gut mass against relative brain mass. (a) Relative brain mass and relative gut mass for each species are determined in relation to the expected brain and gut masses computed on the basis of the anthropoid primate best-fit equations. (b) The relative masses are determined in relation to the expected masses computed on the basis of the general mammalian equations. (c) The relative masses are determined as in (b) but the same species 'average' body mass is used to compute the expected brain mass and the expected gut mass. See text for explanation. Equations are given in Table 3.1 and the data are from Table 3.2. Symbols: X = colobines; diamonds = cebids; open squares = cercopithecids; closed squares = greater and lesser apes; and square with X = humans.

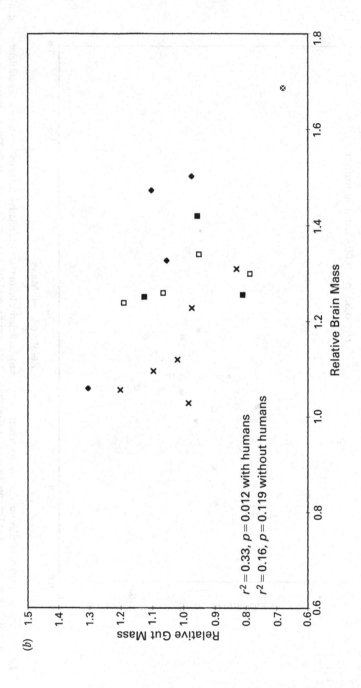

(b)

Relative Gut Mass

Relative Brain Mass

$r^2 = 0.33$, $p = 0.012$ with humans
$r^2 = 0.16$, $p = 0.119$ without humans

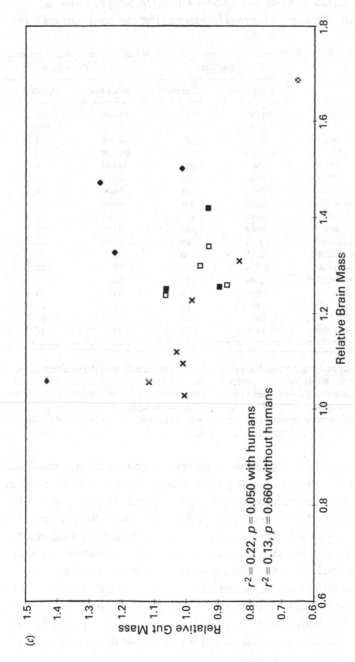

$r^2 = 0.22$, $p = 0.050$ with humans
$r^2 = 0.13$, $p = 0.660$ without humans

Fig. 3-3. (cont.)

Table 3.2. *Data (in grams) for the determination of the best-fit lines for the relationships between gut mass and body mass and between brain mass and body mass*

	Gut data		Brain data	
	Body mass	Gut mass	Body mass	Brain mass
Pongo pygmaeus	64819	1591	53000	413
Hylobates lar	5200	188	5500	108
Hylobates syndactylus	9300	490	10750	122
Homo sapiens	60800	1107	65000	1300
Nasalis larvatus	15880	598	15100	94
Presbytis melalophos	6781	254	6650	80
Presbytis obscura	7580	315	7400	68
Presbytis rubicundus	6350	171	6300	93
Presbytis cristatus	6850	433	8350	64
Colobus polykomos	7662	380	9400	77
Macaca fascicularis	3175	149	5000	69
Cercopithecus cephus	3338	120	3500	64
Erythrocebus patas	11650	280	7800	107
Cercopithecus neglectus	4081	254	5480	71
Cebus apella	2890	110	2480	71
Saimiri sciureus	740	39	665	24
Lagothrix lagothricha	8050	362	6300	96
Alouatta seniculus	4450	360	7250	58

Notes:
For the gut analysis, gut and body masses for the determination of the best-fit line are from Chivers & Hladik (1980: typesetting errors affecting data accuracy in table 6 have been corrected and new species added. Chivers, personal communication, 1990). For the brain analysis, brain and body masses, except for *Homo sapiens,* are from Harvey *et al.* (1987). The *Homo sapiens* data are from the 65-kg 'standard' human male used in the determination of expected organ sizes in Fig. 3.3 and are from Aschoff *et al.* (1971).

species specific 'average' relationship between relative brain size and relative gut size. In Figs. 3.3*a* and 3.3*b* this danger was minimized as much as is currently possible by insuring that gut masses and body masses used to determine the best-fit equation were from the same individuals and that brain masses and body masses were also from the same individuals. See Table 3.2 for the samples used to compute the best-fit equations. Unfortunately there are not many species in common in these two analyses. In order to increase the available sample for the analysis of relative gut mass and relative brain mass (Figs. 3.3*a* and 3.3*b*) species average brain masses and body masses were used from Harvey *et al.* (1980). Relative brain mass was, however, determined on the basis of the more precisely determined best-fit equation.

In Fig. 3.3c the species average body masses from Harvey *et al.* (1987) were also used to compute the best-fit line characterizing the relationship between gut mass and body mass. As might be expected, the inverse relationship between relative brain mass and relative gut mass breaks down further. It is now only barely significant even when humans are included in the relationship ($r^2 = 0.219$, $p = 0.05$ including humans, $r^2 = 0.013$, $p = 0.66$, without humans).

These are only three examples of many possible combinations of data sets and line-fitting techniques that could potentially be applied to the problem of relative brain size and gut size in the anthropoid primates. They do, however, provide a strong caution in relation to drawing conclusions from relatively poor data where species averages are based on small sample sizes. Results are highly dependent both on the particular data employed in the analysis and on the choice of best-fit relationships used to characterize these data.

Until more precise body composition data and BMR data are available for single individuals in a representative sample of anthropoid primates it will not be possible to conclusively test the relationship between BMR and organ size across the anthropoid primates and thereby provide an adequate test for these species of the inverse relationship between brain size and gut size. These problems of data quality and line fitting may also be a concern in recent reports that find no inverse correlation between relative brain size and relative gut mass in other mammals such as bats (Martin, 1996) or pigs (Wrangham, quoted in Gibbons, 1998).

Ecophysiology, energetic challenge and brain evolution

Although data quality poses a problem in testing the inverse relationship between brain size and gut size in the examples given above, where high quality data do exist the general relationship between organ size, metabolic physiology and adaptive strategy is gaining strong support and spawning a new field of evolutionary biology which has been called ecophysiology (e.g. Daan *et al.*, 1990; Piersma & Lindström, 1997; Meerlo *et al.*, 1997; Piersma *et al.*, 1996; Piersma & Gill, 1998; Speakman & McQueenie, 1996; Weber & Piersma, 1996; Konarzewski & Diamond, 1994). For example, Daan and his colleagues (1990) provide good body composition and BMR data from the same individuals representing 22 species of birds distributed over 7 orders (Anseri-, Falconi-, Galli-, Charadrii-, Columbi-, Pici-, and Passeriformes). They also provide daily energy expenditure data (DEE) for free-living parent birds from these same species. These data do not support an inverse relationship between relative gut size and relative brain size in these species of birds ($r = -0.098$, $p = 0.674$)[1]. Even when relative BMR, heart, kidney and liver sizes are held constant, the negative correlation between relative brain size and relative gut size still does not reach significance (partial $r = -0.238$, $p = 0.357$, $d.f. = 15$). These data also do not support any particular relationship between relative brain size and relative basal metabolism ($r = 0.212$, $p = 0.355$). In fact the only thing that relative brain size is significantly correlated with in this sample is the relative size of the leg muscles ($r = 0.623$, $p = 0.003$), a relationship that is awaiting explanation.

The lack of a significant correlation between relative brain size, relative gut size and relative BMR is perhaps not surprising in birds. Birds are not unusually encephalized animals (Bennett & Harvey, 1985) and brain size would not be expected to pose any unusual energetic challenge to adult birds. A bird weighing 500 g, for example, has a much smaller brain (and a smaller gut) than a similarly sized primate, but it has a considerably larger heart and kidneys (Aiello & Wheeler, 1995, in the reply to comments on the lead article). In the data-base provided by Daan and his colleagues (1990), relative BMR is significantly associated both with relative kidney and heart size and with maximal energy turnover during parental care (DEE). In fact, combined heart and kidney lean dry mass explains more of the variation in total body BMR than does total body mass. Daan and his colleagues speculate that, as in mammals, the heart and kidneys of birds may be the most costly of the expensive tissues and that size variation in these organs has a disproportionate effect on total body BMR. Because species with relatively large hearts and kidneys and relatively high BMRs also have relatively high DEEs, they interpret the relatively large organs (kidney and heart) in the context of the evolutionary trade-off between current and future reproduction. Because DEE is related to the intensity of reproductive output, it would be expected to vary with the environmental circumstances. The basal metabolic rate as well as the size of the heart and kidneys (the metabolic engines driving DEE) would then also be expected to vary with the environment and would thus vary between species.

1. Correlations are based on a re-analysis of the data presented in Daan *et al.* (1990). Residual organ sizes and BMR are computed on the basis of reduced major axis equations. The correlation coefficients reported here and their significance levels may, therefore, differ from those reported by the original authors who computed their residuals on the basis of least squares regression equations.

Daan and his colleagues emphasize that these conclusions are speculations and are in need of further testing. The results do emphasize,
however, the growing realization of the potentially highly significant
relationships between metabolic physiology, population biology, reproductive energetics and life history. Other research into eco-physiology
has, to date, concentrated primarily on intraspecific analyses and on the
short-term, sometimes radical, variations in size of internal organs, and
particularly the alimentary tract, in response to the energetic challenge of
required peak performance or resource limitation (Piersma & Lindström,
1997). A notable example is the Burmese python (*Python molurus*) whose
sevenfold increase in BMR within 24 h of having a meal equivalent to 25%
of its body mass is accompanied by a doubling of the size of the small
intestines and a 45% increase in the size of the kidneys and liver (Secor &
Diamond, 1995). Furthermore, considerable reduction in the size of the
digestive organs, and particularly the stomach, has been reported just
prior to migration in shore birds (red knots – *Calidris canutus*; bar-tailed
godwits – *Limosa lapponica*) and in long-distance migrating passerine
birds such as garden warblers (*Sylvia borin*) and thrush nightingales
(*Luscinia luscinia*) (summarized in Piersma & Lindström, 1997). There is
also evidence of a hypertrophy of digestive organs accompanying
increased BMR in migratory red knots over-wintering in temperate as
opposed to tropical climates (Piersma *et al.*, 1996) as well as examples of
general organ hypertrophy in cold stressed laboratory animals (e.g.
Konarzewski & Diamond, 1994) including primates (Chaffee *et al.*, 1966).
Other examples include significant hypertrophy of the guts and other
internal organs accompanying a rise in BMR in gestating and lactating
mice (Speakman & McQueenie, 1996) as well as significant reduction in
size of the internal organs and of BMR in response to food shortage in
birds (Daan *et al.*, 1989) and humans (Keys, 1950; Rivers, 1988). Resource
limitation also has an effect on the differential ontogeny of traits as has
been recently demonstrated in both butterflies (*Precis coenia*) and beetles
(*Onthophagus taurus* and *O. acuminatus*) (Nijhout & Emlen, 1998) and also in
humans (Barker, 1994).

These examples provide illustrations of the relationship between
organ size, metabolic physiology and adaptation during both ontogeny
and adult life. They not only support the relationship between basal
metabolism and the size of the internal organs but also illustrate some of
the ways in which organ size and metabolic physiology can vary in
response to a variety of energetic challenges such as reproduction,

thermoregulation and/or resource limitation. Detailed investigation of these relationships is currently hampered by relatively poor quality data for wider groups of animals, and particularly for larger bodied mammals (Piersma & Lindström, 1997). At present, good quality data are dependent on sacrificing the animals to obtain body composition. The development of non-invasive methods for accurately assessing body composition would not only do away with the necessity of sacrificing animals but would also permit controlled experiments where variation in organ size and in basal metabolic rate could be studied over time in the same individuals. Such advances would be expected to provide the basis for significant contributions to our future knowledge of the general relationship between organ size, metabolic rate and life history adaptation.

Human evolution, the Expensive Tissue Hypothesis and the Maternal Energy Hypothesis

One thing that does emerge from our current knowledge of the relationship between organ size and metabolism is that major changes in organ size occur in response to energetic challenges and that these can take various forms. In the python it is a meal, in migratory birds it is the athletic challenge of the long-distance migration, and in animals living under cold weather conditions it is the thermoregulatory challenge. For some birds it might also be the challenge of reproduction in environments where the risk of mortality may be either high or low.

In humans the growth and maintenance of the large brain is an equivalent major energetic challenge. This is not because the brain, even in humans, is necessarily more expensive than some of the body's other expensive organs (Fig. 3.4). Rather, it is because the pattern of growth of the brain differs from that of any other organ of the body. In all animals the brain grows very rapidly prenatally and in humans it continues along the very steep prenatal growth curve until approximately one year after birth (Martin, 1983). Thereafter the growth velocity decreases and by seven years of age the brain has reached its adult mass (Cabana et al., 1993). While the brain grows very rapidly in early life, the growth of the remaining organs keeps pace with the overall growth of the body. At birth the brain accounts for a phenomenal 60% of overall basal metabolism. This percentage decreases as the other organs steadily grow to reach their adult masses.

The association across mammals in general and primates in particular

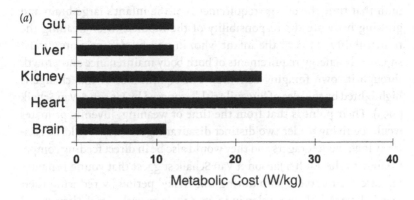

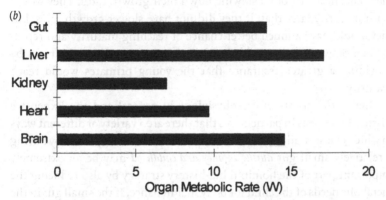

Fig. 3.4. (a) Mass specific metabolic costs (W/Kg) for the five expensive organs in humans. (b) Organ metabolic rate (W) for the five expensive tissues in humans. Data are from Aiello & Wheeler (1995) and are for a 65-kg male with a total BMR of 90.6.

between maternal basal metabolism and/or long gestation times and late weaning reflects the fact that mothers support this brain growth both prenatally during gestation and postnatally during lactation (Martin, 1996; Harvey quoted in Gibbons, 1998). However, this association (the Maternal Energy Hypothesis) does not necessarily negate the Expensive Tissue Hypothesis and particularly the importance of the trade-off between brain size and gut size in human evolution. Alterations in individual metabolic physiology as proposed by the Expensive Tissue Hypothesis, and seen in the larger context of overall life-history strategy, may well provide a means of optimizing the energy budgets of both the infant and the mother.

The critical point in infant ontogeny comes when it is weaned. Up until that time the energy requirements of the infant's large brain and growing body are the responsibility of the mother. After weaning the responsibility shifts to the infant who, in non-human primates, must support the energy requirements of both body maintenance and growth through its own foraging activities. The significance of this change is highlighted by the idea of 'juvenile risk' proposed by Janson & Van Schaik (1993). Their point is that from the time of weaning, juvenile primates would be living under two distinct disadvantages. They would be relatively inefficient foragers and they would also be in direct feeding competition with the adults. Janson & Van Schaik suggest that young primates increase their survivorship during this 'risky' period by reducing their metabolic needs through slowing down their growth rates. They would reach maturity later than if they did not have slower growth rates, but they would have a much better chance of reaching maturity and reproducing. Slow growth would thereby optimize reproductive fitness by providing a greater assurance that the young primates would reach maturity.

One of the points of eco-physiology in general and the Expensive Tissue Hypothesis in particular is that there are a variety of different ways in which energy budgets can be manipulated. The energy saved by having a relatively small gut *during infancy and childhood* may be an extremely important part of the hominin life-history strategy by also reducing the metabolic needs of the child for body maintenance. If the small gut in the infant saved 10% of overall basal metabolism, as it does in the human adult, this would be a considerable energy saving to that infant. Without the reduced gut and corresponding lower maintenance costs to the young hominin, the characteristic long period of hominin growth and development (Bogin & Smith, 1996) may have been even longer. The young hominin would have to compensate for the higher energetic cost of a relatively larger gut by even slower growth. This would have corresponding consequences for overall reproductive fitness.

There is at least one obvious problem with this hypothesis. A small gut requires a high quality diet (Aiello & Wheeler, 1995) and a high quality diet of the type suggested for the early hominins would not have been easily accessible to the young without reducing the feeding competition between adults and young and introducing food sharing or provisioning. There are two main sources of high quality foods that would have been available when the hominin brain increased radically in size during the Plio-Pleistocene. These are roots or tubers (Hatley & Kappelman, 1980;

Conklin-Brittain *et al.*, 1998; O'Connell *et al.*, 1999) and animal-based foods including fish and shell fish (Broadhurst *et al.*, 1998). Both main categories of food would have had a high biomass in the more open, lake-studded habitats in eastern and southern Africa that were occupied by the early hominins during the Plio-Pleistocene. Both would also have had a decreased fiber content and increased nutrient density in relation to other primate foods (Conklin-Brittain *et al.*, 1998) that would be consistent with more rapid digestion and the evolution of relatively smaller guts (Aiello & Wheeler, 1995). And both would require learned skills in food acquisition that would presuppose food sharing between adults and the young who would not have yet acquired these skills or the body strength and/or co-ordination to effectively exploit these resources (e.g. digging for tubers, cracking open shell fish, hunting and scavenging) (Parker & Gibson, 1979).

Exploitation of 'high quality' resources such as roots and tubers or animal-based foods was very probably a necessary prerequisite of hominin occupation of more open African habitats (Williamson & Aiello, 1998). Because of the necessity of provisioning dependent offspring, the net effect of the exploitation of such resources would have been to put an extra energetic strain on mothers. Mothers would not only have had to have expended energy on their own body maintenance and on gestation and lactation but now would also have had to have expended energy on what can be termed as 'extra somatic nursing'. Mothers would have had to provision their dependent, but already weaned, offspring until they acquired the necessary food acquisition skills for themselves.

Solutions to the problem of the increased energetic load on mothers have been seen in changes in social organization and inter-personal inter-action. One of these changes may have been grandmothering, or food sharing by senior females with daughters and grandchildren (Hawkes *et al.*, 1997a,b; O'Connell *et al.*, 1999). This solution may also have had sig-nificant consequences for the evolution of longevity and post-reproduc-tive female life-span (Hawkes *et al.*, 1998). Likewise, modeling has demonstrated that food sharing between unrelated adults of both sexes may have been another solution (Key, 1998; Key & Aiello, 1999, 2000). Another important factor that has generally been overlooked in these socially based arguments is the energetic cost of the maintenance of the mother's own body. A relatively small gut would provide a 10% reduction in the mother's own basal metabolism (Fig. 3.2) and would theoretically allow her to conserve her own energy. The net effect would be to increase her own reproductive output.

A relatively small gut would, therefore, be expected to have fitness benefits not only for the weaned infants and juveniles but also for their mothers. These implications of the Expensive Tissue Hypothesis are at the moment, however, no more than hypotheses themselves. We simply do not have reliable data for humans and non-human primates to adequately look at the relationship between body composition, diet, basal metabolism, daily energy expenditure and reproductive success. What we do know, however, is that the high quality diet available to early hominins would have been consistent with the evolution of relatively small guts and that relatively small guts would help to reduce the overall basal metabolic requirements of the body at the time in human evolution when the energy hungry brain was expanding. We also know that a high quality diet would have had a direct effect on the evolution of a relatively large brain. It would have provided the essential fatty acids to support brain growth and maintenance (Broadhurst *et al.*, 1998) and might also have been at the root of the distinctive human brain lateralization and cognitive differences between males and females. Chimpanzees, and presumably early hominins living on a similar type of diet, would have had a relatively low protein intake (Conklin-Brittain *et al.*, 1998). An increase in protein intake through an increased reliance on animal-based food could have been responsible for earlier fetal maturation and might be directly related to more asymmetric development of the hemispheres of the brain and ultimately to more lateralization of function (Wynn *et al.*, 1996).

Conclusions

The energy requirements of both the growth and maintenance of the relatively large human brain undoubtedly hold important clues in relation to the evolution of modern human adaptation. The Maternal Energy and Expensive Tissue Hypotheses are not mutually exclusive in providing insight into this problem. The Maternal Energy Hypothesis focuses on the question of how we can afford to grow large brains and provides an answer based on the amount of energy the mother diverts to the fetus and infant measured through maternal basal metabolism and the length of gestation and lactation. The Expensive Tissue Hypothesis focuses on a different question. It focuses on the energetic problems of brain growth and maintenance after weaning and suggests answers involving variation in body composition, energy allocation, metabolic efficiency, and in life history pattern. The current challenge is to integrate these various lines of evidence for a better understanding of the human brain and of the unique complex of human life history, social and behavioral adaptations.

We can now bring into focus one point introduced at the beginning of this discussion. Martin (1996) has suggested that the evolution of large brains might be better explained by the metabolic resources allocated by mothers to fetal and postnatal development than by selection for any particular feature or ability. The previous arguments highlight the fact that the growth and maintenance of large brains involves important 'decisions' in relation to resource allocation that go beyond the simple allocation of maternal resources. This is particularly significant in human evolution because of our unusually large brain. It would simply not pay a mother to divert resources into producing infants with large brains, nor would it pay the weanlings to maintain these large brains, if there were not good adaptive reasons to do so. The mother would be better off using any available energy to increase her reproductive output by having more babies and the infant would be better off using any available energy to grow faster, reach maturity sooner and begin reproduction earlier. Energy allocation is undoubtedly important to the growth and maintenance of large brains, but the real issue in human evolution is why we devote so much of our energy budget to the growth and maintenance of large brains. This is a fundamental question that is still awaiting an answer in human evolution.

References

Aiello, L.C. (1996a). Hominine preadaptations for language and cognition. In *Modelling the Early Human Mind*, eds. P. Mellars & K. Gibson, pp. 89–99. Cambridge: McDonald Institute Monograph Series.

Aiello, L.C. (1996b). Terrestriality, bipedalism and the origin of language. In *Evolution of Social Behaviour Patterns in Primates and Man*, ed. J. Maynard-Smith, London: Proceedings of the British Academy, **88**, 269–289.

Aiello, L.C. (1997). Brains and guts in human evolution: the Expensive Tissue Hypothesis. *Brazilian Journal of Genetics*, **20**, 141–148.

Aiello, L.C. (1998a). The Expensive Tissue Hypothesis and the evolution of the human adaptive niche: a study in comparative anatomy. In *Science in Archaeology: an Agenda for the Future*, ed. J. Bayley, pp. 25–36. London: English Heritage.

Aiello, L.C. (1998b). The foundations of human language. In *The Origin and Diversification of Language*, eds. N.G. Jablonski & L.C. Aiello, pp. 15–33. San Francisco: University of California Press.

Aiello, L.C. & Wheeler, P. (1995). The expensive-tissue hypothesis: the brain and the digestive system in human and primate evolution. *Current Anthropology*, **36**, 199–221.

Aiello, L.C. & Wheeler, P. (1996). On diet, energy-metabolism, and brain size in human evolution – Reply. *Current Anthropology*, **37**, 128–129.

Armstrong, E. (1985). Relative brain size in monkeys and prosimians. *American Journal of Physical Anthropology*, **66**, 263–273.

Aschoff, J., Günther, B. & Kramer, K. (1971). *Energie-haushalt und Temperaturregulation*. Munich: Urban and Schwarzenberg.

Barker, D.J.P. (1994). *Mothers, Babies, and Disease in Later Life*. London: BMJ Publishing Group.

Bennett, P.M. & Harvey, P.H. (1985). Brain size, development and metabolism in birds and mammals. *Journal of Zoology*, **207**, 491–509.

Broadhurst, C.L., Cunnane, S.C. & Crawford, M.A. (1998). Rift Valley lake fish and shellfish provided brain-specific nutrition for early *Homo*. *British Journal of Nutrition*, **7**, 3–21.

Bogin, B. & Smith, B.H. (1996). Evolution of the human life cycle. *American Journal of Human Biology*, **8**, 703–716.

Cabana, T., Jolicoeur, P. & Michaud, J. (1993). Prenatal and postnatal growth and allometry of stature, head circumference, and brain weight in Québec children. *American Journal of Human Biology*, **5**, 93–99.

Chaffee, R.R.J., Horvath, S.M., Smith, R.E. & Welsh, R.S. (1966). Cellular biochemistry and organ mass of cold- and heat-acclimated monkeys. *Federation Proceedings*, **25**, 1177–1184.

Chivers, D.J. & Haldik, M. (1980). Morphology of the gastrointestinal tract in primates: Comparisons with other mammals in relation to diet. *Journal of Morphology*, **166**, 337–386.

Conklin-Brittain, N.L., Wrangham, R.W. & Smith, C.C. (1998). Relating chimpanzee diets to potential *Australopithecus* diets. Poster presented at the symposium on Origins and Evolution of Human Diet at the 14th International Congress of Anthropological and Ethnological Sciences in Williamsburg, Virginia (http://www.cast.uark.edu/local/icaes/conferences/wburg/posters/nconklin/conklin.html)

Daan, S., Masman, D., Strijkstra, A. & Verhulst, S. (1989). Intraspecific allometry of basal metabolic rate: relations with body size, temperature, composition, and circadian phase in the kestrel, *Falco tinnunculus*. *Journal of Biological Rhythms*, **4**, 267–283.

Daan, S., Masman, D. & Groenewold, A. (1990). Avian basal metabolic rates: their association with body composition and energy expenditure in nature. *American Journal of Physiology*, **259**, R333–R340.

Foley, R.A. & Lee, P.C. (1991). Ecology and energetics of encephalization in hominid evolution. *Philosophical Transactions of the Royal Society of London* B**334**, 223–232.

Gibbons, A. (1998). Solving the brain's energy crisis. *Science*, **288**, 1345–1347.

Hatley, T. & Kappelman, J. (1980). Bears, pigs, and Plio-Pleistocene hominids: a case for the exploitation of below ground food resources. *Human Ecology*, **8**, 371–387.

Harvey, R.H., Martin, R.D. & Clutton-Brock, T.H. (1987). Life histories in comparative perspective. In *Primate Societies*, eds. B.B. Smuts, D.L. Cheney, R.M. Seyfarth, R.W. Wrangham & T.T. Struhsaker, pp. 181–196. Chicago: University of Chicago Press.

Hawkes, K., O'Connell, J.F. & Rogers, L. (1997a). The behavioral ecology of modern hunter-gatherers, and human evolution. *Trends in Ecology and Evolution*, **12**, 29–32.

Hawkes, K., O'Connell, J.F. & Blurton Jones, N.G. (1997b). Hadza women's time allocation, offspring provisioning, and the evolution of long post-menopausal lifespans. *Current Anthropology*, **38**, 551–578.

Hawkes, K., O'Connell, J.F., Blurton Jones, N.G., Alvarez, H. & Charnov, E.L. (1998). Grandmothering, menopause, and the evolution of human life histories. *Proceedings of the National Academy of Sciences USA*, **95**, 1336–1339.

Janson, C.H. & Van Schaik, C.P. (1993). Ecological risk aversion in juvenile primates: slow and steady wins the race. In *Juvenile Primates: Life History, Development, and Behaviour*, eds. M.E. Pereira & L.A. Fairbanks, pp. 57–74. New York and Oxford: Oxford University Press.

Key, C. (1998). Co-operation, Paternal Care and the Evolution of Hominid Social Groups. PhD Thesis, University of London.

Key, C. & Aiello, L.C. (1999). Dietary change, allocare and the evolution of social organisation. In *The Evolution of Culture*, eds. R.I.M Dunbar, C. Knight & C. Power, pp. 15–33. Edinburgh: Edinburgh University Press.

Key, C. & Aiello, L.C. (2000). A prisoner's dilemma model of the evolution of paternal care, *Folia primatologica*, **71**, 77–92.

Keys, A. (ed.) (1950). *The Biology of Human Starvation*. Minneapolis, MN: University of Minnesota Press.

Konarzewski, M. & Diamond, J. (1994). Peak sustained metabolic rate and its individual variation in cold-stressed mice. *Physiological Zoology*, **67**, 1186–1212.

Leonard, W.R. & Robertson, M.L. (1992). Nutritional requirements and human evolution: A bioenergetics model. *American Journal of Human Biology*, **4**, 179–195.

Leonard, W.R. & Robertson, M.L. (1994). Evolutionary perspectives on human nutrition: The influence of brain and body size on diet and metabolism. *American Journal of Human Biology*, **6**, 77–88.

Leonard, W.R. & Robertson, M.L. (1997). Comparative primate energetics and hominid evolution. *American Journal of Physical Anthropology*, **102**, 265–281.

MacNab, B.K. & Eisenberg, J.F. (1989). Brain size and its relation to the rate of metabolism in mammals. *American Naturalist*, **133**, 157–167.

Martin, R.D. (1983). *Human Brain Evolution in an Ecological Context*. New York: American Museum of Natural History.

Martin, R.D. (1996). Scaling of the mammalian brain: the maternal energy hypothesis. *News in Physiological Sciences*, **11**, 149–156.

Meerlo, P., Bolle, L., Visser, G.H., Masman, D. & Daan, S. (1997). Basal metabolic rate in relation to body composition and daily energy expenditure in the Field Vole, *Microtus agrestis*. *Physiological Zoology*, **70**, 362–369.

Nijhout, H.F. & Emlen, D.J. (1998). Competition among body parts in the development and evolution of insect morphology. *Proceedings of the National Academy of Sciences USA*, **95**, 3685–3689.

O'Connell, J.F.C., Hawkes, K. & Blurton-Jones, N.G. (1999). Grandmothering and the evolution of *Homo erectus*. *Journal of Human Evolution*, **36**, 461–485.

Parker, S.T. & Gibson, K.R. (1979). A model of the evolution of language and intelligence in early hominids. *Behavioral and Brain Sciences*, **2**, 367–407.

Piersma, T. & Gill, R.E. (1998). Guts don't fly: small digestive organs in obese bar-tailed godwits. *The Auk*, **115**, 196–203.

Piersma, T. & Lindström, Å. (1997). Rapid reversible changes in organ size as a component of adaptive behaviour. *TREE*, **12**, 134–138.

Piersma, T., Bruinzeel, L., Drent, R., Kersten, M., Van der Meer, J. & Wiersma, P. (1996). Variability in basal metabolic rate of a long-distance migrant shorebird (Knot *Calidris canutus*) reflects shifts in organ size. *Physiological Zoology*, **69**, 191–217.

Power, C. & Aiello, L.C. (1997). Female proto-symbolic strategies. In *Women in Human Evolution*, ed. L.D. Hager, pp. 153–171. London: Routledge.

Rivers, J.P.W. (1988). The nutritional biology of Famine. In *Famine*, ed. G.A. Harrison, pp. 57–106. Oxford: Oxford University Press.

Secor, S.M. & Diamond, J. (1995). Adaptive responses to feeding in Burmese pythons: pay before pumping. *Journal of Experimental Biology*, **198**, 1313–1325.

Speakman, J.R. & McQueenie, J. (1996). Limits to sustained metabolic rate: the link between food intake, basal metabolic rate, and morphology in reproducing mice, *Mus musculus. Physiological Zoology*, **69**, 746–769.

Stephan, H., Frahm, H. & Baron, G. (1981). New and revised data on volume of brain structures in insectivores and primates. *Folia Primatologica*, **35**, 1–29.

Weber, T.P. & Piersma, T. (1996). Basal metabolic rate and the mass of tissues differing in metabolic scope: migration-related covariation between individual Knots *Calidris canutus. Journal of Avian Biology*, **27**, 215–224.

Williamson, D. & Aiello, L.C. (1998). Modelling the adaptation of early *Homo*. Paper given at the Dual Congress 1998 of the International Association for the Study of Human Palaeontology and the International Association of Human Biologists held in Sun City, South Africa, 28 June – 4 July, 1998.

Wynn, T.G., Tierson, F.D. & Palmer, C.T. (1996). Evolution of sex differences in spatial cognition. *Yearbook of Physical Anthropology*, **39**, 11–42.

Acknowledgements

We would like to thank Dean Falk and Kathleen Gibson for inviting us to participate in the 1997 *American Association of Physical Anthropology* symposium in honor of Harry Jerison. His work opened up the field of allometry and brain evolution to L.C.A., who has benefited from numerous discussions with him in subsequent years. The present contribution would not have been possible without collaboration with Peter Wheeler on the development of the Expensive Tissue Hypothesis or without David Chiver's unique data set on gut size and morphology in the primates. L.C.A. is grateful to Ann MacLarnon for help in getting the gut data set together, to Caroline Ross for explaining the complexities of primate life history variation and to Kristin Hawkes and Jim O'Connell for fascinating discussions on the evolution of human life history strategies. We are also grateful to the following for discussions of the ideas presented in this paper: Barry Bogin, Margaret Clegg, Mark Collard, Claire Imber, Catherine Key, Hartley Odwak, Holly Smith, Volker Sommer, and Helen Wood. And finally L.C.A. is grateful to R.D. Martin who first introduced her to the problems of energetics and the brain and provided the stimulus for this paper by challenging the validity of the Expensive Tissue Hypothesis.

4

Bigger is better: primate brain size in relationship to cognition

Debates between Harry Jerison and Ralph Holloway enlightened and expanded our understandings of the evolution of the human brain and human mind for a period of several decades. Jerison argued that quantitative increases in neural tissue and in neural information processing capacity were the most important determinants of human intelligence (Jerison, 1973). Holloway took a seemingly contradictory stance, that the human brain had been reorganized in relationship to the brains of other primates and that this reorganization was the primary determinant of human mental capacities (Holloway, 1966). These debates have waned in recent years with the realizations that quantitative change and neural reorganization are not mutually exclusive phenomena. Indeed, in mammals, increased brain size correlates with or predicts various forms of brain reorganization including decreased neuronal density, increased ratios of connections to neurons, increased numbers of gyri and fissures, increased neuronal specialization, and increased size of the neocortex, cerebellum, hippocampus, corpus striatum, and diencephalon and other neural structures (Finlay & Darlington, 1995; Gibson & Jessee, 1999; Jerison, 1973, 1982, 1985). Increased numbers of neural processing units or 'modules' would also be expected to result in increased amounts of neural tissue (Preuss, Chapter 7, this volume).

These considerations suggest that among closely related mammalian species those with the larger brains may well have the greatest mental abilities. Not only will they have greater overall information processing capacities, but also, in many cases, they will have increased numbers of neural modules, increased size of the neocortex and of other higher neural processing areas, and increased neural connectivity. Questions remain, however, about which of many possible quantitative measures best reflect species variations in intelligence.

Some investigators consider absolute brain size to be the best predictor of intelligence (Beran *et al.*, 1999; Gibson & Jessee, 1999). It has become almost axiomatic among many scholars, however, that encephalization, i.e. a species' brain size relative to the brain size of other species of similar body size, is a more appropriate measure of intelligence than absolute brain size. For example, although Neanderthals had larger brains than modern humans, they also had greater body mass (Ruff *et al.*, 1997). This has led to the recent interpretation that they were actually less intelligent than modern humans, because their brains were smaller in relationship to their body size (Kappelman, 1997).

Jerison's seminal contributions to this literature derive from his statistical correlations of brain and body size across vertebrate taxa and his concepts that as body size increases, the amount of neural tissue needed to handle body functions also increases (Jerison, 1973, 1985). He, thus, delineated two measures: Encephalization Quotient (EQ) and extra neurons. The mammalian EQ is a measure of the extent to which a mammalian species' brain size exceeds (or falls below) the size that would be expected for a typical mammalian species of similar body size. Thus, a species with an EQ of 1 has the expected brain size of a typical mammal of similar body size. Those with EQs above or below 1 have larger or smaller than expected brain sizes, respectively. Extra neurons are the increased numbers of neurons that large brained species have over those needed to handle the demands of large body size. Extra neurons, thus, are the neurons readily available to mediate intelligence, increased sensorimotor skills, or other advanced functions. Although, for each species, EQ and extra neurons are derived from the same brain and body size data, they do not always provide equivalent predictions of intelligence. In comparison to other Anthropoidea, for instance, gorillas have a relatively low EQ, but relatively large numbers of extra neurons. Bauchot and Stephan defined a parameter very similar to the EQ – the Index of Progression (IP), a measure of brain size relative to the predicted brain size for a basal insectivore of similar body size (Bauchot & Stephan, 1969). Others have attempted to compensate for brain size/body size relationships by defining measures of total brain size or size of the neocortex in relationship to size of other neural structures that are not considered to mediate intellectual functions such as the medulla oblongata (Passingham & Ettlinger, 1974) or to the entire brain other than the neocortex (Dunbar,

1992, 1993, 1997). However, uncertainty remains as to which of these indices best predicts intelligence.

One reason for this remaining uncertainty is that absolute brain size, EQs, IPs, extra neurons, and other measures all provide the expected result that humans are the most intelligent primates. Second, these debates began when animal behavior research was in its infancy and little was known about the intellectual capacities of non-human primates and other animals. This rendered it impossible to test brain size measures against actual performance on behavioral and cognitive tasks. This situation has changed in the last few decades, and we now have a wealth of behavioral data for primates and some other taxa. Third, discussions of brain size in relationship to intelligence can be confounded by attempts to compare distantly-related species with radically different neural and sensorimotor organizations such as elephants, primates, and cetaceans. Such comparisons encounter the major difficulties of devising 'species fair' behavioral tests that fully tap the mental capacities of each taxa and of distinguishing between the relative contributions of highly specific brain organizations versus absolute brain size or encephalization measures. To determine the relative contributions of absolute brain size or measures of encephalization to mental capacities, it is best to begin by comparing related species with relatively similar brain and behavioral organizations.

Primates, particularly the Anthropoidea (monkeys, apes, and humans), share common sensorimotor adaptations in that most have highly developed visual systems and considerable manual dexterity. Most also live in complex social groups. The anatomical and functional organization of the brains of higher primates, such as those of rhesus and squirrel monkeys, are also sufficiently similar to each other and to humans that monkeys have long been used in lieu of humans as experimental subjects by neuroscientists. Hence, higher primates are a logical group in which to examine the relative contributions of absolute brain size versus measures of encephalization to mental capacities. The intense interest in the mental capacities of Neanderthals and other fossil hominids also renders these questions of great importance to anthropologists. This paper explores the issue of whether absolute brain size or measures of encephalization (EQs and IPs) predict differences in mental capacity in the higher primates and can be used to predict intellectual capacities in hominid fossils.

Table 4.1. *Transfer index values for extant primates*

Species*	TI score**
Phaner	−20
Micro	−19
Lemur	−0.5
Samiri	+6
Talapoin	−23
Vervet	+7
Cebus	+0.5
Macaca	+9
Hylobates	+0.9
Pongo	+12
Gorilla	+14
Pan	+12

Notes:
* Species are rank-ordered according to brain complexity which is essentially a dimension of 'extra' brain and neurons (see Beran *et al.*, 1999, and Rumbaugh, 1997, for details).
** Scores that are positive denote positive transfer. Negative scores denote negative transfer.

Performance on the transfer index

The Transfer Index test distinguishes simple stimulus–response learning (e.g. always press the lever in response to a specific stimulus) from tasks that require the mental flexibility to change tactics if the reward system changes (Rumbaugh, 1970, 1997; Rumbaugh & Pate, 1984). In the Transfer Index test, Rumbaugh began by presenting animals of diverse primate species with two stimuli (+ and −) and always rewarding the animals for choosing the +. Animals were trained to two different levels of competency: 67% or 84% correct answers. After the animals reached one of the two competency levels, trial conditions changed, and they were rewarded for choosing the −. Distinct species differences were found (Table 4.1). Some species exhibited negative transfer. They performed more poorly on the reversal learning tasks when trained to 84% correct than when trained to 67% correct. These species appeared to have learned a stimulus–response association which they then had difficulty inhibiting. Other species exhibited positive transfer in that they performed better on the reversal task when trained to an 84% level of competency as compared to a 67% level of competency. They seemed to have learned the conceptual components of the task, i.e. choose the response that is currently rewarded.

Statistically significant correlations were found between performance on this task and body size ($r^2 = 0.87$), cranial capacity ($r^2 = 0.83$), and extra neurons ($r^2 = 0.79$). Statistically significant correlations were also found between cranial capacity and body size ($r^2 = 0.96$) and between cranial capacity and extra neurons ($r^2 = 0.82$). In contrast, no statistical correlation was found between performance on the transfer index task and EQ. Some species with very high EQs, such as cebus monkeys (EQ= 2.54 for *Cebus capuchinus*, 4.79 for *Cebus albifrons*, and 3.49 for *Cebus apella*) and talapoins (EQ= 2.76), performed relatively poorly, and the best performance was exhibited by gorillas who have low EQs (1.76). Rumbaugh and colleagues did not attempt to correlate performance on the Transfer Index task with the Index of Progression. A perusal of the data, however, suggests that these measures would also be unlikely to correlate with performance on this task, because IPs provide similar species rankings to EQs (see Table 4.2). Hence, IPs, like EQs, would predict that gorillas should be poor performers and that cebus and talapoins should be outstanding performers. Although Rumbaugh did not analyze his data according to phylogenetic classifications, his data would be consistent with interpretations that performance varies according to phylogenetic groups, i.e. all prosimians performed poorly on the transfer test, monkeys exhibited intermediate levels of performance, and great apes exhibited the best performance.

Possession of human-like mental capacities

Psychologists and anthropologists often attempt to model the evolution of human mental capacities, particularly those capacities that have sometimes been considered to be unique to the human species including toolmaking, language (especially symbolism and syntax), self-awareness, awareness of the thoughts of others (theory of mind), and deception. Such models require knowledge of the extent to which such capacities are present in other primates and of the extent to which their presence may be reflected in brain size parameters.

Considerable data now exist pertaining to the possible presence or

Table 4.2. *Primate rankings according to EQ and IP*

Primate	IP value*	EQ value**
Homo	28+	7.39–7.79
Miopithecus	12+	2.76
Pan	12+	2.17–2.48
Cebinae	9+	2.54–4.79
Atelinae	9+	2.33–2.48
Hylobatidae	9+	1.93–2.94
Pongo	9−	1.63–1.91
Papioninae	9−	1.73–2.35
Cercopithecinae	8+	1.66–2.18
Pitheciinae	8	
Daubentonia	7	>1.75***
Gorilla	7−	1.53–1.76
Colobidae	6+	
Aotinae	6	
Callitrichinae	6	1.43–1.74
Callimiconinae	6−	1.82–1.92
Alouattinae	5−	0.88–1.38
Other extant prosimians and tarsiers	5–3	0.6–1.39

Notes:
* IP values are from Stephan, H. (1972). Evolution of primate brains: a comparative anatomical perspective. In *The Functional and Evolutionary Biology of Primates*, ed. R. Tuttle, pp. 155–174. Chicago: Aldine.
** EQ values are from Jerison, H. J. (1973). *Evolution of the Brain and Intelligence*. New York: Academic Press.
*** Jerison (1973) does not state the EQ value for Daubentonia, but he does state that it was greater than the value for an extinct prosimian with an EQ of 1.75.

absence of these capacities in great apes (chimpanzee, bonobo, gorilla, and orangutan) and in a number of monkey species. Two major trends have emerged: (1) great apes possess the rudiments of each of these behavioral capacities (Byrne, 1995; Gibson, 1996; Parker, 1996); (2) monkey capacities in each of these behavioral domains are either absent, or they fall below the capacities of the great apes (Byrne, 1995; Tomasello & Call, 1997).

Members of all great ape species, for example, have mastered elements of gestural or visually based symbolic communication in captive settings and have exhibited the ability to combine symbols in a rule-like, syntactic, fashion (Gardner & Gardner, 1969; Miles, 1990; Patterson & Linden, 1981; Premack & Premack, 1983; Rumbaugh, 1977; Savage-Rumbaugh, 1986; Savage-Rumbaugh & Lewin, 1994; Savage-Rumbaugh *et al.*, 1980, 1986, 1998). Members of at least two great ape species (bonobo and chimpanzee) have also demonstrated comprehension of English words (Beran *et al.*, 2000; Savage-Rumbaugh *et al.*, 1993). To date, no monkeys have exhibited these language-like skills. Similarly, some members of all great ape species have exhibited mirror self-recognition capacities (Gallop, 1970, 1977, 1982; Parker *et al.*, 1994; Povinelli *et al.*, 1993; Suarez & Gallop, 1981), but no monkeys have clearly demonstrated such abilities (Gallop & Suarez, 1991; Suarez & Gallop, 1986). Great ape deceptive and imitative capacities also exceed those of monkeys, and great apes appear to have greater abilities to understand others' thoughts (Byrne, 1995; Byrne & Whiten, 1988; Whiten & Byrne, 1997).

The one possible exception to this general trend relates to tool-behavior. Chimpanzees make tools in the wild (Boesch & Boesch, 1983, 1990; Goodall, 1986; McGrew, 1974, 1992), and all great apes can make and use tools in captivity (Bard *et al.*, 1995; Call & Tomasello, 1994; Tomasello & Call, 1997; Toth *et al.*, 1993). Cebus monkeys also use and make tools in captivity (Anderson, 1996; Gibson, 1990; Parker & Gibson, 1977; Visalberghi, 1987, 1990, 1993; Westergard & Suomi, 1994). However, cebus monkey performance on complex tool-using tasks lags behind that of chimpanzees (Visalberghi *et al.*, 1995).

Great apes also more closely resemble humans than do monkeys in other object manipulation behaviors. Humans, chimpanzees, and bonobos routinely group objects into sets of four to 12, but cebus monkeys and macaques only form sets of up to three objects. By the end of the second year, humans routinely form three to four contemporaneous sets of objects (Langer, 1980, 1986, 1989, 2000). Apes are more developmentally delayed in this respect than humans, but do eventually begin to compose multiple simultaneous sets of objects (Spinozzi, 1993). In contrast, the monkeys never compose more than one set of objects at a time (Langer 1989, 1993, 2000; Spinozzi & Natale, 1989). These differences in set composition indicate that young apes and humans apply greater amounts of information processing capacity to their object manipulation endeavors than do monkeys. Langer has demonstrated that, in humans, the composition of objects into sets precedes and contributes to the development of mathematical, classificatory, and causal thought. Hence, these species differences have strong implications for the development of higher intellectual capacities.

To the extent that tool-making, other forms of object manipulation, language, self-awareness and theory of mind reflect cognitive skills similar to those possessed by humans, animals who possess these capacities would be expected to perform better on human-like intelligence tests than those who do not. Jean Piaget described the developing human infant and child as progressing through a series of stages of intelligence: sensorimotor (birth to 18–24 months), preoperational (2 to 7 years), concrete operations (7 to 12 years) and formal operations (from 12 years). Analyses of the behavioral performances of non-human primates using Piagetian measures support the view that ape performance on intelligence tests exceeds that of monkeys (Parker & McKinney, 1999). Adult great apes perform at the early preoperational stage (equivalent to that of a 3 to 4 year old human child) on varied object manipulation, imitative, social, and symbolic tasks. Cebus monkeys reach substages 5 or 6 of the sensorimotor stage in the tool-using domain, but only stage 4 in the imitative and object concept domain. Macaques reach substage 4 of the sensorimotor stage, and lemurs appear to reach only substage 2 of the sensorimotor stage (Antinucci, 1989; Antinucci *et al.*, 1986; Chevalier-Skolnikoff, 1977, 1983, 1989; Mathieu & Bergeron, 1983; Mathieu *et al.*, 1976; Natale *et al.*, 1986; Parker, 1977, 1990; Parker & McKinney, 1999; Parker & Gibson, 1979; Vauclair, 1982). Hence, performance on Piagetian tasks mirrors performance on tests for the presence of human-like behavioral capacities: humans exhibit the best performance followed by great apes. Cebus monkeys perform better on tool-using than on other tasks, and they may outperform other monkeys in the tool-using domain.

These data imply that if our search is for a primate brain size measure most predictive of the presence of human-like mental capacities, we should choose a measure that differentiates great apes on the one hand, from monkeys and prosimians on the other. Absolute brain size yields this distinction (Table 4.3) as do a number of other measures that strongly correlate with absolute brain size (r^2 ranging from 0.92 to 0.99; Finley & Darlington, 1995; Gibson & Jessee, 1999) including extra neurons, body size, and the size of many neural processing areas including the neocortex, cerebellum, corpus striatum, diencephalon, and hippocampus (Tables 4.3 and 4.4). In contrast, EQs and IPs do not yield these distinctions.

Discussion

These findings counter the common view that the best predictors of primate intelligence are measures of encephalization. Rather, absolute brain size, extra neurons, and body size predict performance on the transfer test whereas EQ does not. Absolute brain size, extra neurons, body

Table 4.3. *Absolute brain size and extra neurons distinguish great apes from monkeys*

	Brain sizes in grams	Extra neurons
Humans	~1300	~8.5
Great apes	287–570	2.59–3.86
Hylobatids	87–105	1.17–1.42
Papionae	179–222	1.76–2.19
Other Old World monkeys	41–140	0.76–1.45
New World monkeys	9.5–118	0.24–1.50

Notes:
The data in this table are from Jerison, H. J. (1973), *Evolution of the Brain and Intelligence*, New York: Academic Press. The human data represent an approximate mean of male and female values. The great ape data represent the range from the smallest (female orangutan) to largest (male gorilla) brains. The hylobatid and monkey values represent the range of brain sizes reported for the diverse species in these groups, most of which are delineated according to sex.

Table 4.4. *Absolute sizes of higher neural processing areas distinguish great apes from monkeys*

	Neocortex	Corpus striatum	Cerebellum	Hippocampus
Humans	1006525	28689	137421	10287
Great apes	291592–341444	12246–14567	43663–69249	31.2–86.8
Hylobatids	65800	4784	12078	2673
Papionae	140142	7182	18683	3398
Other Old World Monkeys	26427–68733	1908–4146	3374–12113	707–2295
New World Monkeys	2535–70856	174–4950	468–12438	133–1586

Notes:
Data in this table are from Stephan *et al.* (1981), New and revised data on volumes of brain structures in insectivores and primates. *Folia Primatologica*, **35**, 1–39. All weights are expressed in grams. When two numbers are given, they represent the range of values reported by Stephan *et al.*

size, and the size of a number of neural structures including the neocortex, cerebellum, corpus striatum, diencephalon, and hippocampus also distinguish great apes from monkeys. Each of these measures, thus, corresponds to current behavioral findings that great apes possess greater capacities than monkeys in a variety of cognitive domains including symbolic, deceptive, and mirror self-recognition capacities, and the abilities to understand the minds of others. In contrast, EQ and other measures of relative encephalization do not predict these results, but rather predict that many monkeys and some prosimians would match or exceed great apes in their cognitive skills.

The finding that absolute brain size better predicts mental capacities than does EQ is not entirely unexpected based on current understandings of brain function and current hypotheses of the neural mediation of language and other higher mental capacities. The brain is a computational organ, and the power of all known computational systems reflects the numbers of units in the system (Byrne, 1996). It is also known that the amount of neocortex devoted to sensorimotor functions for diverse body parts does not correspond to the actual size of the body parts. Rather, those body areas with the greatest motor dexterity and greatest sensory acuity command the greatest amount of sensorimotor cortex. In humans, for example, the amount of neocortical sensory and motor tissue devoted to the tongue is far larger than that devoted to the thoracic body wall, and the amount of tissue devoted to the macula (retinal area of greatest visual acuity) is greater than that devoted to the larger, peripheral retina. Similar phenomena characterize other species. The hands of racoons, the tails of spider monkeys, the snouts of coatimundis, and the lips of llama all command unusually large amounts of neural tissue (Pubols & Pubols, 1972; Welker & Seidenstein, 1959; Welker et al., 1976). Hence, increased size of sensorimotor processing areas corresponds primarily to increased sensorimotor capacities, rather than to increased body size. To the extent, then, that increased mental capacities rely upon enhanced sensorimotor skills, one would expect such capacities to reflect absolute brain size rather than indices of encephalization. Although not all complex mental capacities necessarily demand advanced sensorimotor skills, some clearly do, such as speech, motor imitation, and the fine motor skills needed for tool-making and drawing. In this regard, it also pertinent to note that the only qualitative reorganization yet demonstrated for the human brain involves the primary visual cortex (Preuss et al., 1999).

Currently, two dichotomous hypotheses are frequently invoked to explain the neural basis of higher cognitive capacities. The first postulates that qualitatively unique, genetically-determined, mental modules underlie distinct behavioral domains such as language, theory of mind, and self-awareness (Fodor, 1983; Tooby & Cosmides, 1992; Pinker, 1997). This interpretation implies that the evolution of each new behavioral capacity requires the addition of new neural modules – that is, an increase in brain size. The second posits that these behavioral abilities reflect the enhanced hierarchical mental constructional and information processing capacities provided by the enhanced computational powers of enlarged brains (Gibson, 1988, 1990; Greenfield, 1991). More research is needed to determine the extent to which the addition of new mental modules or increased mental constructional capacities may have led to the evolution of specific human and great ape abilities, and it is, of course, possible that both processes were involved. The essential point, however, is that both theoretical models lead to the same expectation – increased mental capacities require additional neural tissue. Hence, both theories would imply that absolute amounts of neural tissue are more pertinent to the emergence of language and other higher cognitive skills than amounts of neural tissue relative to body size.

Although EQs and other measures of encephalization do not predict cognitive capacities in non-human primates, they do correlate with feeding behaviors in varied mammalian taxa. Specifically, carnivores have larger EQs than herbivores, and fruit eating bats and primates have larger EQs than insectivores or foliovores (Jerison, 1973; Clutton-Brock & Harvey, 1980; Milton, 1988). Also, the prosimians, New World monkeys, and great apes with the largest IPs are all omnivorous extractive foragers who use complex manipulative techniques to obtain embedded high energy food resources (e.g. *Daubentonia*, *Cebus*, and *Pan*) (Gibson, 1986). Fruit eaters and extractive foragers would be expected to require enhanced neural capacities for the cognitive mapping of widely dispersed food resources and for the sensorimotor skills needed to obtain difficult to process foods. These factors may partially explain why they have larger absolute brain sizes than others of similar body size. Such abilities, however, would not automatically lead to increases in higher cognitive capacities such as theory of mind or language. Also, EQ confounds two variables: body size and brain size. Mammalian herbivores tend to have large body sizes and large gut sizes compared to mammals that eat higher quality, more readily digestible diets. Their smaller EQs may simply be an artifact of their enlarged bodies and guts (Byrne, 1996). Moreover, as Aiello, Bates & Joffe note (Chapter 3, this volume) a metabolic trade-off may exist between gut size and brain size. This would allow mammals with small guts to have relatively larger brains than other mammals. Consequently, the enlarged EQs and IPs of frugivores may primarily reflect metabolic and dietary factors rather than mental capacities. These relationships between diet and measures of encephalization may also explain why tool using primates tend to have large IPs and EQs. Primate tool-users extract embedded, high quality, readily digestible foods, such as nuts and insects (Parker & Gibson, 1977). Hence, they tend to have small digestive tracts.

The measures discussed here are, of course, not the only potential quantitative measures of brain expansion. An alternative measure, neo-cortical ratio, has often been used in recent years (Dunbar, 1992). Neocortical ratio is the ratio of the size of the neocortex to the size of the remainder of the brain. In non-human primates, neocortical ratio corre-lates with neocortical size. Neocortical ratio and neocortical size are not the same measures, however, and they do not always yield the same pre-dictions of intelligence. The enlargement of any portion of the brain other than the neocortex will automatically decrease the neocortical ratio, and, hence, result in lower estimates of intelligence than the use of neo-cortical size alone. Gorillas, for example have the largest neocortices of any non-human primates, but their neocortical ratios are relatively small (Dunbar, 1992, 1993; Stephan, 1972, Stephan et al., 1981). The reason for this seeming discrepancy is that, in gorillas, the cerebellum is dispropor-tionately enlarged compared to the neocortex.

The neocortical ratio has achieved popularity, because in a sample of non-human primates that excluded some species with very small (oran-gutans) and very large (colobus) group sizes, neocortical ratio correlated more strongly with social group size than did absolute neocortical size (Dunbar, 1992, 1993). Neocortical ratio also correlates with rates of tactical deception in nonhuman primates (Byrne, 1996), but absolute brain size would also be likely to correlate with this measure given that the large brained apes and baboons exhibit the greatest frequencies of deception. Further, as delineated by Byrne (1996), deception can entail greater or lesser degrees of understanding of the minds of the deceived on the part of the deceiver. Baboons, who have large neocortical ratios and high rates of deception, nonetheless appear to have lesser degrees of under-standing of others minds than do the great apes (Byrne, 1996). There is also considerable overlap in neocortical ratios between monkeys and apes (Gibson & Jessee, 1999). Hence, neocortical ratio does not predict mental differences between apes and monkeys. Nor have any theoretical explana-tions been advanced to explain why enlargement of other neural process-ing centers should decrease the mental capacities provided by the neocortex. Quite the contrary, many additional neural structures includ-ing the cerebellum, amygdala, hippocampus, and basal ganglia are known to contribute to learning and memory processes. Moreover, the neocortex does not function in isolation, but rather as part of several major neural circuits involving both cortical and subcortical structures. Given these considerations, it is not surprising that neocortical ratio, like EQ, fails to predict the cognitive differences between great apes and other non-human primates. Hence, neocortical ratio can be considered a better predictor of intelligence than the absolute size of the neocortex or brain, only if social group size is considered a better measure of intelligence than performance on cognitive tasks. No theoretical justification for such an interpretation has been presented.

The finding that absolute brain size and body size predict key aspects of intellectual performance in non-human primates is a welcome one. Absolute brain size is readily estimated from cranial capacity, and, thus, is one of the easiest measures to determine from the fossil record. It is also an important finding, because it indicates that quantum increases in brain size are likely to be accompanied by increases in intellectual capacity, even when accompanied by increased body size. For example, this finding strongly suggests that the large brained, large bodied, Neanderthals were highly intelligent beings, despite previous suggestions that they lacked intelligence because their brain sizes were smaller in relationship to body mass than is the case for modern humans (Kappelman, 1997).

This paper has focused primarily on neural and mental differences between great apes and monkeys. It is evident, however, from the data in Tables 4.3 and 4.4 that monkeys vary considerably in absolute brain size and in the size of many neural processing areas. If the thesis of this paper is correct, behavioral data should eventually document major cognitive and sensorimotor differences among the monkeys. In particular, this paper would predict that the large-brained baboons should have the greatest mental capacities of the monkeys. Some major sensorimotor differences do occur among monkeys and appear to relate to brain size. The prehensile-tailed New World monkeys, for instance, have larger brains than other New World monkeys. Little data, however, exist on the comparative cognitive capacities of monkeys. Hence, at this point, it is not possible to test the thesis of this paper based on behavioral data from diverse monkey species.

Summary and conclusions

Body size, absolute brain size and extra neurons all correlate with performance of non-human primates on a test of mental flexibility – the

Transfer Index. These measures all correlate with each other. Brain size also correlates with size of the neocortex, hippocampus, cerebellum, and corpus striatum, each of which also distinguishes great apes from monkeys. Each of these measures, thus, corresponds to emerging findings that the great apes possess greater mental constructional capacities and greater cognitive abilities in realms once thought to be uniquely human than do monkeys. Such capacities include symbolism, syntax, imitation, theory of mind, mirror recognition, deception, and tool-making. In contrast, EQ does not correlate with performance on the transfer test and neither EQ nor neocortical ratio distinguish great apes from monkeys. These findings suggest that the most practical measure for distinguishing intelligence and predicting the presence of human-like mental skills in hominid fossils is absolute brain size. EQ does not predict intelligence in primates and should not be used to determine intelligence in fossil hominids. EQ, however does correlate with dietary strategies and, thus, may reflect a combination of metabolic and intellectual strategies.

References

Anderson, J.R. (1996). Chimpanzee and capuchin monkeys: comparative cognition. In *Reaching into Thought: The Minds of Great Apes*, eds. A. Russon, K. Bard & S. Parker, pp. 23–56. Cambridge: Cambridge University Press.

Antinucci, F. (1989). *Cognitive Structures and Development in Nonhuman Primates*. Hillsdale, NJ: Erlbaum.

Antinucci, F., Spinozzi, G. & Natale, F. (1986). Stage V cognition in an infant gorilla. In *Current Perspectives in Primate Social Dynamics*, eds. D. Taub & F.A. King, pp. 403–415. New York: Van Nostrand Reinhold.

Bard, K.A., Fragaszy, D.M. & Visalberghi, E. (1995). Acquisition and comprehension of a tool-using behavior by young chimpanzee (*Pan troglodytes*): Effects of age and modelling. *International Journal of Comparative Psychology*, 8, 47–68.

Bauchot, R. & Stephan, H. (1969). Encephalisation et niveau evolutif chez les Simiens. *Mammalia*, 33, 225–275.

Beran, M.J., Gibson, K.R. & Rumbaugh, D.M. (1999). Predicting hominid intelligence from brain size. In *The Descent of Mind: Psychological Perspectives on Hominid Evolution*, eds. M.C. Corballis & S.E.G. Lea, pp. 88–97. New York: Oxford University Press.

Beran, M.J., Savage-Rumbaugh, E.S., Brakke, K.E., Kelley, J.W. & Rumbaugh, D.M. (1998). Symbol comprehension and learning: A 'vocabulary' test of three chimpanzees (*Pan troglodytes*). *Evolution of Communication*, 2, 171–188.

Boesch, C. & Boesch, H. (1983). Optimisation of nut-cracking with natural hammers by wild chimpanzees. *Behaviour*, 83, 265–286.

Boesch, C. & Boesch, H. (1990). Tool use and tool making in wild chimpanzees. *Folia Primatologica*, 43, 86–99.

Byrne, R. (1995). *The Thinking Ape: Evolutionary Origins of Intelligence*. New York: Oxford University Press.

Byrne, R. (1996). Relating brain size to intelligence in primates. In *Modelling the Early Human Mind*, eds. P. Mellars & K.R. Gibson, pp. 49–57. Cambridge: The McDonald Archaeological Institute.

Byrne, R.W. & Whiten, A. (1988). *Machiavellian Intelligence*. New York: Oxford University Press.

Call, J. & Tomasello, M. (1994). The social learning of tool use by orangutans (*Pongo pygmeaus*). *Human Evolution*, 9, 297–313.

Chevalier-Skolnikoff, S. (1977). A Piagetian model for describing and comparing socialization in monkey, ape, and human infants. In *Primate Biosocial Development*, eds. S. Chevalier-Skolnikoff & F. Poirier, pp. 159–188. New York: Garland Press.

Chevalier-Skolnikoff, S. (1983). Sensorimotor development in orangutans and other primates. *Journal of Human Evolution*, 12, 545–561.

Chevalier-Skolnikoff, S. (1989). Spontaneous tool use and sensorimotor intelligence in Cebus compared with other monkeys and apes. *Behavioral and Brain Sciences*, 12, 561–627.

Clutton-Brock, T.H. & Harvey, P.H. (1980). Primates, brains and ecology. *Journal of Zoology*, 190, 309–323.

Dunbar, R.I.M. (1992). Neocortex size as a constraint on group size in primates. *Journal of Human Evolution*, 20, 469–493.

Dunbar, R.I.M. (1993). Coevolution of neocortical size, group size, and language in humans. *Behavioral and Brain Sciences*, 16, 681–735.

Dunbar, R.I.M. (1997). *Grooming, Gossip, and the Evolution of Language*. London: Faber & Faber Limited.

Finlay, B.L. & Darlington, R.B. (1995). Linked regularities in the development and evolution of mammalian brains. *Science*, 268, 1570–1584.

Fodor, J.A. (1983). *The Modularity of Mind*. Cambridge, MA: MIT Press.

Gallop, G.G. (1970). Chimpanzees: Self-recognition. *Science*, 167, 86–87.

Gallop, G.G. (1977). Self-recognition in primates. *American Psychologist*, 32, 329–338.

Gallop, G.G. (1982). Self-awareness and the emergence of mind in primates. *American Journal of Primatology*, 2, 237–248.

Gallop, G.G. & Suarez, S.D. (1991). Social responding to mirrors in rhesus monkeys: Effects of temporary mirror removal. *Journal of Comparative Psychology*, 105, 376–379.

Gardner, R.A. & Garnder, B. (1969). Teaching sign language to a chimpanzee. *Science*, 165, 664–672.

Gibson, K.R. (1986). Cognition, brain size and the extraction of embedded food resources. In *Primate Ontogeny, Cognition, and Social Behaviour*, eds. J.G. Else & P.C. Lee, pp. 93–103. Cambridge: Cambridge University Press.

Gibson, K.R. (1988). Brain size and the evolution of language. In *The Genesis of Language: a Different Judgment of Evidence*, ed. M. Landsberg, pp. 149–172. Berlin: Mouton de Gruyter.

Gibson, K.R. (1990). New perspectives on instincts and intelligence: Brain size and the emergence of hierarchical mental constructional skills. In *'Language' and Intelligence in Monkeys and Apes: Comparative Developmental Perspectives*, eds. S.T. Parker & K.R. Gibson, pp. 197–228. Cambridge: Cambridge University Press.

Gibson, K.R. (1996). The biocultural human brain, seasonal migrations, and the emergence of the Upper Paleolithic. In *Modelling the Early Human Mind*, eds. P. Mellars & K. Gibson, pp. 33–46. Cambridge: The McDonald Institute for Archaeological Research.

Gibson, K.R. & Jessee, S. (1999). Language evolution and the expansion of multiple neurological processing areas. In *The Origins of Language: What Nonhuman Primates Can Tell Us*, ed. B.J. King, pp. 189–227. Santa Fe: SAR Press.

Goodall, J. (1986). *The Chimpanzees of Gombe*. Cambridge, MA: Harvard University Press.

Greenfield, P.M. (1991). Language, tools, and the brain: The development and evolution of hierarchically organized sequential behavior. *Behavioral and Brain Sciences*, 14, 531–595.

Holloway, R. (1966). Cranial capacity, neural reorganization and hominid evolution: a search for more suitable parameters. *American Anthropologist*, 68, 103–121.

Jerison, H.J. (1973). *Evolution of the Brain and Intelligence*. New York: Academic Press.

Jerison, H.J. (1982). Allometry, brain size, cortical surface, and convolutedness. In *Primate Brain Evolution: Methods and Concepts*, eds. E. Armstrong & D. Falk, pp. 77–84. New York: Plenum Press.

Jerison, H.J. (1985). On the evolution of mind. In *Brain and Mind*, ed. D.A. Oakley, pp. 1–31. London: Metheun.

Kappelman, J. (1997). They might be giants. *Nature*, 387, 126–127.

Langer, J. (1980). *The Origins of Logic: Six To Twelve Months*. New York: Academic Press.

Langer, J. (1986). *The Origins of Logic: One To Two Years*. New York: Academic Press.

Langer, J. (1989). Comparisons with the human child. In *Cognitive Structures and Development in Nonhuman Primates*, ed. F. Antinucci, pp. 229–242. Hillsdale, NJ: Erlbaum.

Langer, J. (1993). Comparative cognitive development. In *Tools, Language and Cognition in Human Evolution*, eds. K.R. Gibson & T. Ingold, pp. 300–313. Cambridge, Cambridge University Press.

Langer, J. (2000). The descent of cognitive development. *Developmental Science*, 3, 361–378.

Mathieu, M. & Bergeron, G. (1983). Piagetian assessment on cognitive development in chimpanzees (*Pan troglodytes*). In *Primate Behavior and Sociobiology*, eds. A.B. Chiarelli & R. Corruccini, pp. 142–147. New York: Springer-Verlag.

Mathieu, M., Bouchard, M., Granger, L. & Herscovitch, J. (1976). Piagetian object permanence in *Cebus capuchinus, Lagothrica flavicauda* and *Pan troglodytes. Animal Behaviour*, 24, 575–588.

McGrew, W.C. (1974). Tool use in wild chimpanzees in feeding upon driver ants. *Journal of Human Evolution*, 3, 501–508.

McGrew, W.C. (1992). *Chimpanzee Material Culture: Implications for Human Evolution*. London: Cambridge University Press.

Miles, H.L.W. (1990). The cognitive foundations for reference in a signing orangutan. In *'Language' and Intelligence in Monkeys and Apes: Comparative Developmental Perspectives*, eds. S.T. Parker & K.R. Gibson, pp. 511–539. Cambridge: Cambridge University Press.

Milton, K. (1988). Foraging behaviour and the evolution of primate intelligence. In *Machiavellian Intelligence*, eds. R. Byrne & A. Whiten, pp. 285–305. Oxford: Clarendon Press.

Natale, F., Antinucci, F., Spinozzi, G. & Poti, P. (1986). Stage 6 object concept in nonhuman primate cognition: A comparison between gorilla (*Gorilla gorilla gorilla*) and Japanese macaque (*Macaca fascata*). *Journal of Comparative Psychology*, **100**, 335–339.

Parker, S.T. (1977). Piaget's sensorimotor series in an infant macaque: A model for comparing unstereotyped behavior and intelligence in human and nonhuman primates. In *Primate Biosocial Development*, eds. S. Chevalier-Skolnikoff & F. Poirier, pp. 43–112. New York: Garland Press.

Parker, S.T. (1990). Origins of comparative developmental evolutionary studies of primate mental abilities. In *'Language' and Intelligence in Monkeys and Apes: Comparative Developmental Perspectives*, eds. S.T. Parker & K.R. Gibson, pp. 3–74. Cambridge: Cambridge University Press.

Parker, S.T. (1996). Apprenticeship in tool-mediated extractive foraging: the origins of imitation, teaching, and self-awareness in apes. In *Reaching into Thought: The Minds of the Great Apes*, eds. A.E. Russon, K. Bard & S.T. Parker, pp. 348–370. Cambridge: Cambridge University Press.

Parker, S.T. & Gibson, K.R. (1977). Object manipulation, tool use, and sensorimotor intelligence as feeding adaptations in cebus monkeys and great apes. *Journal of Human Evolution*, **6**, 623–641.

Parker, S.T. & Gibson, K.R. (1979). A developmental model for the evolution of language, intelligence and the brain. *Behavioral and Brain Sciences*, **2**, 367–408.

Parker, S.T. & McKinney, M.L. (1999). *Origins of Intelligence: the Evolution of Cognitive Development in Monkeys, Apes, and Humans*. Cambridge: Cambridge University Press.

Parker, S.T., Mitchell, R.W. & Boccia, M.L. eds. (1994). *Self-awareness in Animals and Humans*. Cambridge: Cambridge University Press.

Passingham, R.E. & Ettlinger, G. (1974). A comparison of cortical function in man and other primates. *International Review of Neurobiology*, **16**, 233–299.

Patterson, F.L. & Linden, E. (1981). *The Education of Koko*. New York: Holt, Rinehart & Winston.

Pinker, S. (1997). *How the Mind Works*. New York: W.W Norton and Company.

Povinelli, D.J., Rulf, A.B., Landau, K.R. & Bierschwale, D.T. (1993). Self-recognition in chimpanzees: Distribution, ontogeny, and patterns of emergence. *Journal of Comparative Psychology*, **107**, 347–372.

Premack, D. & Premack, A.J. (1983). *The Mind of an Ape*. New York: Norton.

Preuss, T.M., Qi, H.-S & Kaas, J.H. (1999). Distinctive compartmental organization of human primary visual cortex. *Proceedings of the National Academy of Sciences USA*, **96**, 11601–11606.

Pubols, B.H. & Pubols, L.M. (1972). Neural organization of somatosensory representation in the spider monkey. *Brain, Behavior, and Evolution*, **5**, 342–346.

Ruff, C.B., Trinkaus, E. & Holliday, T.W. (1997). Body mass and encephalization in Pleistocene *Homo*. *Nature*, **387**, 173–176.

Rumbaugh, D.M. (1970). Learning skills of anthropoids. In *Primate behavior: Developments in Field and Laboratory Research*, ed. L. Rosenblum, pp. 1–70. New York: Academic Press.

Rumbaugh, D.M. (1977). *Language Learning by a Chimpanzee: The LANA Project*. New York: Academic Press.

Rumbaugh, D.M. (1997). Competence, cortex, and primate models: A comparative primate perspective. In *Development of the Prefrontal Cortex: Evolution, Neurobiology, and Behavior*, eds. N.A. Krasnegor, G.R. Lyon & P.S. Goldman-Rakic, pp. 117–139. Baltimore, MD: Paul H. Brookes.

Rumbaugh, D.M. & Pate, J.L. (1984). The evolution of cognition in primates: A comparative perspective. In *Animal Cognition*, eds. H.L. Roitblat, T.G. Bever & H.S. Terrace, pp. 569–587. Hillsdale, NJ: Erlbaum.

Savage-Rumbaugh, E.S. (1986). *Ape Language: From Conditioned Response to Symbol*. New York: Columbia University Press.

Savage-Rumbaugh, E.S. & Lewin, R. (1994). *Kanzi: The Ape at the Brink of the Human Mind*. New York: Wiley.

Savage-Rumbaugh, E.S., Murphy, J., Sevcik, R.A., Brakke, K.E., Williams, S.L. & Rumbaugh, D.M. (1993). Language comprehension in ape and child. *Monographs of the Society for Research in Child Development*, **58**, (3–4, Serial No. 233).

Savage-Rumbaugh, E.S., McDonald, K., Sevcik, R.A., Hopkins, W.D. & Rubert, E. (1986). Spontaneous symbol acquisition and communicative use by pygmy chimpanzees (*Pan paniscus*). *Journal of Experimental Psychology: General*, **115**, 211–235.

Savage-Rumbaugh, E.S., Rumbaugh, D.M., Smith, S.T. & Lawson, J. (1980). Reference: The linguistic essential. *Science*, **210**, 922–925.

Savage-Rumbaugh, E.S., Shanker, S. & Taylor, T.J. (1998). *Apes, Language, and the Human Mind*. New York: Oxford University Press.

Spinozzi, G. (1993). Development of spontaneous classificatory behavior in chimpanzees (*Pan troglodytes*). *Journal of Comparative Psychology*, **107**, 193–200.

Spinozzi, G. & Natale, F. (1989). Classification. In *Cognitive Structure and Development in Nonhuman Primates*, ed. F. Antinucci, pp. 163–187. Hillsdale, NJ: Erlbaum.

Stephan, H. (1972). Evolution of primate brains: a comparative anatomical perspective. In *The Functional and Evolutionary Biology of Primates*, ed. R. Tuttle, pp. 155–174. Chicago: Aldine.

Stephan, H., Frahm, H. & Baron, G. (1981). New and revised data on volumes of brain structures in insectivores and primates. *Folia Primatologica*, **35**, 1–39.

Suarez, S.D. & Gallop, G.G. (1981). Self-recognition in chimpanzees and orangutans, but not gorillas. *Journal of Human Evolution*, **10**, 175–188.

Suarez, S.D. & Gallop, G.G. (1986). Social responding to mirrors in rhesus macaques: Effects of changing mirror locations. *American Journal of Primatology*, **11**, 239–244.

Terrace, H.S. (1979). *Nim*. New York: Knopf.

Tomasello, M. & Call, J. (1997). *Primate Cognition*. New York: Oxford University Press.

Tooby, J. & Cosmides, L. (1992). The psychological foundations of culture. In *The Adapted Mind*, eds. J.H. Barkow, L. Cosmides & J. Tooby, pp. 20–136. New York: Oxford University Press.

Toth, N., Schick, K.D., Savage-Rumbaugh, E.S., Sevcik, R.A. & Rumbaugh, D.M. (1993). Pan the tool-maker: Investigations into the stone tool-making and tool-using capabilities of a bonobo (*Pan paniscus*). *Journal of Archaeological Science*, **20**, 81–91.

Vauclair, J. (1982). Sensorimotor intelligence in human and nonhuman primates. *Journal of Human Evolution*, **11**, 257–264.

Visalberghi, E. (1987). Acquisition of nut-cracking behavior by two capuchin monkeys (*Cebus apella*). *Folia Primatologica*, **49**, 168–181.

Visalberghi, E. (1990). Tool use in cebus. *Folia Primatologica*, **54**, 146–154.

Visalberghi, E. (1993). Tool use in a South American monkey species: An overview of the characteristics and limits of tool use in Cebus apella. In *The Use of Tools by Human and Non-human Primates*, eds. A. Berthelet & J. Chavaillon, pp. 247–273. New York: Oxford University Press.

Visalberghi, E., Fragaszy, D.M. & Savage-Rumbaugh, E.S. (1995). Performance in a tool-using task by common chimpanzees (*Pan troglodytes*), bonobos (*Pan paniscus*), an orangutan (*Pongo pygmaeus*), and capuchin monkeys (*Cebus apella*). *Journal of Comparative Psychology*, **109**, 52–60.

Welker, W.I., Adrian, H.O., Lifschutz, W., Kaulen, R., Caviedes, E. & Gutman, W. (1976). Somatic sensory cortex of llama (*Lama glama*). *Brain, Behavior and Evolution*, **13**, 184–193.

Welker, W.I. & Seidenstein, S. (1959). Somatic sensory representation in the cerebral cortex of the racoon (*Procyon lotor*). *Journal of Comparative Neurology*, **111**, 469–501.

Westergard, G. & Suomi, S. (1994). A simple stone tool technology in monkeys. *Journal of Human Evolution*, **27**, 399–404.

Whiten, A. & Byrne, R.W. (1997). *Machiavellian Intelligence II: Extensions and Evaluations*. New York: Cambridge University Press.

5
_____

The evolution of sex differences in primate brains

Although it has long been recognized that, around the world, adult men have larger brains on average than adult women (Pakkenberg & Voigt, 1964; Pakkenberg & Gundersen, 1997), many workers have traditionally viewed men's larger brains as simple correlates of their larger mean body masses. Other findings which suggest that the internal structure of the brains of men and women are, on average, organized differently (summarized in Kimura, 1992), and that the two sexes perform differently on certain cognitive tasks (Kimura, 1992; Falk, 1997) have traditionally been minimized with the latter being attributed largely to variations in developmental experience, as noted by Kimura (1992). Recent reports in the neurosciences, however, underscore the differences between the brains of men and women in gross volume adjusted for body size (Ankney, 1992; Falk *et al.*, 1999), and in internal anatomy that reflects neurological wiring (Gur *et al.*, 1999; Giedd *et al.*, 1996b). Furthermore, convincing arguments are emerging which support the hypothesis that the neuroanatomical differences between the sexes form the substrates for their differences in average cognitive processing (Andreasen *et al.*, 1993; Gur *et al.*, 1999). The purpose of this chapter is to outline some of these new findings and to interpret them within an evolutionary framework.

Sex differences in brain size at equivalent body masses

Humans

Ankney (1992) plotted bivariate regression equations that relate brain weight to body height and body surface area for men and women from data provided in the literature (Ho *et al.*, 1980a,b). He found that, for any

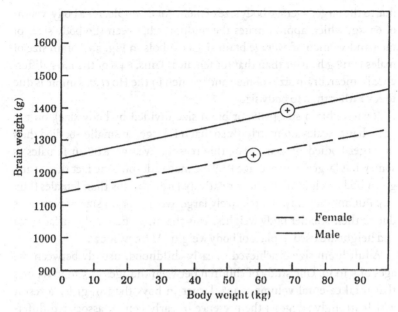

Fig. 5.1. Regressions of brain weight (g) against body weight (kg) using data from Ho *et al.* (1980b) for Caucasian females (*n* = 390) and Caucasian males (*n* = 414). The equation for males (top line) is brain weight (g) = 1242 + 2.19 body weight (kg). That for females is brain weight (g) = 1138 + 1.96 body weight (kg). For each sex, the mean values for brain size are indicated in their bivariate position with body weight (circle + symbol). Note that at any given body weight, brains are larger in males than females. Reproduced from Falk *et al.* (1999).

given stature or body surface area, brain size is approximately 100 g larger in men than in women (Ankney, 1992). Although stature is more stable than body weight during an individual's lifetime and is therefore preferred by some workers as the independent variable in regressions pertaining to brain size (Pakkenberg & Voigt, 1964), body weight is the classic measure of body size that is used for a variety of taxa including primates (Jerison, 1973, 1991; Smith & Leigh, 1998; Smith & Jungers, 1997). Following Ankney's lead, Falk *et al.* (1999) therefore plotted regressions from Ho *et al.* (1980a,b) for 414 men and 390 women that relate brain weight to body weight (Fig. 5.1), and obtained results that appear very similar to the regressions for men and women when body surface area or height are the independent variables (Ankney, 1992).

The difference between the mean male (1392 g) and the mean female (1252 g) brain weights in Fig. 5.1 is 140 g, only a small fraction of which is due to the larger average body size of men. For example, for a body weight of 63 kg, which approximates the midpoint between the body sizes of men and women of average brain size (symbols in Fig. 5.1), brain size of males is 118 g heavier than that for females. Thus, 84% of the 140 g difference in mean brain sizes of men and women in the Ho *et al.* sample is due to sex rather than to body size.

Relative brain size (RBS, or brain size divided by body size), on the other hand, scales allometrically so that it is larger in smaller-bodied than in larger-bodied primates. For this reason, average RBS in females is somewhat larger than average RBS for males, despite the fact that at any given body weight males have relatively larger brains than females (Fig. 5.1). Put another way, the relatively large average brain size of women is due to their smaller body weights, as is the case when body surface area and height are used in place of body weight (Ankney, 1992).

Adult brain size is achieved in early childhood, usually between the ages of 5 to 10. One study of children between the ages of 5 to 17 reports that total cerebral volume is 10% larger in boys than in girls, 'a result which strongly suggests the presence of early gender-associated differences in cerebral development and organization' (Reiss *et al.*, 1996, p. 1770). The bottom line from numerous studies is that by the time of early childhood (if not earlier), males at any given body weight have brains that are around 10% larger than those of females (Falk *et al.*, 1999). It would be interesting to learn the extent (if any) to which sexual dimorphism in brain size develops prenatally in humans, since sex differences in brain size begin developing prenatally in rhesus monkeys (see below).

Rhesus monkeys

Falk *et al.* (1999) plotted bivariate least squares regression equations that relate brain volume (cm³) to body weight (kg) for 39 male and 44 female rhesus monkeys (*Macaca mulatta*) (Fig. 5.2). Brain volumes were determined with mustard seed and, as is traditional, 1 cm³ assumed to equal 1 g of brain tissue. The data for male and female rhesus monkeys exactly parallel the situation for humans, both with respect to allometric scaling of RBS and the fact that males have absolutely and relatively larger brains than females at any given body weight.

Data concerning brain growth during postnatal development are also available for a larger sample of rhesus macaques that contains the specimens included in Fig. 5.2 (Konigsberg *et al.*, 1990). Cranial capacity was regressed on age for 90 male and 93 female macaques 5 years of age or

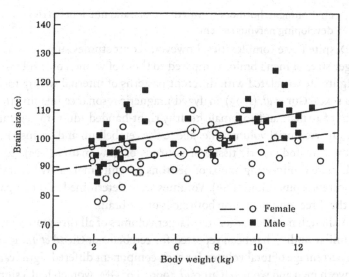

Fig. 5.2. Least squares regressions of brain volume (cm³) against body weight (kg) for 44 female and 39 male rhesus monkeys using data from Falk *et al.* (1999). Brain size was measured as a volume using mustard seed, and 1 cm³ is assumed to be equivalent to 1 g. The equation for males (top line) is brain volume (cm³) = 94.6 + 1.20 body weight (kg); that for females is brain volume (cm³) − 88.7 + 0.95 body weight (kg). For each sex, the mean values for brain volume are indicated in their bivariate position with body weight (circle + symbol). Note that, as is the case for humans, at any given body weight, brains are larger in males than females. Reproduced from Falk *et al.* (1999).

older, and for 71 male and 76 female macaques less than 5 years of age. In these analyses, the slopes for the two sexes did not differ significantly but the intercepts were significantly higher for the males in both age ranges (Konigsberg *et al.*, 1990). It therefore appears that, because the intercept (cranial capacity at birth) was significantly higher for males than for females, the development of sexual dimorphism in brain size is at least partly a prenatal event (see Falk *et al.*, 1999, for further discussion).

Sex differences in gross wiring of human brains

Giedd *et al.* noted that, with respect to brain size (1996b, p. 228):

The interpretation of volumetric changes is complicated by the myriad of factors contributing to structure size, including the number and size of neurons and glial cells, packing density, vascularity, and matrix composition. These parameters, in turn, are affected by genetics, environment, hormones, growth factors, and nutrients in the developing nervous system.

Despite these complexities, however, recent studies suggest that the larger sizes of men's brains compared to those of women of similar body weights are correlated with different patterns of internal wiring for the two sexes. Gur *et al.* (1999) analyzed magnetic resonance imaging (MRI) scans of 40 male and 40 female healthy right-handed adults to determine the supertentorial volumes (i.e. above the cerebellum and brainstem) of (1) the somatodendritic tissue of neurons or gray matter (GM), (2) the myelinated connecting axons of neurons or white matter (WM), and (3) the cerebrospinal fluid (CSF). Volumes were determined and compared for the three components on both sides of the brain.

Although men had absolutely larger volumes of all three components (a similar finding has been reported for cerebellum; Giedd *et al.*, 1996a), the percentage of total volume for each component differed significantly between men and women (Gur *et al.* 1999). For GM, women had a significantly higher percentage (about 55%) than men (about 51%); for WM, on the other hand, men had a significantly greater percentage of total volume (about 40%) than women (about 38%). Men also had significantly more CSF in their sulci (about 8%) than women (6%). (Ventricular CSF, on the other hand, measured about 1% for each sex.)

Some of these differences are apparent in Gur *et al.*'s (1999) scatterplots and regression lines of the three components against total supertentorial volumes for men and women (Fig. 5.3). The slopes for GM for men and women are identical, but that for WM is much steeper in men than women (Gur *et al.*, 1999). Consequently, increased cranial volume in men is associated with proportional increases in GM and WM, whereas GM increases at a greater rate than WM as brain size increases in women (Fig. 5.3). In a comparison of the 21 men and 14 women in their study that had overlapping supertentorial volumes (1100–1350 ml), Gur *et al.* found the same significant difference in GM that characterized the larger sample, indicating that the sex difference is not due to scaling effects associated with different brain volumes for the sexes.

The findings of Gur *et al.* pertaining to different relative proportions of GM and WM in the sexes contradict an earlier study that focused on children and contained only 21 males, one of whom was discarded from the analysis because he had a WM volume that was over 2 SDs above the mean for males (Reiss *et al.*, 1996). Reiss *et al.* found that as age increased between 5 and 17 years, GM volume decreased and WM volume increased for both sexes. Because WM increases at a steeper rate when plotted

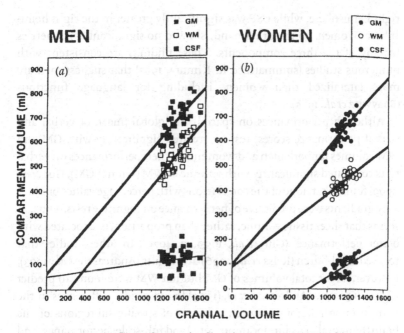

Fig. 5.3. Scatterplots and regression lines for gray matter (GM), white matter (WM), and CSF against supertentorial cranial volumes for men (squares) and women (circles) (from Gur *et al.*, 1999, with permission).

against cranial volume in men than women (Gur *et al.*, 1999), it is possible that the wiring differences between the sexes detected by Gur *et al.* but not by Reiss *et al.* do not become statistically significant until adulthood. Along these lines, Reiss *et al.* noted that (1996, p. 1770) 'increase in brain myelinization in the first and second decades of life is likely to be a primary contributor to expansion of the volume of the white matter compartment in the age group sampled in this study.' They also observed that WM expansion was particularly prominent in the prefrontal region of the brain. With respect to the sex differences in proportions of GM and WM, Gur *et al.* concluded that the higher percentage of GM in women makes relatively more tissue available for computation as opposed to (WM) transfer of information across distant regions. This observation will be returned to below.

Relationship to brain lateralization and cognition

Interestingly, Gur *et al.* (1999) reported that men and women were lateralized differently for the three components of supertentorial cranial volume. For men, GM was significantly greater in the left than in the right hemisphere, while CSF was significantly greater in the right hemisphere. Women, on the other hand, showed no significant asymmetries for any of the three components. These findings are consistent with numerous studies (summarized in Kimura, 1992) that suggest men are more lateralized than women, including for language functions (Shaywitz *et al.*, 1995).

Although performances on spatial, and global (mean of verbal and spatial performance scores) tests correlated significantly with GM and WM volumes for both men and women and their performances on verbal tests correlated significantly with volume of WM (but not GM), Gur *et al.* (1999) found that none of the correlations with percentage values or laterality gradients were predictive of performance on cognitive tests. Thus, 'it seems that sheer tissue volume, rather than proportion, is associated with better performance' (Gur *et al.*, 1999, p. 4070). In other studies that focused on children (Reiss *et al.*, 1996) and adults (Andreasen *et al.*, 1993), however, larger total volumes of GM but not WM were found to predict higher IQ scores. Andreasen *et al.* (1993) found gender differences in the pattern of correlations between volumes of specific subregions of the brain (temporal lobe, hippocampus, etc.) and full-scale, performance, and verbal IQs.

Differential roles of parental genomes for brain development and evolution

During mammalian development, certain genes are expressed from either the paternal or maternal genome due to silencing of autosomal alleles of the opposite parent through genomic imprinting. In recent years, the differential contributions of maternal and paternal genomes have been quantified for brain development in mice (Keverne *et al.*, 1996b). Because imprinted genes are also important for certain genetic disorders that influence human brain development and function, the authors applied their findings from rodents to formulate a novel basis for studying primate brain evolution (Keverne *et al.*, 1996a). A review of these studies may shed light on the evolution of the sexually dimorphic primate brains described in previous sections.

By comparing the effects of imprinted genes on brain development in chimeric mice embryos formed from duplicated paternal and duplicated maternal genomes, Keverne *et al.* (1996b) found that cells from the duplicated paternal genomes contributed substantially to development of the basal forebrain (including hypothalamus and septum) but not the cortex.

Cells from the duplicated maternal genomes, on the other hand, contributed substantially to the cortex, striatum and hippocampus but not to the basal forebrain. Cells from the maternal but not paternal chimeric embryos also enhanced brain growth. (Body growth, however, is enhanced by paternally expressed genes.) Keverne *et al.* (1996b, p. 91) therefore hypothesized that 'genomic imprinting may have facilitated a rapid non-linear expansion of the brain, especially the cortex, during development over evolutionary time.'

This hypothesis was explored by comparing the structures of the brain to which maternal and paternal genomes contribute differentially in rodents across different phylogenies of primates (Keverne *et al.*, 1996a). (See Keverne *et al.*, 1996a,b, for discussion of clinical evidence for humans that supports this leap.) Because of their roles in planning ahead and execution of actions, the neocortex and striatum were grouped together as the 'executive' brain (Keverne *et al.*, 1996a) which, as noted, is differentially influenced by the maternal genome. The 'emotional' brain (which is under strong hormonal influence), on the other hand, consisted of the hypothalamus and septum which are differentially influenced by paternal genes (Keverne *et al.*, 1996a). Keverne *et al.* found that, unlike structures to which paternal genomes make substantial contributions, the executive brain shows grade shifts across groupings with simians having the largest executive brain, prosimians the next largest, and insectivores the smallest when regressed against brain stem and controlling for body weight (Fig. 5.4).

According to Keverne *et al.*, the fact that increased executive brain coincided with decreased emotional brain during primate evolution does not imply that primarily motivated behavior declined, but rather that (1996a, p. 694) 'the controlling mechanisms for the behaviour have shifted away from neuroendocrine determinants in favour of intelligent behavioural strategies.' The authors speculated that differences in parental lifestyles of primates placed different selective pressures on brain evolution in the sexes, thus favoring remodeling through genomic imprinting. Keverne *et al.* enumerated various factors that may have contributed to the evolution of an increased executive brain in primates: increased group size, increased numbers of females in groups, female bonding and centrality to groups, and females as primary care-givers. They also noted that males more often migrate from their natal groups, usually have more overt male dominance hierarchies, and are frequently characterized by higher levels of sexual promiscuity and aggression than females.

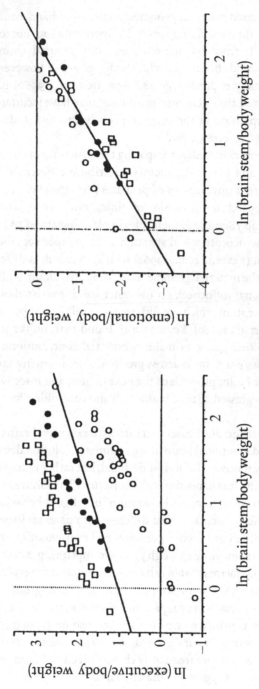

Fig. 5.4. Structures to which (left) maternally imprinted genomes make a substantial contribution (executive brain = neocortex + striatum) and those to which (right) paternally imprinted genomes contribute substantially (emotional brain = hypothalamus + septum) regressed against brain stem and controlling for body weight. The executive brain is positively correlated with phylogenetic groupings, showing grade shifts across groupings with simians having the largest and insectivores the smallest executive brains. The reverse is true for the emotional brain. Hollow circles, insectivores; filled circles, prosimians; hollow squares, simians (from Keverne et al., 1996a, with permission).

Keverne *et al.* conclude with a caveat that is important for the present paper (1996a, p. 695): 'Although differential selection pressures may have operated on the maternally and paternally imprinted genes, such is the nature of genomic imprinting that the advantages are transmitted to both daughters and sons. Males are therefore at liberty to progressively take advantage of their cortical enlargement, ...' The differences in the sizes of the brains of male and female macaques and humans of equivalent body sizes, and the differences in gross wiring of the brains of men and women discussed above, suggest that the sexes in at least some species of primates have remodeled (and taken advantage of) their enlarged brains in different ways. But why?

A possible evolutionary explanation

Before attempting to explain the sexual dimorphism that characterizes gross size and internal wiring of human brains, it is worthwhile to review current thinking about the high degree of sexual dimorphism in body size that characterizes some, but by no means all, primate species. A large number of studies (reviewed in Falk, 2000) converge on the interpretation that sexually dimorphic body sizes in some primates (e.g. baboons, orangutans) are associated with different strategies by which males and females maximize their reproductive fitness. According to this interpretation, females use their calories to conceive, gestate, and nurse offspring rather than to build and support (their own) bigger bodies. Male primates in sexually dimorphic species, on the other hand, tend to maximize their reproductive fitness by siring as many offspring as possible. To do so, they must compete with other males for breeding females (a limited resource). As a result of this intrasexual selection, males convert their calories to larger bodies and bigger teeth. This interpretation is strengthened by the fact that, among primates, the species in which males attempt to monopolize sexual access to the greatest number of females (e.g. that live in so-called 'harems') are characterized by the greatest degree of sexual dimorphism in canine and body sizes (Falk, 2000). Put another way, competition among males for sexually receptive females favors larger anatomical weaponry.

As reviewed in this paper, sexual dimorphism also characterizes the brains of some species of primates. At given body weights, male rhesus monkeys and men have larger brains than conspecific females. Furthermore, at similar total volumes, the internal wiring of human brains is also sexually dimorphic. (Unfortunately, comparable data on internal wiring are not presently available for nonhuman primates.) In seeking an evolutionary explanation for neurological sexual dimorphism in (at least) humans, it seems reasonable to focus on the differential reproductive strategies that appear to be the basis of sexual dimorphism in body size for highly dimorphic primates. To do so, one must explore how differentially greater volumes of GM might have facilitated reproductive fitness in the early ancestors of women on the one hand, and how differentially greater volumes of WM could have enhanced reproductive fitness in the early ancestors of men on the other. Furthermore, such an explanation should incorporate the known functional/cognitive correlates of brain size, GM, and WM; and should be consistent with the different average cognitive performances on standard tests that distinguish men and women (Kimura, 1992). Ideally, the explanation should also accord with what is known about genomic imprinting (Keverne *et al.*, 1996a,b) and the physical constraints associated with increasing the size and extent of internal connections of the brain (see Hofman, Chapter 6, this volume). With these criteria in mind, a preliminary explanation that accounts for the evolution of sexually dimorphic brains is outlined below along with suggestions for future research.

Keverne *et al.* suggest that genomic imprinting in primates is an evolutionary retention that serves different maternal and paternal reproductive interests in their developing offspring, and that it is (1996a, p. 695) 'perfectly compatible with the two genomes cooperating to produce viable whole brain function.' Thus the differential maternal genetic contributions to the executive brain are related, in part, to behaviors that have been emancipated from gonadal hormonal control (in both sexes) and that enable, among other activities, maternal investment in offspring. Such behaviors include anticipation, forward planning, and the execution of plans (Keverne *et al.*, 1996a). It is reasonable to assume that because of its important role for maternal tracking and interacting with offspring, vocal communication was under strong selective pressure in the ancestors of females ranging at least from rodents (contact calls) to people (speech) (reviewed in Falk, 1997). Keverne *et al.*'s hypothesis is therefore concordant with the conclusion of Gur *et al.* (1999) that the higher percentage of GM in women compared with men makes relatively more tissue available for computation and may in some way be related to their superior performance on language tasks.

The male imprinted emotional brain, on the other hand, constitutes a target area for hormonal action and is concerned primarily with motivated behaviors (in both sexes), including those such as aggression that enable intrasexual competition in nonhuman male primates (Keverne *et al.*, 1996a). Specifically, Keverne *et al.* suggest that the differential selection pressures that may have favored remodeling of brains in males of various primate species are related to the fact that, compared to females, males in many Old World primate societies frequently 'show greater mobility from the natal group, are more exploratory and their hierarchies are more overt, with high levels of sexual promiscuity and aggression' (1996a, p. 695). This suggestion is similar to the one we offered as a possible explanation for the sexual dimorphism in brain sizes of rhesus monkeys and humans (Falk *et al.*, 1999, p. 237):

> It may be that visuospatial skills were differentially selected in a polygynous common ancestor of rhesus monkeys and humans in conjunction with extensive navigating that occurs only in males, as was suggested to explain differential spatial abilities in male and female polygynous voles (Gaulin & Fitzgerald, 1989). If our evolutionary hypothesis is correct, further cognitive testing of rhesus monkeys should reveal significant sex differences in the processing of visuospatial information.

At the time we offered the above hypothesis, we were unaware of the fact that men have proportionally more WM than women, a finding which turns out to be consistent with our explanation. Thus according to Gur *et al.* (1999), spatial tasks at which men excel may require greater intrahemispheric transfer than the verbal tasks at which women excel, which could explain why men have greater proportions of WM than women. As noted by Kimura (1992), the spatial tasks at which men excel include mental rotation of objects, navigating their ways through routes, and guiding or intercepting projectiles. Because all of these tasks involve both vision and movement, transfer of information over long myelinated axons (WM) that connect posterior visual areas with the frontal lobe of a hemisphere (i.e. association fibers) seems plausible.

As detailed by Hofman (Chapter 6, this volume), however, the proportions of GM and WM in large-brained primates are governed by certain design principles, one of which is that increased WM is associated with certain costs (in terms of monopolizing available space and reducing conduction efficiency) that need to be balanced by other design features. Compared to GM, WM increases disproportionately with brain size across monkeys, apes and humans (see Fig. 6.2 of Hofman, Chapter 6, this volume) and, as Hofman observes (pp. 116–117), 'the evolutionary process of neocorticalization in primates is mainly due to the progressive expansion of the axonal mass, rather than to the increase in the number of cortical neurons.' As brain size increases across anthropoid primates, the number of distinct cortical areas is also reported to increase, possibly as a mechanism for minimizing the lengths of axons and therefore their conduction time, thus optimizing processing efficiency (Hofman, Chapter 6, this volume). Because of these design principles, the greater proportion of WM in men's compared with women's brains is consistent with their greater degree of cortical lateralization compared to women (e.g. for language; Shaywitz *et al.*, 1995) which may be viewed as a form of cortical specialization.

The visuospatial hypothesis: suggestions for future research

At the moment, the best hypothesis regarding sexual dimorphism in human brain size and internal wiring is that men's and women's different neurological 'Bauplans' are due to evolutionary histories that maximized reproductive fitness in each sex, perhaps through genomic imprinting. Thus women's brains reflect selection in their ancestors for skills that enhanced successful mothering including, of course, vocal communication (see Falk, 1997, for review). Similarly, men's brains reflect earlier selection for abilities that increased their success at finding and competing for mates. Visuospatial skills such as those related to navigating the environment (and those used to accurately aim projectiles?) would have been plausible targets for natural selection that ultimately left their marks on the underlying neurological substrates.

One can begin to explore this hypothesis by carrying out comparative neurological and behavioral studies on nonhuman primates. Of the two broad categories of behavior associated with differentially high performance on tests by women and men, communication skills and visuospatial processing respectively, the latter is easiest to compare across a range of primates including humans for the simple reason that, while only *Homo sapiens* has humanlike language, visuospatial skills such as mental rotation have been reported for nonhuman primates (Falk *et al.*, 1999). Thus one hopes that, in the future, performances on visuospatial tasks will be assessed in the two sexes and the results evaluated in terms of socioecological variables (e.g. residence and mating patterns) across a variety of primate species. The results of such studies should also be analyzed in light of (future) comparative studies that assess the extent of sexual dimorphism in brain sizes and proportions of GM and WM. Towards that end in my laboratory, John Redmond (Redmond & Sansone, 2000) has begun quantifying gross brain size relative to body mass for males and females of several primate species including owl monkeys (*Aotus*), baboons (*Papio*), gibbons and siamangs (*Hylobates*), and chimpanzees (*Pan*); and Arthur Sansone (Redmond & Sansone, 2000) is conducting similar analyses on tamarins (*Saguinus*), capuchin monkeys (*Cebus*), howler monkeys (*Alouatta*), leaf monkeys (*Presbytis*), red colobus monkeys (*Procolobus*), and a variety of macaques (*Macaca*). We expect the results of these studies to raise new questions that will be pursued in an ongoing effort to untease the evolutionary correlates of sexually dimorphic primate brains.

References

Andreasen, N.C., Flaum, M., Swayze, V., O'Leary, D.S., Alliger, R., Cohen, G., Ehrhardt, J. & Yuh, W.T.C. (1993). Intelligence and brain structure in normal individuals. *American Journal of Psychiatry*, **150**, 130–134.

Ankney, C.D. (1992). Sex differences in relative brain size: The mismeasure of woman, too? *Intelligence*, **16**, 329–336.

Falk, D. (1997). Brain evolution in females: An answer to Mr. Lovejoy. In *Women in Human Evolution*, ed. L. Hager, pp. 114–136. London: Routledge.

Falk, D. (2000). *Primate Diversity*. New York: W.W. Norton.

Falk, D., Froese, N., Sade, D.S. & Dudek, B.C. (1999). Sex differences in brain/body relationships of rhesus monkeys and humans. *Journal of Human Evolution*, **36**, 233–238.

Gaulin, S.J.C. & Fitzgerald R.W. (1989). Sexual selection for spatial-learning ability. *Animal Behavior*, **37**, 322.

Giedd, J.N., Snell, J.W., Lange, N., Rajapakse, J.C., Casey, B.J., Kozuch, P.L., Vaituzis, A.C., Vauss, Y.C., Hamburger, S.C., Kaysen, D. & Rapoport, J.L. (1996a). Quantitative magnetic resonance imaging of human brain development: ages 4–18. *Cerebral Cortex*, **6**, 551–560.

Giedd, J.N., Vaituzis, A.C., Hamburger, S.D., Lange, N., Rajapakse, J.C., Kaysen, D., Vauss, Y.C. & Rapoport, J.L. (1996b). Quantitative MRI of the temporal lobe, amygdala, and hippocampus in normal human development: Ages 4–18 years. *The Journal of Comparative Neurology*, **366**, 223–230.

Gur, R.C., Turetsky, B.I., Matsui, M., Yan, M., Bilker, W., Hughett, P. & Gur, R.E. (1999). Sex differences in brain gray and white matter in healthy young adults: Correlations with cognitive performance. *The Journal of Neuroscience*, **19**, 4065–4072.

Ho, K.-C., Roessmann, U., Straumfjord, J.V. & Monroe, G. (1980a). Analysis of brain weight. Adult brain weight in relation to sex, race, and age. *Archives of Pathology and Laboratory Medicine*, **104**, 635–639.

Ho, K.-C., Roessmann, U., Straumfjord, J.V. & Monroe, G. (1980b). Analysis of brain weight. Adult brain weight in relation to body height, weight, and surface area. *Archives of Pathology and Laboratory Medicine*, **104**, 640–645.

Jerison, H.J. (1973). *Evolution of the Brain and Intelligence*. New York: Academic Press.

Jerison, H.J. (1991). *Brain Size and the Evolution of Mind, Fifty-Ninth James Arthur Lecture on the Evolution of the Human Brain*. New York: The American Museum of Natural History.

Keverne, E.B., Fran, L.M. & Nevison, C.M. (1996a). Primate brain evolution: Generic and functional considerations. *Proceedings of the Royal Society of London*, B**262**, 689–696.

Keverne, E.C., Fundele, R., Narasimha, M., Barton, S.C. & Surani, M.A. (1996b). Genomic imprinting and the differential roles of parental genomes in brain development. *Developmental Brain Research*, **92**, 91–100.

Kimura, D. (1992). Sex differences in the brain. *Scientific American*, **267**, 119–125 .

Konigsberg, L., Falk, D., Hildebolt, C., Vannier, M., Cheverud, J. & Helmkamp, R.C. (1990). External brain morphology in rhesus macaques (*Macaca mulatta*). *Journal of Human Evolution*, **19**, 269–284.

Pakkenberg, B. & Gundersen, J.G. (1997). Neocortical neuron number in humans: Effect of sex and age. *Journal of Comparative Neurology*, **384**, 312–320.

Pakkenberg, H. & Voigt, J. (1964). Brain weight of the Danes. *Acta Anatomica*, **56**, 297–307.

Redmond, J. & Sansone, A. (2000). Brain/body relationships in New and Old World monkeys and apes. *American Journal of Physical Anthropology Supplement*, **30**, 295.

Reiss, A.L., Abrams, M.T., Singer, H.S., Ross, J.L. & Benckla, M.B. (1996). Brain development, gender and IQ in children: A volumetric imaging study. *Brain*, **119**, 1763–1774.

Shaywitz, B.A., Shaywitz, S.E., Pugh, K.R., Constable, R.T., Skudlarski, P., Fulbright, R.K., Bronen, R.A., Fletcher, J.M., Shankweller, D.P., Katz, L. & Gore, J.C. (1995). Sex differences in the functional organization of the brain for language. *Nature*, **373**, 607–609.

Smith, R.J. & Jungers, W.L. (1997). Body mass in comparative primatology. *Journal of Human Evolution*, **32**, 523–559.

Smith, R.J. & Leigh, S.R. (1998). Sexual dimorphism in primate neonatal body mass. *Journal of Human Evolution*, **34**, 173–201.

6
_____

Brain evolution in hominids: are we at the end of the road?

A progressive enlargement of the hominid brain started about 2 million years ago, probably from a bipedal, australopithecine form with a brain size comparable to that of a modern chimpanzee. Since then, a threefold increase in endocranial volume has taken place, leading to one of the most complex and efficient structures in the animated universe, the human brain. In view of the central importance placed on brain evolution in explaining the success of our species, one may wonder whether there are physical limits that constrain its processing power and evolutionary potential.

In this paper I will explore some of the design principles and operational modes that underlie the information processing capacity of the cerebral cortex in primates, and I will argue that with the evolution of the human brain we have nearly reached the limits of biological intelligence.

Biological limits to brain size

The human brain contains about 100 billion neurons, more than 100 000 km of interconnections, and has an estimated storage capacity of 1.25×10^{12} bytes (Cherniak, 1990; Hofman, 2000). These impressive numbers have led to the idea that our cognitive capabilities are virtually without limit. The human brain, however, has evolved from a set of underlying structures that constrain its size, and the amount of information it can store and process. In fact, there are a number of related factors that interact to limit brain size, factors that can be divided into two categories: (1) energetic constraints, and (2) neural processing constraints (Fig. 6.1).

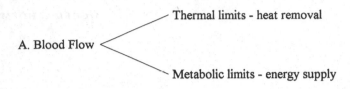

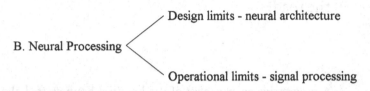

Fig. 6.1. Biological limits to brain size.

Energetic limits

The human brain generates about 15 watts (W) in a well-insulated cavity of about 1500 cm³. From an engineering point of view, removal of sufficient heat to prevent thermal overload could be a significant problem. But the brain is actively cooled by blood and not simply by heat conduction from the surface of the head. So the limiting factor is how fast the heat can be removed from the brain by blood flow. It has been suggested by Falk (1990) and others that the evolution of a 'cranial radiator' in hominids helped provide additional cooling to delicate and metabolically expensive parts of the brain, such as the cerebral cortex. This vascular cooling mechanism would have served as a 'prime releaser' that permitted brain size to increase dramatically during human evolution. So, to increase cooling efficiency in a larger brain, either the blood must be cooler when it first enters the structure, or the flow-rate must be increased above current levels.

Another factor related to blood flow has to do with the increasing energy requirements of a larger brain, a problem that is exacerbated by the high metabolic cost of this organ. It is unlikely, however, that the rate of blood flow or the increasing volume used by the blood vessels in the brain – in human about 4% – constrain its potential size. A bigger brain is metabolically possible because our cardiovascular system could evolve to transport more blood at greater pressure to meet the increased demand. This should not be taken to imply that thermal and metabolic mechanisms play no role at all in setting limits to brain size. Ultimately, energetic considerations will dictate and restrict the size of any neuron-based system, but as theoretical analyses indicate, thermal and metabolic factors alone are unlikely to constrain the potential size of our brain until it has increased to at least ten times its present size (Cochrane *et al.*, 1998).

Neural-processing limits

If the ability of an organism to process information about its environment is a driving force behind evolution, then the more information a system, such as the brain, receives, and the faster it can process this information, the more adequately it will be able to respond to environmental challenges and the better will be its chances of survival. The limit to any intelligent system therefore lies in its abilities to process and integrate large amounts of sensory information and to compare these signals with as many memory states as possible, and all that in a minimum of time. It implies that the functional capacity of a neuronal structure is inherently limited by its neural architecture and signal processing time. In the next section I will examine some of the design principles and operational modes that constrain the potential size and processing power of the human brain.

Evolution and geometry of the cerebral cortex

The evolution of the brain in mammals has been accompanied by a reorganization of the brain as a result of differential growth of certain brain regions. Consequently, the geometry of the brain, and especially the size and shape of the cerebral cortex, have changed notably since the late Cretaceous (Jerison, 1973). The evolutionary expansion of the cerebral cortex, indeed, is among the most distinctive morphological features of mammalian brains (Fig. 6.2). Particularly in species with large brains, and most notably in great apes, dolphins and whales, the brain becomes disproportionately composed of this cortical structure (Welker, 1990; Northcutt & Kaas, 1995).

The principal mathematical method for identifying and formalizing these changes in the brain's geometry is allometry. Using this method, analyses of the cerebral cortex in anthropoid primates revealed that the volume of the neocortex is highly predictable from absolute brain size. The volume of the neocortical gray matter is basically a linear function of brain volume, whereas the mass of interconnections, forming the

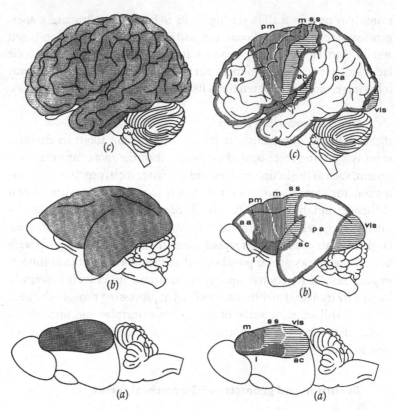

Fig. 6.2. Lateral views of the brains of the hedgehog (*a*), the prosimian *Galago*
(*b*), and human (*c*), to show the progressive increase and evolutionary
differentiation of the neocortex. In the hedgehog almost the entire neocortex
is occupied by sensory (ss, vis, ac) and motor (m) areas. In the prosimian *Galago*
the sensory cortical areas are separated by an area occupied by association
cortex (pa). A second area of association cortex (aa) is found in front of the
premotor cortex (pm). In humans the association areas are strongly developed.
Abbreviations: aa, anterior association area; ac, acoustic area; i, insular cortex;
m, motor cortex; pa, posterior association area; pm, premotor cortex; ss,
somatosensory cortex; vis, visual cortex (from Nieuwenhuys, 1994, with
permission).

underlying white matter volume, increases disproportionately with
brain size (Fig. 6.3). As a result, the volume of gray matter expressed as a
percentage of total brain volume is about the same for all anthropoid primates. The relative white matter volume, on the other hand, increases
with brain size, from 9% in pygmy marmosets (*Cebuella pygmaea*) to 34% in
humans, the highest value in primates (Hofman, 1989). In fact, the evolutionary process of neocorticalization in primates is mainly due to the pro-

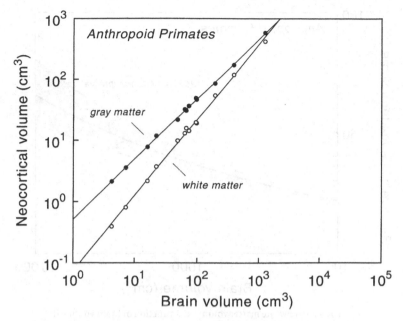

Fig. 6.3. Volumes of cerebral gray and white matter as a function of brain volume in anthropoid primates, including humans. Logarithmic scale. The slopes of the regression lines are 0.985 ± 0.009 (gray matter) and 1.241 ± 0.020 (white matter). Note the difference in the rate of change between gray matter ('neural elements') and white matter ('neural connections') as brain size increases.

gressive expansion of the axonal mass, rather than to the increase in the number of cortical neurons.

The non-linear nature of this process is further emphasized by plotting the relative volume of white matter as a function of brain size (Fig. 6.4). The exceptionally high correlation between both variables ensures that the curve, and its confidence limits, can be used for predictive purposes to estimate the volume of white matter relative to brain volume for a hypothetical primate. The model, for example, predicts a white matter volume of about 1470 cm³ for an anthropoid primate with a brain volume of 3000 cm³. In other words, in such a large brained primate, white matter would comprise about half of the entire brain volume, compared to one-third in modern man.

Computer simulation of the growth of the neocortex at different brain sizes, using a conservative scenario, revealed that with a brain size of about 3500 cm³ the total volume of the subcortical areas (i.e. cerebellum,

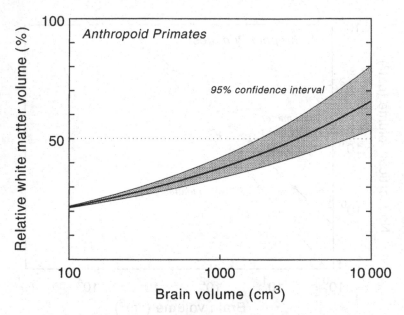

Fig. 6.4. Relative white matter volume as a function of brain volume in anthropoid primates. Semilogarithmic scale. The proportion of white matter ('neural connections') increases with brain size, from 22% in a monkey brain of 100 cm³ to about 65% in a hypothetical primate with a brain size of 10 000 cm³.

brain stem, diencephalon, etc.) reaches a maximum value (Fig. 6.5). Increasing the size of the brain beyond that point, following the same design principle, would lead to a further increase in the size of the neocortex, but to a reduction of the subcortical volume. Consequently, primates with very large brains (e.g. over 5 kg) may have a declining capability for neuronal integration despite their larger number of cortical neurons. In other words, the larger the brain grows beyond this critical size, the less efficient it will become, thus limiting any improvement in processing power. The model also predicts an absolute upper limit to primate brain size. Without a radical change in the macroscopic organization of the brain, however, this hypothetical limit will never be approached, because at that point (c. 8750 cm³) the brain would consist entirely of cortical neurons, and their interconnections, leaving no space for any other brain structure.

Of course, extrapolations based on brain models, such as the one used in the present study, implicitly assume a continuation of brain developments that are on a par with growth rates in the past. One cannot exclude

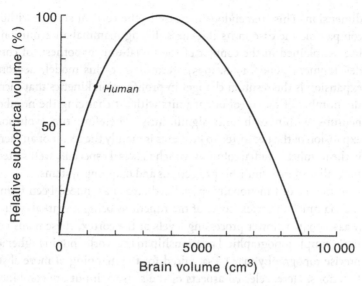

Fig. 6.5. Relative subcortical volume as a function of brain volume. The predicted subcortical volume (i.e. brain volume − predicted neocortex volume) must be zero at zero brain size. Likewise, the subcortical volume will be zero when the brain is exclusively composed of cortical matter. At a brain size of 3575 cm³ the subcortical volume has a maximum. The maximum simulated value for the subcortical volume (366 cm³) is then taken as 100%. The larger the brain grows beyond this critical size, the less efficient it will become. Assuming constant design, it follows that this model predicts an upper limit to the brain's processing power.

the possibility of new structures evolving in the brain, or a higher degree of specialization of existing brain areas, but within the limits of the existing 'Bauplan' there does not seem to be an incremental improvement path available to the human brain. At a point, corresponding to a brain volume two to three times that of modern man, the brain reaches its maximum processing power.

Design principles of neuronal organization

Comparisons among mammals show that the surface area of the cortical sheet varies by more than five orders of magnitude, while the thickness of the cortex varies by less than one order of magnitude (Hofman, 1989; Allman, 1990; Welker, 1990). Therefore, evolutionary changes in the cerebral cortex have occurred mainly parallel to the cortical surface (tangentially) and have been sharply constrained in the vertical (radial) dimension. This tremendous increase in the cortical surface without a comparable increase in its thickness during mammalian evolution has been explained in the context of the radial-unit hypothesis of cortical development (Rakic, 1988, 1995). According to this model, neocortical expansion is the result of changes in proliferation kinetics that increase the number of radial columnar units without changing the number of neurons within each unit significantly. Therefore the evolutionary expansion of the neocortex in primates is mainly the result of an increase in the number of radial columns, which makes it especially well suited for the elaboration of multiple projections and mapping systems.

A mosaic of functionally specialized areas has indeed been found in the mammalian cortex, some of the functions being remarkably diverse (Kaas, 1993). At lower processing levels of the cortex, these maps bear a fairly simple topographical relationship to the world, but in higher areas precise topography may be sacrificed for the mapping of more abstract functions. Here, selected aspects of the sensory input are combined in ways that are likely to be relevant to the animal. Over the past 20 years the use of modern anatomical tracing methods and physiological recording has established that small-brained mammals, such as rats and opossums, typically have about 15 well-differentiated neocortical areas, whereas monkeys and humans have well over 50. In fact, the maps differ in the attributes of the stimulus represented, in how the field is emphasized and in the types of computations performed. Clearly, the specifications of all these representations mean that functional maps can no longer be considered simply as hard-wired neural networks. They are much more flexible than previously thought, and are continually modified by feedback and lateral interactions. These dynamic changes in maps, which seem likely to result from local interactions and modulations in the cortical circuits, provide the plasticity necessary for adaptive behavior and learning.

Although species vary in the number of cortical areas they possess, and in the patterns of connections within and between areas, the structural organization of the cerebral cortex is remarkably similar. It has been estimated, for example, that within 1 mm³ of human cortex there are about 50 000 neurons that contain 150 m of dendrites and 100 m of axons, and that these neurites have about 50×10^6 synapses (Cherniak, 1990). The basic structural uniformity of the neocortex suggests that there are general architectural principles governing its growth and evolutionary development (Rakic, 1988). It is now well established that the cerebral cortex forms as a smooth sheet populated by neurons that proliferate at the ventricular surface and migrate outwards along radial glial fibers, forming distinct neural networks that are organized in columnar arrays stretched out through the depth of the cortex (Leise, 1990; Malach, 1994; Krubitzer, 1995). It has been postulated that these modular units have spatial dimensions depending on the number of local circuit neurons and that both the number and size of modules increase with increasing brain size (Hofman, 1985; Prothero, 1997). Scaling models, furthermore, indicate that the difference in modular diameter among mammals is only minor compared to the dramatic variation in overall cortex size. Thus it seems that the main cortical change during evolution has presumably been an increase in the number, rather than in the size of these units.

Although the details of the interpretation of the columnar organization of the cortex are still controversial, it is evident that the cerebral cortex is characterized by the hierarchical organization of groups of neurons. To group neurons into clusters interacting over relatively short distances allows these groups to inform as many adjacent clusters of neurons about the state of the 'emitting' cluster with as little as possible redundancy of information. Figure 6.6 shows a simple schematic diagram illustrating the effect of increasing the number of functional units on the number of interconnections. When the modular units are connected to all others by separate fibers and when each additional unit becomes connected with each of the already existing ones, then the number of connections (C) is related to the number of units (U) according to the equation: $C = U(U-1)$, which is nearly equivalent to $C = U^2$. In such a system the number of connections increases much faster than the number of units. Generally, the growth of connections to units is a factorial function of the number of units in a fully connected network and a linear function of the number of units in a minimally connected network. Recently we have shown that in species with convoluted brains the mass of interconnective nerve fibers, forming the underlying white matter, is proportional to the 1.5 power of cortical surface area (Hofman, 1991). In other words, the fraction of mass devoted to wiring seems to increase much slower than that needed to maintain a high degree of connectivity between the modular units.

These findings are in line with a model of neuronal connectivity (Deacon, 1990; Ringo, 1991) which says that as brain size increases there must be a corresponding fall in the fraction of neurons with which any neuron communicates directly. The reason for this is that if a fixed percentage of interconnections is to be maintained in the face of increased

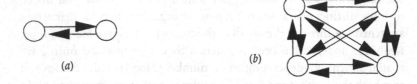

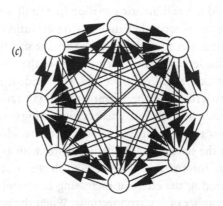

Fig. 6.6. The problem of network allometry is represented by three neural circuits that exhibit maximum connectivity. These diagrams depict that the number of connections (C) grows much faster than the number of units (U) in a fully connected network: $C = U(U-1)$ (from Ringo, 1991, with permission).

neuron number, then a large fraction of any brain size increase would be spent maintaining such a degree of wiring while the increasing axon length would reduce neural computational speed (Ringo *et al.*, 1994). The human brain, for example, has an estimated interconnectivity of the order of 10^3, based on data about the number of modular units and myelinated nerve fibers (Fig. 6.7). This implies that each cortical module is connected to a thousand other modules and that the mean number of processing steps, or synapses, in the path interconnecting these modules, is about two.

Once the brain has grown to a point where the bulk of its mass is in the form of connections, then further increases (as long as the same ratio in interconnectivity is maintained) will be unproductive. Increases in number of units will be balanced by decreased performance of those units due to the increased conduction time. This implies that large brains may tend to show more specialization in order to maintain processing capac-

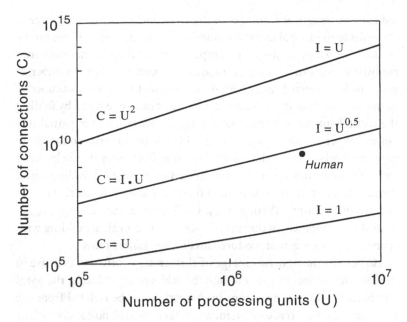

Fig. 6.7. Number of connections (C) as a function of number of processing units (U) in a neural network. Logarithmic scale. In a binary system, with an interconnectivity of $I = 1$, the growth of connections is a linear function of the number of units, and in a fully connected network ($I = U$) both variables are related according to a power function (cf. Fig. 6.6). The human cerebral cortex, with an estimated interconnectivity of about 10^3, lies somewhere between these extremes, and close to the line for $I = U^{0.5}$. It implies that in humans the number of myelinated axons scales to the 1.5 power of the number of modular units.

ity. Indeed, an increase in the number of distinct cortical areas with increasing brain size has been reported (Kaas, 1987; Welker, 1990). It may even explain why large-brained species may develop some degree of brain lateralization as a direct consequence of size. If there is evolutionary pressure on certain functions that require a high degree of local processing and sequential control, such as linguistic communication in human brains, these will have a strong tendency to develop in one hemisphere (Aboitiz, 1996).

Biological limits to information processing

The processing or transfer of information across cortical regions, rather than within regions, in large-brained primates can only be achieved by reducing the length and number of the interconnective axons in order to set limits to the axonal mass. The *number* of interconnective fibers can be reduced, as we have seen, by compartmentalization of neurons into modular circuits in which each module, containing a large number of neurons, is connected to its neural environment by a small number of axons. The *length* of the interconnective fibers can be reduced by folding the cortical surface and thus shortening the radial and tangential distances between brain regions. Local wiring – preferential connectivity between nearby areas of the cortex – is a simple strategy that helps keep cortical connections short. In principle, efficient cortical folding could further reduce connection length, in turn reducing white matter volume and conduction times (Young, 1993; Griffin, 1994; Scannell *et al.*, 1995). Thus the development of the cortex does seem to coordinate folding with connectivity in a way that produces smaller and faster brains.

However, a major disadvantage of this strategy is that an increase in the relative number of gyri can only be achieved by reducing the gyral width. At the limit, the neurons in the gyri would be isolated from the remainder of the nervous system, since there would no longer be any opening for direct contact with the underlying white matter. Prothero & Sundsten (1984) therefore introduced the concept of the gyral 'window', which represents the hypothetical plane between a gyrus and the underlying white matter through which nerve fibers running to and from the gyral folds must pass. According to this hypothesis, there would be a brain size where the gyral 'window' area has an absolute maximum. A further increase in the size of the brain beyond that point, i.e. at 2800 cm³, would increase the cortical surface area, but the 'window' would decrease, leading to a lower degree of neuronal integration and an increase in response time.

Recently, Cochrane and his colleagues (1998) looked at the different ways in which the brain could evolve to process more information or work more efficiently. They argue that the human brain has (almost) reached the limits of information processing that a neuron-based system allows and that our evolutionary potential is constrained by the delicate balance maintained between conduction speed, pulse width, synaptic processing time, and neuron density. By modeling the information processing capability per unit time of a human-type brain as a function of interconnectivity and axonal conduction speed they found that the human brain lies about 20%–30% below the optimal, with the optimal processing ability corresponding to a brain about twice the current volume.

Concluding remarks

The design of the human brain is such that it may perform a great number of complex functions with a minimum expenditure of energy and material, both in the performance of the functions and in the construction of the system. The similarity in brain design among primates indicates that brain systems among related species are morphologically constrained and that there are potential limits to the size of the brain and to the amount of information it can store and process. When the brain's geometry is considered in combination with the processing and transmission time of axons and dendrites, the degree of neuronal interconnectivity is near the capability limits of a neuron-based system. Once the brain has grown to a point where the bulk of its mass is in the form of connections, further increases will be unproductive, due to the declining capability of neuronal integration and increased conduction time. At this point, corresponding to a brain size two to three times that of modern man, the brain reaches its maximal processing power. The larger the brain grows beyond this critical size, the less efficient it will become.

Any significant enhancement of brain power or intelligence would require a simultaneous improvement of neural organization, signal processing (pulse width, transmission time and processing speed) and thermodynamics. Such a scenario, however, is an unrealistic biological option and must be discarded because of the trade-off that exists between these factors. It seems that within the limits of the existing 'Bauplan' there is no incremental improvement path available to the human brain. This implies that, as a species, *Homo sapiens* is nearly at the end of the road for brain evolution. Any further step in the evolution of intelligence will then have to take place outside our nervous system, in a technological world where the selection mechanisms and forces are radically different from those operating in nature.

References

Aboitiz, F. (1996). Does bigger mean better? Evolutionary determinants of brain size and structure. *Brain, Behavior and Evolution*, 47, 225–245.

Allman, J.M. (1990). Evolution of neocortex. In *Cerebral Cortex*, vol. 8A, eds. E.G. Jones & A. Peters, pp. 269–283. New York: Plenum Press.

Cherniak, C. (1990). The bounded brain: toward quantitative neuroanatomy. *Journal of Cognitive Neuroscience*, 2, 58–66.

Cochrane, P., Winter, C.S. & Hardwick, A. (1998). Biological limits to information processing in the human brain. British Telecommunications Publications, http://www.labs.bt.com/papers/index.htm

Deacon, T.W. (1990). Rethinking mammalian brain evolution. *American Zoologist*, 30, 629–705.

Falk, D. (1990). Brain evolution in *Homo*: The 'radiator' theory. *Behavioral and Brain Sciences*, 13, 333–381.

Griffin, L.D. (1994). The intrinsic geometry of the cerebral cortex. *Journal of Theoretical Biology*, 166, 261–273.

Hofman, M.A. (1985). Neuronal correlates of corticalization in mammals: a theory. *Journal of Theoretical Biology*, 112, 77–95.

Hofman, M.A. (1989). On the evolution and geometry of the brain in mammals. *Progress in Neurobiology*, 32, 137–158.

Hofman, M.A. (1991). The fractal geometry of convoluted brains. *Journal für Hirnforschung*, 32, 103–111.

Hofman, M.A. (2000). Evolution and complexity of the human brain: some organizing principles. In: *Evolution of Brain and Cognition*, eds. G. Roth & M. Wullimann, pp. 501–521. Heidelberg: Spektrum Verlag/Wiley.

Jerison, H.J. (1973). *Evolution of the Brain and Intelligence*. New York: Academic Press.

Kaas, J.H. (1987). The organization of neocortex in mammals: implications for theories of brain function. *Annual Review of Psychology*, 38, 129–151.

Kaas, J.H. (1993). Evolution of multiple areas and modules within neocortex. *Perspectives in Developmental Neurobiology*, 1, 101–107.

Krubitzer, L. (1995). The organization of neocortex in mammals: are species differences really so different? *Trends in Neurosciences*, 18, 408–417.

Leise, E.M. (1990). Modular construction of nervous systems: a basic principle of design for invertebrates and vertebrates. *Brain Research Reviews*, 15, 1–23.

Malach, R. (1994). Cortical columns as devices for maximizing neuronal diversity. *Trends in Neurosciences*, 17, 101–104.

Nieuwenhuys, R. (1994). The neocortex: an overview of its evolutionary development, structural organization and synaptology. *Anatomy and Embryology*, 190, 307–337.

Northcutt, R.G. & Kaas, J.H. (1995). The emergence and evolution of mammalian cortex. *Trends in Neurosciences*, 18, 373–379.

Prothero, J.W. (1997). Cortical scaling in mammals: a repeating units model. *Journal of Brain Research*, 38, 195–207.

Prothero, J.W. & Sundsten, J.W. (1984). Folding of the cerebral cortex in mammals: a scaling model. *Brain, Behavior and Evolution*, 24, 152–167.

Rakic, P. (1988). Specification of cerebral cortical areas. *Science*, 241, 170–176.

Rakic, P. (1995). A small step for the cell, a giant leap for mankind: a hypothesis of neocortical expansion during evolution. *Trends in Neurosciences*, 18, 383–388.

Ringo, J.L. (1991). Neuronal interconnection as a function of brain size. *Brain, Behavior and Evolution*, 38, 1–6.

Ringo, J.L., Doty, R.W., Demeter, S. & Simard, P.Y. (1994). Time is of the essence: a conjecture that hemispheric specialization arises from interhemispheric conduction delay. *Cerebral Cortex*, 4, 331–343.

Scannell, J.W., Young, M.P. & Blakemore, C.J. (1995). Analysis of connectivity in the rat cerebral cortex. *Journal of Neuroscience*, 15, 1463–1483.

Welker, W. (1990). Why does cerebral cortex fissure and fold? A review of determinants of gyri and sulci. In *Cerebral Cortex*, vol. **8A**, eds. E.G. Jones & A. Peters, pp. 3–136. New York: Plenum Press.

Young, M.P. (1993). The organization of neural systems in the primate cerebral cortex. *Proceedings of the Royal Society of London*, B**252**, 13–18.

Neurological substrates of species-specific adaptations

Introduction to Part II

Despite the emphasis on brain size in the classic paleoneurological literature, it has long been recognized that species-specific adaptations have neurological substrates that depend on more than just overall brain size. This concept is embodied in Harry Jerison's principle of proper mass (1973, p. 8): 'The mass of neural tissue controlling a particular function is appropriate to the amount of information processing involved in performing the function.' Thus brains do not merely enlarge globally as they evolve, their cortical and internal organization also changes in a process known as reorganization. The chapters in Part II explore the neurological underpinnings of some of the senses, adaptations, and cognitive abilities that are important for primates.

It is fitting that this section opens with a chapter on cerebral diversity by Todd Preuss that provides a clear synopsis of mammalian cortical anatomy, thus laying the groundwork for the rest of the volume. Preuss details the tension between classical studies that emphasize the microanatomical similarities between brains of different mammals and therefore highlight brain size as a main focus of natural selection, and more recent investigations that reveal a remarkable diversity in mammalian cortical organization and therefore emphasize neurological reorganization as a driving force during brain evolution (Preuss, 1993, 1995). There is no doubt where Preuss comes down in this debate, as is clear from his observation that 'to focus exclusively on the ancestral features of cortical organization that mammals share, however, is to ignore those features of cortical organization that distinguish one group of mammals from another and provide the basis for their particular behavioral and cognitive abilities.' In Chapter 7, Preuss provides a welcome synthesis of new findings regarding cortical specializations in mammals including

primates. Although he views the cortex as 'a veritable hotbed of evolutionary reorganization' and advocates future evolutionary studies of cortical microanatomy, in the end Preuss recognizes the importance of brain
size with a thoughtful and entertaining description of how the evolutionary enlargement of the human brain may have related to modifications in
cortical microanatomy in conjunction with new cognitive functions.

It is almost received wisdom among evolutionary biologists that, as
ancestral primates adapted to arboreal habitats, the sense of smell
decreased in importance in conjunction with a greater reliance on vision.
Chapters 8 and 9 by Brunetto Chiarelli and Ralph Holloway *et al.* address
the evolution of certain neurological substrates related to processing
odors and visual information, respectively. Although most primates
including humans have a poorly developed sense of smell (i.e. they are
microsmatic), Chiarelli describes the neuroanatomical and neurochemical substrates for perception of odorants and pheromones in a variety of
mammals including primates (Keverne, 1983), and then asks whether or
not sensitivity to biological smells correlates positively with the emission
of pheromones and with hormone development in humans. Chiarelli
answers affirmatively, citing research that confirms 'strong interactions
between olfactory, endocrine, and reproductive systems' in humans. For
example, women can discriminate the odor of their own offspring from
those of other infants, simply by smelling garments previously worn by
the infants (Schaal *et al.*, 1980); and adult men and women are able to identify gender, self odor, and the odor of their partners by smelling garments
that have been worn for some time without use of deodorants or perfumes. In reference to the frequently cited fact that menstrual cycles of
women who are roommates tend to converge over time, Chiarelli specu-
lates that some factor that is related to social closeness and interaction
must exist that shifts the timing of the biological clock in the brain thus
causing a change in ovulation and cycling (Stern & McClintock, 1998).
Chiarelli further suggests that humans may be influenced by genetically
based pheromonal communication when they select mates. This chapter
is particularly interesting because pheromone research has traditionally
received little attention in the field of human brain evolution, despite its
recognized importance for mammals in general.

As noted by Holloway *et al.* in Chapter 9, although there is not serious
disagreement about the fact that the brain became reorganized as well as
enlarged during hominid evolution, there is considerable controversy
about when reorganization related to reduction in primary visual striate

cortex (Brodmann's area 17) took place. In order to re-examine this tick-lish question, new comparative data from chimpanzees and humans are provided in this chapter. In particular, photographs of the brains of two chimpanzees, 'Frank' and 'Chuck', illustrate the positions of the lunate sulci that form the anterior borders of area 17 in each hemisphere. Significantly, Holloway *et al.* observe that, in three of the four hemi-spheres, the lunate sulci are 'clearly in a more posterior position than found in most other chimpanzee hemispheres.' The authors also docu-ment a high degree of variation of primary visual striate cortex for humans (Gilissen & Zilles, 1995; Klekamp *et al.*, 1994), and conclude that 'given that this variability is shared between *Homo* and *Pan*, it would appear possible that some of the australopithecine ancestors of *Homo* could have expressed these variations also, given a pongid–hominid divergence of 5–7 MYA.' As an extra bonus, the last section of this chapter, which predicts the state of brain studies in the year 2010, is especially interesting.

In addition to focusing on specific modalities such as olfaction or vision, neurological reorganization may also be investigated by compara-tive studies of broader areas of the cerebral cortex. In Chapter 10, Emmanuel Gilissen reviews and analyzes symmetries and asymmetries of the cerebral cortices of chimpanzees and humans by comparing the extents of their intra- and interspecific variation in overall cortical shape, asymmetrical projections of specific lobes (petalia patterns), and morphology of the planum temporale (PT) and parietale (PP). Gilissen shows that both species share a common pattern in which the shape of the cortical surface is highly variable in certain association cortices and, con-cordant with Holloway *et al.* (Chapter 9, this volume), the region of the occipital pole. It is noteworthy, however, that for both chimpanzees and humans the cortical regions of highest intraspecific variability have not been uniformly progressive during primate brain evolution (Armstrong, 1990; Gilissen & Zilles, 1995). Like humans, chimpanzees tend to manifest asymmetries in PT and PP, but they lack the combination of obvious right frontal and left occipital petalias that, according to Gilissen, 'remain the only human specific pattern of asymmetry'. Gilissen concludes with the important observation that 'patterns of asymmetries are not intercorre-lated and that humans show an extreme state of "mosaic" structural asymmetries, when compared to chimpanzees and probably gorillas'. Chapter 10 is must-reading for anyone interested in the evolution of brain lateralization.

The important discovery that chimpanzees are characterized by a humanlike L > R planum temporale, reported recently by Patrick Gannon and colleagues (Gannon *et al.*, 1998) is followed-up in Chapter 11 with a comparative study of this region in macaques, apes and humans. Based on their findings, Gannon *et al.* propose that the distinguishable suite of neurological features that is related to receptive language in humans began a gradual evolution 20 million years ago, resulting in the first appearance of an asymmetrical gross anatomy for the planum temporale 10 million years later in the common ancestor of gorillas and humans. The authors discuss the potential functional significance of this cortical area for nonhuman primates, and suggest that chimpanzees, at least, possess a complex polymodal communicative repertoire that humans have yet to decipher. This raises the important question of whether language areas in the human brain are 'hard wired' for vocal/auditory (speaking/hearing) modes of communication, or whether they are equipotential and plastic with respect to combining these modes with gestural/visual modalities. In discussion about language-trained apes (Savage-Rumbaugh, 1998; Savage-Rumbaugh & Lewin, 1994), Gannon *et al.* note that it would be 'educational to see whether we, as a more cognitively sophisticated species, would be better qualified to comprehend natural chimpanzee "language" than they are at comprehending ours'. Comparative research on the planum temporale is sure to continue, and future investigators will benefit greatly from this interesting and synthetic chapter.

In addition to imaging the brains of living primates, noninvasive medical imaging techniques are currently being applied to the study of braincases and their corresponding 'virtual endocasts', from fossil primates including early hominids. In Chapter 12, Phillip Tobias provides an historical overview that details pioneering work in the application of computerized tomography (CT) to fossil skulls, much of which was carried out on australopithecine specimens from South Africa. For example, Tobias describes CT analysis of the famous Taung child (Conroy *et al.* 1990), which contributed to reassessment of its age at death (based on revelations about dentition), and the more recent application of 3D-CT technology to the skull of an adult male *Australopithecus africanus* specimen, Stw 505 ('Mr. Ples'), that yielded a provocative estimate of its endocranial capacity (Conroy *et al.*, 1998). As background for this discussion, the chapter begins with lucid descriptions of the processes that result in traditional natural and artificial (as opposed to virtual) endocasts. Mean endocranial capacity is also reassessed for *Australopithecus africanus*, and new data are provided that shed light on the extent of variation in brain size that characterized this species. At the conclusion of this chapter, Tobias brings readers back full circle to the evolution of brain size (Part I) by posing a series of hypotheses about how demography, diet, nutrition, and paleoecological variables may have constrained the phylogenetic increase in brain size.

One of the most exciting advances in the study of brain evolution is the application of noninvasive medical imaging technology to comparative neuroanatomical studies of living primates. In Chapter 13, Katerina Semendeferi summarizes recent research that uses magnetic resonance imaging (MRI) and 3D reconstruction to image parts of the brains of living apes and humans in order to elucidate the neurological reorganization that took place in hominids after their split from other hominoids. Much of the MR research on apes was pioneered by Semendeferi and her colleagues, and with exciting results. For example (and contrary to expectation), Semendeferi and colleagues found that the frontal lobes of humans are not disproportionately enlarged compared to apes (Semendeferi & Damasio, 2000), leading to the conclusion that 'it is possible that the frontal lobes increased after the split of the Miocene hominoids from the line leading to the extant lesser apes'. Similarly (and, again, surprisingly), Semendeferi reports that the human cerebellum is statistically significantly smaller than expected for an ape brain of human size. As she notes, however, 'it remains to be seen if subdivisions of the frontal lobe and other regions of the brain into sub-sectors reveal differences in their relative size' (see also, Preuss, Chapter 7, this volume). Semendeferi also briefly reviews pilot work of other investigators using positron emission tomography (PET) (Kaufman et al., 1999) and functional magnetic resonance imaging (fMRI) (Dubowitz et al., 1998; Vanduffel et al., 1998) to assess the neurological substrates of certain sensory, motor, and cognitive tasks in monkeys. Although the application of these techniques to comparative evolutionary studies is in its infancy, Semendeferi concludes that their contributions are already significant and that 'the future looks promising'.

Just as studies of brain evolution are advancing because of medical imaging technology, they are also benefiting from experimental applications of geometric morphometrics for analyzing variation in the shapes and sizes of brains, skulls, and endocasts. In the final chapter, Katrin Schäfer et al. use both traditional metric techniques and geometric morphometrics to analyze and compare changes in the external and internal (braincase) surfaces in median sagittal planes of skulls representing mid-Pleistocene and modern humans. Results confirm and extend earlier findings that the size and shape of the exocranium changed from the mid-Pleistocene to the present. In the thicker fossil skulls, the area enclosed by the midsagittal contour of the exocranium is larger, and the position of nasion is more anterior and that of inion is more posterior and superior. On the other hand, the size and shape of the endocranium in the midsagittal plane remained remarkably stable. Since Bookstein *et al.* (1999) have shown that size of the inner frontal bone increased by ~11%, questions about exactly which regions of cortex contributed to this increase remain to be answered by future geometric morphometric studies that will invariably include sliding landmarks. Apart from the frontal bone, other cranial regions such as the occipital bone are worth analyzing in the midsagittal plane with these techniques. The next step would be to extend geometric morphometric analyses to regions beyond the midsagittal plane. Meanwhile, the changes and invariances detected by Schäfer *et al.* raise serious questions about associating specific cognitive abilities (or lack thereof) with morphologies of the skull or face that characterize different species of early hominid (e.g., Neandertals). As Harry Jerison elucidated in his classic book, *Evolution of the Brain and Intelligence* (1973), we must turn to the braincase of such skulls and the endocasts that they yield to even begin such an undertaking.

References

Armstrong, E. (1990). Evolution of the brain. In *The Human Nervous System*, ed. G. Paxinos, pp. 1–16. New York: Academic Press.

Bookstein, F., Schäfer, K., Prossinger, H., Fieder, M., Seidler, H., Stringer, C., Weber, G.W., Arsuaga, J.L., Slice, D., Rohlf, F.J., Recheis, W., Mariam, A.J. & Marcus, L.F. (1999). Comparing frontal cranial profiles in archaic and modern *Homo* by morphometric analysis. *The Anatomical Record (New Anatomist)*, **257**, 217–224.

Conroy, G.C., Vannier, M.W. & Tobias, P.V. (1990). Endocranial features of *Australopithecus africanus* revealed by 2- and 3-D computed tomography. *Science*, **247**, 838–841.

Conroy, G.C., Weber, G.W., Seidler, H., Tobias, P.V., Kane, A. & Brunsden, B. (1998). Endocranial capacity in an early hominid cranium from Sterkfontein, South Africa. *Science*, **280**, 1730–1731.

Dubowitz, D.J., Chen, D., Atkinson, D.J., Grieve, K.L., Gillikin, B., Bradley, W.G. & Anderson, R.A. (1998). Functional magnetic resonance imaging in macaque cortex. *Neuroreport*, **9**(10), 2213–2218.

Gannon, P.J., Holloway, R.L., Broadfield, D.C. & Braun, A.R. (1998). Asymmetry of chimpanzee planum temporale: humanlike pattern of Wernicke's brain language area homolog. *Science*, **279**, 220–222.

Gilissen, E. & Zilles, K. (1995). The relative volume of the primary visual cortex and its intersubject variability among humans: a new morphometric study. *Comptes Rendus Académie des Sciences (Paris) Série 2a*, **320**, 897–902.

Jerison, H.J. (1973). *Evolution of the Brain and Intelligence*. New York: Academic Press.

Kaufman, J.A., Phillips-Conroy, J., Black, K.J. & Perlmutter, J.S. (1999). Regional cerebral blood flow in anaesthetized baboons (*Papio anubis*): The use of Positron Emission Tomography in anthropology. *American Journal of Physical Anthropology*, n.SUPPL., **28**, 166.

Keverne, E.B. (1983). Pheromonal influences on the endocrine regulation of reproduction. *Trends in Neuroscience*, **6**, 381–384.

Klekamp, J., Reidel, A., Harper, C. & Kretschmann, H.J. (1994). Morphometric study on the postnatal growth of the visual cortex of Australian Aborigines and Caucasians. *Journal of Brain Research*, **35**, 541–548.

Preuss, T.M. (1993). The role of the neurosciences in primate evolutionary biology: Historical commentary and prospectus. In *Primates and their Relatives in Phylogenetic Perspective*, ed. R.D.E. MacPhee, pp. 333–362. New York: Plenum Press.

Preuss, T.M. (1995). The argument from animals to humans in cognitive neuroscience. In *The Cognitive Neurosciences*, ed. M.S. Gazzaniga, pp. 1227–1241. Cambridge, MA: MIT Press.

Savage-Rumbaugh, S. (1998). Nyota.http://www.gsu.edu/~wwwlrc/biographies/nyota.html: Language Research Center.

Savage-Rumbaugh, S. & Lewin, R. (1994). *Kanzi: An Ape at the Brink of the Human Mind*. New York: John Wiley & Sons Inc.

Schaal, B., Montagner, H., Hertling, E., Bolzoni, D., Moyse, R. & Quichon, R. (1980). Les stimulations olfactives dans les relations entre l'enfant et la mere. *Reproduction, Nutrition, Development*, **20**, 843–858.

Semendeferi, K. & Damasio, H. (2000). The brain and its main anatomical subdivisions in living hominoids using magnetic resonance imaging. *Journal of Human Evolution*, **38**, 317–332.

Stern, K. & McClintock, M.K. (1998). Regulation of ovulation by human pheromones. *Nature*, **392**, 177–179.

Vanduffel, W., Beatse, E., Sunaert, S., Van Hecke, P., Tootell, R.B.H. & Orban, G.A. (1998). Functional magnetic resonance imaging in an awake rhesus monkey. *Society for Neuroscience*, **24**, 10–12.

7

The discovery of cerebral diversity: an unwelcome scientific revolution

Studies of mammalian and primate brain evolution have traditionally focused on changes in encephalization, that is, changes in brain size statistically adjusted to compensate for changes in body size, rather than on changes in the internal organization of the brain. There are some very sound reasons for stressing size. Mammals do indeed vary dramatically in absolute and relative brain size: at a given body weight, brain weight can vary more than five-fold across species (Stephan *et al.*, 1988). Moreover, brain size changes can have profound consequences for the developmental biology and ecology of mammalian taxa, because larger-brained taxa grow more slowly and live longer than do smaller-brained taxa of comparable body size (Sacher, 1982; Finlay & Darlington, 1995) and because brain tissue is energetically very demanding (Aiello & Wheeler, 1995). Conveniently, brain size is relatively tractable empirically, which is to say that one can measure it with reasonable precision in all sorts of living and extinct taxa, whereas the internal features of brain organization can be examined only with difficulty in extant taxa and not at all in extinct forms. Finally, there can be little doubt that variations in brain size are in some way related to variations in cognitive and behavioral abilities.

But in precisely *what* ways are brain size, cognition, and behavior related? Harry Jerison has ably articulated the view that encephalization serves as an index of general animal intelligence (see especially Jerison, 1961, 1973), and in doing so has provided the underpinning for modern brain allometry studies. His approach has not been universally embraced, however, Ralph Holloway (see especially Holloway, 1966a,b) being notable among those who have questioned whether there is a straightforward relationship between brain size and cognitive capacity, emphasizing instead that evolutionary changes in cognitive and behavioral capacities reflect reorganization of systems internal to the brain.

How one reckons the relative importance of size and reorganization in brain evolution depends on one's conception of mammalian brain structure and how that structure varies between mammalian groups. If the internal organization of the brain remains constant as brain size varies, or if brain organization changes in regular and predictable ways as brain size varies, then knowing a species' level of encephalization tells us something significant about the status of that species' brain relative to the brains of other species, because all species are regular variants of a common plan of brain organization. Under this view, it is reasonable to regard more encephalized animals as having more of some general information-processing substrate than less encephalized animals. If brains vary significantly in their internal organization, however, encephalization indices can not reasonably be considered as proxies for general cognitive ability across a wide variety of mammalian species. The task of understanding the brain organization of any one species becomes much more difficult, as does the business of relating brain to behavior and cognition.

The controversy over quantitative versus qualitative change did not begin with Jerison and Holloway: it goes back to the very beginnings of evolutionary biology and of the neurosciences (Preuss, 1993, 1995a). The proponents of quantity have generally held the upper hand. Darwin and Huxley strongly defended the idea that the human mind and brain are extensions of the minds and brains of our close relatives – that the difference between us and them are matters of degree rather than of kind (Huxley, 1863; Darwin, 1871). The consensus view among neuroscientists in the late 1800s and early 1900s seems to have been that brain evolution was mainly a matter of progressive encephalization and differentiation within the bounds of a common brain plan (Preuss, 1995a). The concept of differentiation was invoked because workers believed that in larger brains, one could distinguish more cell types, the cellular laminae of the cerebral cortex appeared to be more sharply defined, and one could distinguish more subdivisions (areas) of the cortex. It is important to appreciate that these neuroscientists did not necessarily regard the appearance of additional cell types, cellular strata, and areas, as tantamount to the evolution of new structural elements within the brain. Rather, these were regarded as the products of differentiation, by which was meant an unfolding of structural tendencies or potentialities latent in the basic mammalian brain plan (see, for example, Elliot Smith, 1924, and Le Gros Clark, 1959). That is, as brains got bigger, existing components become more refined and better sorted out, but nothing new was added. This view of brain evolution accorded well with the popular view that the course of evolution was linear and progressive. Thus, the early neuroscientific literature is filled with references to the 'phylogenetic scale' and to 'higher' and 'lower' mammals, concepts that modern evolutionists regard as problematic. One gets little sense that there is a diversity of mammalian brain organization – that different groups of mammals (primates, rodents, cetaceans, and so forth) evolved their own distinctive specializations of brain organization (for a conspicuous exception, see Brodmann, 1909).

The view that the internal histological and connectional organization of mammalian brains are fundamentally conservative crystallized at an early point in the history of neuroscience, when knowledge of brain structure was quite rudimentary by modern standards. In the early 1970s there began a revolution in neuroscientific methodology that continues to this day. The fruits of this revolution include new techniques for studying the physiology and molecular biology of neurons, and – for the first time – reliable and sensitive methods for studying the connections between neurons. Our understanding of the structure of cerebral cortex, in particular, has been profoundly affected by these developments. Once regarded by some as a relatively homogenous neural net, today cerebral cortex is recognized as perhaps the most complex entity known to science. Moreover, since the cortex is the largest component of mammalian brains (Stephan *et al.*, 1981), undergoes enormous evolutionary changes in absolute and relative size, and provides much of the neural substrate for cognitive processing, cortical organization and its phyletic variations are matters of vital importance to students of brain evolution. How does our new and detailed understanding of the organization of cerebral cortex bear on the question of encephalization versus reorganization? The answer to this depends on what you read. If you read the neuroscience textbooks and review papers, you get the impression that there is very little variation in the internal organization of cerebral cortex, and that brain evolution must be mainly about size. A careful perusal of the primary literature, however, suggests that the cortex is a veritable hotbed of evolutionary reorganization.

Cortical organization and evolution: the doctrine of basic uniformity

In this section, I give a synopsis of mammalian cortical anatomy as it is presented in modern textbooks and review papers (for example, Eccles, 1984; White, 1988; Churchland & Sejnowski, 1992; Shepherd, 1994; Hendry, 1996), and then consider some contemporary ideas about cortical evolution. Cerebral cortex is a bilateral structure that caps the brainstem. It consists of a thin, outer shell of cells (the gray matter) overlying a mass of axons (the white matter) passing to and from the cortex. Cortex is divided into two broad regions, the neocortex (or isocortex) and the allocortex. Allocortex includes the hippocampus, olfactory cortex, and related regions situated along the margins of the cortical sheet. Neocortex, which makes up the largest part of the cerebral mantle in most mammals, includes regions devoted to vision, somatosensation, audition, equilibrium, motor cortex, and higher-order cognitive functions. The main subdivisions of the cortex are called *areas*. Cortical areas are distinguished from one another by their appearance in tissue stained for cell bodies ('cytoarchitecture') and for myelinated fibers ('myeloarchitecture'), as well as by their connections and functional properties. Neuroscientists do not yet have a complete accounting of cortical areas for any mammalian species, although there is reason to think that the number of cortical areas is phyletically variable. Cortical areas receive inputs from subcortical structures, the most numerous inputs arising from the thalamus. Groups of functionally related areas tend to be located close to one another and to form strongly interconnected networks. Cortex exerts its influence on behavior by means of projections to deep brain structures and to the spinal cord.

Cerebral cortex consists of a variety of neurons, which can be grouped broadly into pyramidal and non-pyramidal classes (Fig. 7.1). Pyramidal cells are generally large cells with a distinctive, elongated apical dendrite that extends towards the cortical surface, several basal dendrites, and a long axon that may branch repeatedly and which makes synaptic contacts that release an excitatory transmitter (glutamate or aspartate). Pyramidal cells are the main extrinsic cells of the cortex, giving rise to projections to distant cortical areas as well as to subcortical structures. Non-pyramidal cells are mainly intrinsic neurons (also known as interneurons or local-circuit neurons), with axons that synapse on cells close to the parent cell body. Non-pyramidal cells consist of both excitatory and inhibitory

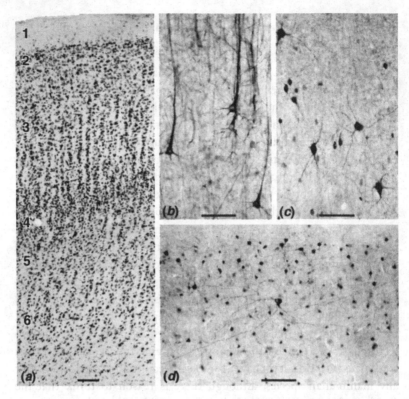

Fig. 7.1. At low magnification (*a*), the stratification of cortex into layers can be discerned, as in this Nissl-stained section from the extrastriate cortex of a chimpanzee. In this section, the clustering of cells into vertical aggregates or columns can also be seen (especially in layers 3, 4, and 5), although other cortical regions are not so obviously columnar. The Nissl stain only shows cell bodies; immunocytochemical techniques can often reveal more of the distinctive morphologies of cortical cell types. Pyramidal cells stained for neurofilament protein are shown in (*b*); the tall, broad apical dendrites and the finer basal dendrites of these cells are clearly visible in this preparation. Presumed inhibitory interneurons immunoreactive for parvalbumin and calbindin are shown in (*c*) and (*d*), respectively. Figs. 7.1 (*b*), (*c*), and (*d*), were taken from the motor cortex of a chimpanzee. Scale bars = 100 μm.

classes. The main excitatory cells are the so-called spiny stellate cells, upon which thalamic fibers synapse. Inhibitory interneurons, which express the transmitter γ-amino butyric acid (GABA), display a remarkable variety of morphological, connectional, and biochemical phenotypes (Figs. 7.1*c,d*). Interneurons are subdivided into classes based on differences in morphology and biochemistry. Much current interest focuses on identifying the morphological and connectional properties of neurons that express specific calcium-binding proteins (CBPs; especially parvalbumin, calbindin, or calretinin), cells that are readily stained with immunocyto-chemical techniques (Andressen *et al.*, 1993). Calcium-binding proteins regulate intracellular calcium concentrations, and thereby influence cel-lular excitability; thus, cells that express different calcium-binding pro-teins may have different physiological properties (Baimbridge *et al.*, 1992).

Cortical neurons are arrayed through the thickness of the gray matter in several more-or-less distinct layers (laminae), which are distinguished on the basis of cell size and packing density. In the neocortex, most workers enumerate six layers (following Brodmann, 1909), although sub-divisions of these layers can be recognized in some cortical areas. Inputs to the cortex tend to be layer specific. For example, in many mammals, a major afferent projection from the thalamus terminates in layer 4 and deep layer 3 of neocortex (Fig. 7.2). Afferents from other sources terminate in other layers. Similarly, projections from the cortex to sites in other parts of the brain tend to arise from layer-specific populations of pyrami-dal cells. For example, the projections to the spinal cord arise from large pyramidal cells, the cell bodies of which reside in layer 5. Projections to other neocortical areas can arise from any combination of the layers that contain pyramidal cells, namely layers 2, 3, 5, and 6.

Within a neocortical area, the flow of information has a strong vertical component. There are strong connections between neurons and the cells located immediately above and below them, and indeed in some cortical regions, examination of sections stained to show cell bodies suggest that cells are grouped into vertical clusters that span the thickness of the cortex (Fig. 7.1a). These vertical aggregations are called *columns*. As a result of the vertical organization of connections, information conveyed by tha-lamic fibers terminating in layer 4 is transformed and conveyed to deeper and more superficial layers, where further transformations are effected and from which output projections arise. In addition to vertical connec-tions, the cells of a given column may have horizontally directed connec-tions with nearby columns of the same area.

Students of evolution will naturally want to know what happens to the structure of the neocortex over the course of evolutionary history. Not much, would seem to be the answer implied by textbook and review-paper accounts of cortical organization. I say 'implied' because textbook accounts rarely have much to say about evolution, presenting their subject matter in a nearly species-free fashion. When results are related to particular species, the point is usually to illustrate allegedly *general* principles of organization rather than species- or taxon-specific characteristics. This is not merely a matter of convenience or simplification. Hand in hand with recent progress in the study of cortical organization has come a new interpretation – or more accurately, a family of kindred interpretations – of cortical evolution. These interpretations share the view that there is a 'basic uniformity of structure' of the neocortex across species, as Rockel *et al.*, (1980) expressed it.

The doctrine of basic uniformity is founded on the concept that neocortex is comprised of cell columns, which are viewed as the basic structural-functional units of cortical organization (see especially Szentágothai, 1975, 1978; Creutzfeldt, 1977, 1978; Goldman & Nauta, 1977; Hubel & Wiesel, 1977; Mountcastle, 1978; Rockel *et al.*, 1980; Eccles, 1984). One of the key tenets of this doctrine is the idea that columns preserve a nearly invariant cellular composition. In their seminal paper, Rockel *et al.* (1980) reported the number of neurons in columns of specific neocortical areas in different species. They took as their working unit of tissue a volume measuring 25×30 μm across the surface of the cortex (reflecting their estimate of typical column width) and extending through the thickness of the cortex (which varies between areas and species). Rockel *et al.* reported that columns have nearly the same number of cells, approximately 110, in whatever area of the cortex they are located, and they reported this number to be nearly constant across species. They found only one major exception to this rule – the primary visual cortex of primates, in which cell number was found to be much higher, approximately 270 cells per column.

Basic uniformity extends also to the cellular and connectional organization of the neocortex. There is thought to be a basic complement of cell types, distributed in a particular laminar pattern, and with a stereotyped set of interconnections so as to constitute a 'basic cortical circuit' (see especially Shepherd, 1988, and White, 1988, and also Creutzfeldt, 1977, 1978). Also, the laminar organization of extrinsic inputs and outputs conforms to a common plan. In one version of this theory (Creutzfeldt, 1977, 1978), each cortical column performs the same transformation on incoming information. As a result, differences in the functions of particular cortical areas arise from differences in their input sources and output targets, rather than from differences in the information-processing functions of the columns that comprise the areas. Differences in input and output parameters are also invoked to explain variations in the histological appearance (i.e. cyto- and myeloarchitecture) of areas (Creutzfeldt, 1977,

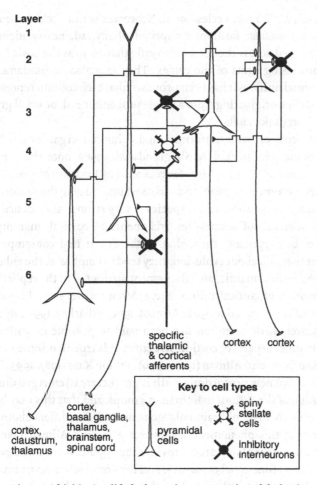

Fig. 7.2. A highly simplified schematic representation of the laminar organization and local circuitry of cerebral cortex, abstracted from diagrams presented in modern textbooks and review papers (see especially, Shepherd, 1988, White, 1988, and Douglas & Martin, 1998). The major excitatory inputs to the cortex arise from the thalamus and cortex and terminate at middle levels of the cortex (layer 4 and deep 3), synapsing on spiny stellate cells and on portions of pyramidal cells that lie within these layers. Excitation is then passed to more superficial layers and to deeper layers by means of the excitatory outputs of the spiny stellate cells and by local collaterals of pyramidal cell axons. Excitation of pyramidal cells is constrained by strong projections from inhibitory interneurons, which are themselves activated by collateral fibers arising from excitatory neurons. Pyramidal cells are the major output neurons of the cortex and the most numerous cell type, comprising about 70% of the neuronal population of the cortex. In addition to inputs to the middle layers from the thalamus and cortex, other layers receive afferents from a variety of cortical and subcortical sources.

1978; Rockel, *et al.*, 1980; Eccles, 1984). Neocortex is thus held to be constructed in a *modular* fashion, comprised of myriad, nearly identical columns arrayed across the cerebral mantle that serve as the basic information-processing units of the cortex. They may also be fundamental developmental units, as it has been proposed that each column represents a clonal cell line originating from a single progenitor cell, or small group of progenitors (Rakic, 1988).

The concepts of basic uniformity and columnar organization have been enormously influential. As Skoglund *et al.* (1996a) note, the number of cells in a cortical column – 110 – as reckoned by Rockel *et al.* (1980) 'has more or less become a neuroanatomical constant.' Faith in the uniformity of columnar organization across species is very strong, as evidenced by the preponderance of species-free treatments of cortical anatomy. It should not be surprising, then, that to the extent that contemporary neuroscientists talk about evolution, they tend to emphasize the enlargement of the cortical mantle, an enlargement attributed to the replication or proliferation of cortical columns (e.g. Mountcastle, 1978; Bugbee & Goldman-Rakic, 1983; Rakic, 1988; Allman, 1990; Killackey, 1995). By contrast, relatively little attention has been paid to possible evolutionary changes in other aspects of cortical structure. It is true that some neuroscientists such as John Allman (1977, 1990) and Jon Kaas (1987, 1995) have emphasized that new neocortical subdivisions (i.e. areas) emerged during the evolution of the various mammalian groups, and that this may be an important mechanism of brain enlargement. Opinion differs about the significance of this phenomenon, however. Kaas and Allman take the view that the advent of new areas provides the opportunity for the evolutionary of novel functional capacities, and thus represent important evolutionary innovations. Other workers, however, are inclined to view the advent of new areas in terms of differentiation, in the sense of an elaboration, refinement, or segregation of preexisting structural characteristics and functional capacities (as discussed in Preuss, 1995a).

The remarkable diversity of mammalian cortical organization

The modern, canonical view of cortical organization, with its emphasis on the microanatomical similarities among mammalian species, would seem to provide strong justification for the view that brain evolution is mainly or exclusively a matter of size, and that one can downplay changes in the internal organization of the brain. If one goes beyond the text-books and review papers to the primary literature, however, one quickly discovers that mammalian cortical organization is remarkably diverse: neuroscientists have documented differences at virtually every level of cortical organization that has been examined. What follows is merely a sampler.

Variations in columnar and cellular organization

It is increasingly clear that the strong claims made by Rockel *et al.* (1980) concerning the constancy of cell number in a column, or alternatively, under a unit area of neocortical surface, cannot be sustained. Beaulieu (1993) and Skoglund *et al.* (1996b) have reported large differences in column cell number between different areas of rat cortex (as high as 45% in the Skoglund study). Although comprehensive comparisons of differ-ent species have yet to be carried out using modern quantitative tech-niques, there is also evidence for major phyletic differences in column cell number. In cetaceans, it has been reported that there are only 20% as many cortical neurons below a unit area of cortical surface as indicated by Rockel *et al.* (Garey & Leuba, 1986; see also Haug, 1987). Among primates, Zilles and colleagues (1986) found that layer 4 of the posterior cingulate cortex was less densely packed with small cells in prosimians than in anthropoids. The observations of Preuss & Goldman-Rakic (1991) suggest that the differences in layer 4 cell density between prosimians and anthro-poids extend throughout much of the parietal and temporal cortex.

Rockel *et al.* (1980) evidently assumed that column width was essen-tially invariant (~30 μm) across species and did not actually identify dis-crete columns before counting cells. Peters & Yilmaz (1993) attempted to do just this. They noted that the apical dendrites of pyramidal cells form bundles, and thus defined a column as the set of cells associated with a single dendritic bundle. They used this approach to compare the colum-nar organization of the primary visual area (V1) of cats with that of macaque monkeys (Peters & Sethares, 1991), and reported that cat V1 columns are wider than those of macaques (56 μm vs. 31 μm) and con-tained more neurons (203 vs. 142). In addition, they reported lamina-specific differences in neuron number between cats and macaques, cats having for example a very cell-rich layer 6.

There are many additional phyletic differences in the laminar organ-ization of isocortex that can be observed with Nissl-stained material. For example, as shown in Fig. 7.3, cetaceans have an extremely thick layer 1

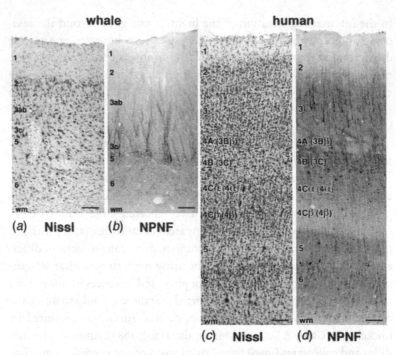

Fig. 7.3. Comparative histology of the primary visual area (V1) of a pygmy
sperm whale (*Kogia breviceps*) and a human (*Homo sapiens*). Sections were cut
frozen at 50 μm thickness and stained for Nissl or for nonphosphorylated
neurofilament protein (NPNF) using the SMI-32 antibody. All sections are
shown at the same magnification. In humans, and most other mammals, there
is a preponderance of very small cells in cortical layer 4; in primates, layer 4 is
very well developed in area V1, and subdivisions have been distinguished
(there are alternative numbering schemes). By contrast, cetaceans have
virtually no small-celled layer 4 in visual cortex or in any other part of the
cortex. Layer 1 is relatively very broad in cetaceans, although the cortex is very
narrow overall. Note also that in cetaceans, nonphosphorylated neurofilament
is expressed only in a restricted set of pyramidal cells, forming a narrow band
in the middle of the cortex, whereas in humans, this protein is expressed by a
variety of pyramidal cell populations in both the superficial and deep cortical
layers. Photographs of the whale material were kindly supplied by Dr Patrick
Hof. Scale bars = 150 μm.

and a prominent layer 2, and lack a well-developed, small-celled layer 3
(Morgane *et al.*, 1985; Glezer *et al.*, 1988). Only in the primary visual cortex
of cetaceans has an incipient layer 4 been described (Garey *et al.*, 1985;
Morgane *et al.*, 1988). The cortex of some bats and insectivores bears at
least a superficial resemblance to that of cetaceans in these and other features. It has been suggested that the prominence of layers 1 and 2 in ceta-

ceans, bats, and insectivores, and the poor development of layer 4, represent the primitive, reptile-like condition of mammalian cortex (Sanides, 1970; Morgane et al., 1985; Glezer et al., 1988). The peculiar traits of cetaceans, bats, and insectivores are lacking, however, in the outgroups of the main eutherian radiation (specifically edentates, marsupials, and monotremes), and therefore it is more likely that they represent independently evolved specializations rather than primitive retentions. There is some evidence that the unusual features of cortical lamination in these mammals reflect unusual patterns of connectivity. Specifically, it has been argued (on the basis of indirect histochemical evidence) that thalamic projections terminate primarily in layers 1 and 3 in cetaceans (Glezer et al., 1988; Revishchin & Garey, 1996), rather than layer 4 and the deep part of layer 3, as they do in animals such as primates.

Few studies have attempted to compare the intrinsic connectivity of homologous cortical areas in different species or to compare the local connections of different areas within a taxon. There is, nonetheless, evidence of variation in these aspects of organization. LaChica et al. (1993) noted differences in the interlaminar connections of the primary visual cortex of the primates Galago and Saimiri. Kritzer and colleagues have reported differences in the intrinsic connectivity of prefrontal cortex and primary visual cortex in macaque monkeys (Kritzer et al., 1995) as well as differences between the primary visual area and higher-order visual areas (Kritzer et al., 1992).

By contrast to the paucity of dedicated comparative studies of local circuitry, there are numerous studies comparing the neuronal phenotypes of different cortical regions and different taxa. These studies are pertinent to the claim of a basic cortical circuit, because the functions of local cortical circuits must depend on the morphology and physiology of the pyramidal and non-pyramidal cells that comprise them. All mammalian groups that have been examined possess cells that can be classified with confidence as pyramidal cells on morphological groups. This said, some mammals have morphologically distinctive subsets of pyramidal cells. In cetaceans, and in at least some bat and insectivore species, layer 2 contains numerous large, dark cells with distinctive, bifurcating apical dendrites that ramify within layer 1, as well as poorly developed basal dendrites; these cells are believed to be modified pyramidal cells (Sanides & Sanides, 1972; Valverde, 1983, 1986). Ceteceans also exhibit a variety of other unusual morphologies among pyramidal cells located in deeper layers (Garey et al., 1985). Whereas most mammalian taxa have pyramidal cells with a single main apical dendrite trunk, in one marsupial species, the quokka (*Setonix brachyurus*), most pyramidal cells in the primary visual cortex have paired apical dendrites (Tyler *et al.*, 1998). In rats, layer 4 of primary visual cortex contains small 'star pyramidal' cells, which have an apical dendrite; these cells are probably homologous to the spiny stellate cells found in layer 4 of macaques and cats, which lack an apical dendrite (Peters & Yilmaz, 1993).

Cortical neurons are biochemically variable across taxa. For example, there is abundant evidence that the pyramidal cells of rats do not express parvalbumin (Celio, 1990), while many of the layer 5 pyramidal cells of Mongolian gerbils do (Brückner *et al.*, 1994). The primates *Galago* and *Macaca* also possess parvalbumin-positive pyramidal cells, although possibly only in somatic sensorimotor areas (Preuss & Kaas, 1996). As illustrated in Fig. 7.3, there are also phyletic differences in the expression of a cytoskeletal protein (neurofilament) by pyramidal cells (Campbell & Morrison, 1989; Hof *et al.*, 1992; Preuss *et al.*, 1999). Among inhibitory interneurons, there appear to be important phyletic distributions of cells expressing particular calcium-binding proteins. In a broad comparative study that included cetaceans (whales and dolphins), primates, rodents, bats, and insectivores, Glezer and colleagues (Glezer *et al.*, 1993) noted layer-specific differences in the numbers of cells expressing a particular CBP as well as differences in the morphologies of interneurons expressing a particular CBP (see also Glezer *et al.*, 1992). There are also reports indicating that primate species vary in the laminar organization of interneurons and neuropil expressing parvalbumin or calbindin in homologous cortical areas (Blümcke *et al.*, 1990; Hendry & Carder, 1993; Preuss & Kaas, 1996; del Río & DeFelipe, 1997).

Variations in long connections and large-scale organization

Mammalian groups display a number of differences in the connections of the cortex with subcortical structures and in the connections among cortical areas. In all mammals that have been examined, the primary visual area (V1) receives a strong projection from the lateral geniculate nucleus (LGN), which in turn receives projections arising from the retina. The precise sources and laminar distribution of these inputs vary across taxa, however (Casagrande & Kaas, 1994). In all prosimian and anthropoid primates that have been examined, LGN afferents terminate in a broad band in the middle of the cortical thickness corresponding to Brodmann's layer

4C. In most Old World and New World monkeys that have been examined, there is an additional, more superficial tier of projections that terminate in layer 4A of Brodmann. However, this projection is reported to
be absent in *Aotus* (Horton, 1984), the only nocturnal anthropoid, and
there is indirect evidence from histochemical studies suggesting that this
projection may be reduced or absent in apes (Preuss *et al.*, 1998, 1999) and
in humans (Horton & Hedley-Whyte, 1984; Wong-Riley *et al.*, 1993). Tree
shrews exhibit a different, and evidently unique, distribution of geniculate terminations within V1 (Hubel, 1975). Whereas the LGN projects
exclusively (almost) to area V1 in primates and tree shrews, this nucleus
sends strong projections to the second visual area (V2) as well as to V1 in at
least some carnivores (Dreher, 1986) and probably also in bats (Funk &
Rosa, 1998).

Some of the most remarkable connectional variants found in
mammals involve the somatic sensorimotor cortex. In most mammals
that have been examined (including a variety of eutherians, marsupials,
and monotremes), the projections from the thalamus to the cortex are
almost entirely uncrossed or ipsilateral; that is, the right thalamus projects to the right cortex and the left thalamus to the left cortex. However,
in hedgehogs (*Erinaceus europaeus*), the thalamus of each hemisphere sends
a major projection to the somatic sensorimotor cortex of *both* hemispheres (Regidor & Divac, 1992; Dinopoulos, 1994). Moreover, the cortical
projections to the spinal cord are largely uncrossed in hedgehogs,
whereas in most other mammals the largest contingent of corticospinal
fibers are crossed (Nudo & Masterton, 1990). These specializations are not
found in all insectivores: tenrecs (*Echinops telfairi*) are reported to have
mainly uncrossed thalamocortical projections (Künzle, 1995) and least
shrews (*Cryptotis parva*) display predominantly crossed corticospinal projections (Nudo & Masterton, 1990), similar to most other mammals.
Clearly, the somatic cortex of hedgehogs is remarkably specialized – a
point worth bearing in mind given that hedgehogs have often been cast in
the role of *ur*-mammals.

Inputs to the cortex arise from nuclei in the brainstem that contain the
monoaminergic transmitters dopamine, norepinephrine, and serotonin.
These substances are thought to modulate the responsiveness of cortical
neurons to other kinds of inputs, rendering some classes of inputs more
effective than others (e.g. Arnsten, 1997). An important series of comparative studies has revealed remarkable differences between rats and anthropoid primates (specifically macaques and humans) in the laminar

organization of projections to the frontal lobe arising from the dopamine-containing nuclei of the brainstem (Berger et al., 1991; Berger & Gaspar, 1995). In rats, for example, the dopaminergic projections to the medial frontal cortex are distributed mainly to the deep cortical layers (5 and 6), while in primates these projections are preferentially distributed to the superficial layers (1–3). There are important regional differences in dopamine innervation as well: the primary motor area (M1) of rats is nearly devoid of dopaminergic fibers, while M1 is among the areas most densely innervated by dopaminergic fibers in macaques and humans (Gaspar et al., 1989; Williams & Goldman-Rakic, 1998). In view of these differences, it is not surprising that laminar and regional distribution of receptor molecules specific for dopamine (D1 and D2 receptors) varies widely across taxa (Richfield et al., 1989; Berger et al., 1990). There is much additional evidence of phyletic variation in the distribution of neurotransmitters and receptors between the different orders of mammals (Berger et al., 1988; Zilles et al., 1993; Hof et al., 1995) as well as within orders (Kosofsky et al., 1984; Gebhard et al., 1995; Dupouy et al., 1996; Wang et al., 1997).

The systems of long corticocortical connections that link cortical areas into functional networks have been studied in only a few taxa (mainly primates, carnivores, and rodents, with some limited investigations of bats and tree shrews), yet some intriguing differences stand out. In all primates and carnivores that have been examined (and in bats and tree shrews also, as far as is known), the primary sensory areas are connected only to areas of the same sensory modality. For example, the first (V1) and second visual areas (V2) are connected with other visual areas, but not with the primary somatosensory (S1) or auditory cortex (A1); there are no connections between V1 and the frontal lobe. Rats are different. In rats, V1 and V2 are both interconnected with a variety of frontal areas, and furthermore, there are direct connections between V2 and the primary somatosensory and primary auditory areas (Vogt & Miller, 1983; Miller & Vogt, 1984; Sukekawa, 1988; Reep et al., 1990; Paperna & Malach, 1991; van Eden et al., 1992; Condé et al., 1995).

It is now widely accepted that mammals vary in the number of cortical areas they possess. It seems likely that larger-brained mammals generally possess more cortical areas than do smaller-brained taxa (Kaas, 1987). For example, primates evidently possess on the order of 50–100 cortical areas (Felleman & Van Essen, 1991; Preuss & Goldman-Rakic, 1991), while there is good reason to believe that rats possess only a small fraction of that number (Zilles & Wree, 1985). Once we account for the areas that primates and rodents both possess (which are mainly lower-order sensory and motor areas, such as V1, and certain limbic areas such as orbital, insular, and cingulate cortex), we have accounted for most of rodent cortex but for only a small part of anthropoid cortex. Primates therefore have many areas that have no obvious counterparts in rodents or in other relatively small-brained mammals, including animals such as bats and tree shrews, which are thought to be close relatives of primates (Preuss & Kaas, 1999). It is very likely that primates possess many unique cortical areas, including a number of higher-order sensory areas (Allman, 1977; Kaas, 1987) as well as the classical higher-order association regions – the dorsolateral prefrontal, posterior parietal, and inferotemporal cortex (Preuss, 1995b; Preuss & Kaas, 1999). It is interesting that the higher-order association regions of primates are strongly connected with each other and these regions are all connected with a prominent thalamic structure, the medial pulvinar, which has no obvious counterpart in other mammals (Preuss, 1993). Thus, not only do primates possess primate-specific higher-order cortical territories, but these territories form a distinctive connectional system.

The evidence presented in this section belies the claim that there is a basic uniformity of cortical organization among mammals. The existence of extensive variation in cortical organization does not, of course, preclude the possibility that there are some features of cortical biology that are widely or even universally shared among mammals (see, e.g., Tyler et al., 1998). For example, all mammalian groups that have been examined possess a cortical mantle, and this structure receives inputs from the thalamus, gives rise to descending projections, and is comprised of neurons with recognizably pyramidal morphologies as well as non-pyramidal, GABA-containing neurons. Furthermore, even if columns are not the immutable modules depicted in some theories, many cortical areas from a diverse range of taxa do display some sort of columnar organization. To focus exclusively on the ancestral features of cortical organization that mammals share, however, is to ignore those features of cortical organization that distinguish one group of mammals from another and provide the basis for their particular behavioral and cognitive abilities. Among other things, such a focus leaves one with little to say about the distinctively human characteristics of the human brain (Preuss, 2000).

New approaches to human brain evolution

The discovery of cortical diversity could not be more inconvenient. For neuroscientists, the fact of diversity means that broad generalizations about cortical organization based on studies of a few 'model' species, such as rats and rhesus macaques, are built on weak foundations. To obtain better-founded generalizations about widely shared characteristics, and to better understand the remarkable modifications of cortical organization produced by evolution, neuroscience needs to adopt a genuinely comparative methodology based on modern phylogenetic principles (Nishikawa, 1997).

The fact of cortical diversity is perhaps even more inconvenient for those anthropologists and paleontologists wanting to investigate brain evolution. To acknowledge the diversity of cerebral organization is to acknowledge that the issue of reorganization versus encephalization has been settled in favor of reorganization. There is no longer a good reason to consider encephalization as an index of some general functional capacity (intelligence) that is common to all mammals. We must face up to the fact that encephalization is largely uninterpretable in terms of cognitive or behavioral processes. Having said this, I want to emphasize that I am not proposing that we ignore brain size. After all, mammals do vary enormously in brain size, and the peculiarly large size of the human brain demands explanation. I suggest, rather, that we treat evolutionary changes in brain size as symptoms of changes in internal organization. Thus, among the questions we must consider about human brain evolution are, what kinds of changes in internal organization could result in massive increases in brain size?

One plausible account of human brain evolution involves the differential enlargement of particular brain subdivisions. Given the enormous enlargement of the brain that occurred during human phylogeny, we might expect that certain regions of the human brain are differentially enlarged compared to their ape homologues. Classically, human brain enlargement has been linked to the expansion of the higher-order association regions of the frontal, temporal, and parietal lobes (Brodmann, 1909, 1912; Blinkov & Glezer, 1968). Recently, the idea that the frontal lobe expanded during human evolution has been challenged (Semendeferi et al., 1997). In my view, however, there are sound empirical grounds (reviewed in Preuss, 2000) for supposing that the *prefrontal* portion of the frontal lobe was enlarged during human evolution in comparison to primary sensorimotor structures, as were portions of posterior association cortex. Nevertheless, it would be very useful to have additional information about the absolute and relative sizes of homologous brain structures in humans, apes, and other primates, and advancements in this area are being made (Matano & Hirasaki, 1997; Rilling & Insel, 1998; Semendeferi *et al.*, 1998).

As noted above, it appears that larger-brained mammals tend to have more cortical areas than smaller-brained taxa. For this reason, it is very tempting to suppose that the expansion of human cortex was accompanied by the addition of new areas, and the classical language-related territories (Broca's and Wernicke's areas) have been cited as likely neomorphic structures (Brodmann, 1909; Crick & Jones, 1993; Killackey, 1995). At the present time, however, there is no good evidence that humans possess species-specific cortical areas, and furthermore, there are well-founded claims that homologues of Broca's and Wernicke's areas are present in nonhuman primates (Preuss, 2000). Once again, however, we must also confess that the data currently available for addressing the possibility of human-specific cortical areas are very deficient: we simply do not possess maps of human and ape cortical areal organization that are of sufficient detail and reliability to determine which cortical fields are shared by apes and humans and which are unique to one group or another. Developing such maps should be a major priority for research in the near future, as much progress could be made on this front using histochemical and immunocytochemical techniques currently available.

Although the enormous size of the human brain constitutes its most conspicuous characteristic, there are good reasons to think that human brain evolution was not exclusively a matter of enlargement. If it is the case, as has been suggested, that homologues of at least some of the human cortical language areas are present in apes and monkeys, then we must suppose that the evolution of language entailed changes in the internal organization of the language areas and perhaps also changes in the interconnections of human cortical areas. While there is as yet no direct evidence regarding the nature of changes in the classical language-related areas, there is evidence bearing on other cortical regions. We have recently found histological evidence suggesting that the human primary visual area differs from that of both apes and monkeys in the way it segregates information arising from the magnocellular (M) and parvocellular (P) layers of the lateral geniculate nucleus (Preuss *et al.*, 1999). Humans also possess structural and functional characteristics of higher-order visual cortical areas that distinguish them from monkeys (Tootell & Taylor, 1995; Tootell *et al.*, 1997), although as yet the higher-order visual areas of apes have not been examined with comparable techniques. The functional significance of these changes are unclear, but their character suggests that humans have enhanced capacities for analyzing moving stimuli (Preuss *et al.*, 1999). It is tempting (if very premature) to speculate that these changes occurred in response to the challenge of visually decoding the rapid mouth movements of speech, stimuli that can exert a strong influence on the interpretation of speech in face-to-face interactions (McGurk & MacDonald, 1976), and in addition the task of monitoring the manual gestures that normally accompany speech (McNeill, 1992).

The evidence that the visual system was modified in human evolution comes as quite a surprise (to me, at least), as it is axiomatic among neuroscientists and psychologists that the visual abilities of humans and monkeys (macaque monkeys, anyway) are virtually identical. One wonders whether this is just the tip of the iceberg: if the human visual system shows such specializations, what surprises await us when we explore the microanatomy of brain regions more commonly identified with human-specific psychological abilities, such as the classical language areas and the prefrontal cortex?

In advocating evolutionary studies of cortical microanatomy, I want to emphasize that I am not proposing that we ignore brain size. Indeed, there are reasons to suspect that the evolutionary enlargement of the human brain may have been related to modifications of cortical microanatomy. Consider the changes in the structure of cortical areas that would likely have accompanied the evolution of new functional capacities. Functional imaging studies in humans indicate that higher-order cognitive tasks engage multiple cortical areas dispersed across the cortical mantle (Roland, 1993; Frackowiack *et al.*, 1997), areas that are probably linked by direct corticocortical connections. The evolution of new cognitive abilities might involve the enhancement of existing links between areas, or even the establishment of links between previously unconnected areas. In either case, the proliferation of connections would produce a cascade of effects. In the areas giving rise to new projections, existing pyramidal cells would have to be enlarged to support new axon collaterals or new pyramidal cells would need to be generated. On the receiving end of the projections, the dendrites of cells upon which the new axons terminate would enlarge to accommodate the additional synapses. These increases in gray matter would be accompanied by increases in white matter as new fibers are generated. Furthermore, the size-increasing effects of all these kinds of changes would be multiplied because cortical areas tend to be reciprocally connected. Finally, in addition to size changes resulting from the generation of new connections, the intrinsic information-processing demands imposed on cortical areas by the evolution of new functions could also promote their enlargement. If the processing demands of a new cognitive function were incompatible with older (but still important) functions carried out by cortical areas, the cell populations mediating the new function might become spatially segregated from populations supporting the old function. This would result in the formation of separate compartments within the original area, each specialized for different tasks. Cortical areas commonly display internal compartmentation, the best known example being the ocular dominance columns of area V1 of primates, in which projections from the left and right eyes terminate in alternating compartments within area V1 (for a description, see Casagrande & Kaas, 1994). It is reasonable to think that the evolutionary addition of functionally specialized territories within existing areas would result in the enlargement of those areas.

References

Aiello, L.C. & Wheeler, P. (1995). The expensive-tissue hypothesis – the brain and the digestive-system in human and primate evolution. *Current Anthropology*, **36**, 199–221.

Allman, J. (1990). Evolution of neocortex. In *Cerebral Cortex. Volume B: Comparative Structure and Evolution of Cerebral Cortex, Part II*, eds. E.G. Jones & A. Peters, pp. 269–283. Plenum.

Allman, J.M. (1977). Evolution of the visual system in the early primates. In *Progress in Psychology and Physiological Psychology*, eds. J.M. Sprague & A.N. Epstein, pp. 1–53. New York: Academic.

Andressen, C., Blümcke, I. & Celio, M. (1993). Calcium-binding proteins: selective markers of nerve cells. *Cell and Tissue Research*, **271**, 181–208.

Arnsten, A. (1997). Catecholamine regulation of the prefrontal cortex. *Journal of Psychopharmacology*, **11**, 151–162.

Baimbridge, K.G., Celio, M.R. & Rogers, J.H. (1992). Calcium-binding proteins in the nervous system. *Trends in Neurosciences*, **15**, 303–308.

Beaulieu, C. (1993). Numerical data on neocortical neurons in adult rat, with special reference to the GABA population. *Brain Research*, **609**, 284–292.

Berger, B., Febvret, A., Greengard, P. & Goldman-Rakic, P.S. (1990). DARPP-32, a phosphoprotein enriched in dopaminoceptive neurons bearing dopamine D1 receptors: Distribution in the cerebral cortex of the newborn and adult rhesus monkey. *Journal of Comparative Neurology*, **299**, 327–348.

Berger, B. & Gaspar, P. (1995). Comparative anatomy of the catecholaminergic innervation of rat and primate prefrontal cortex. In *Phylogeny and Ontogeny of Catecholamine Systems in the CNS of Vertebrates*, eds. W. J. A. J. Smeets & A. Reiner, pp. 293–324. Cambridge: Cambridge University Press.

Berger, B., Gaspar, P. & Verney, C. (1991). Dopaminergic innervation of the cerebral cortex: Unexpected differences between rodent and primate. *Trends in Neuroscience*, 14, 21–27.

Berger, B., Trottier, S., Verney, C., Gaspar, P. & Alvarez, C. (1988). Regional and laminar distribution of the dopamine and serotonin innervation in the macaque cerebral cortex: A radioautographic study. *Journal of Comparative Neurology*, 273, 99–119.

Blinkov, S. & Glezer, I. (1968). *The Human Brain in Figures and Tables*. New York: Basic Books.

Blümcke, I., Hof, P. R., Morrison, J. H. & Celio, M. R. (1990). Distribution of parvalbumin immunoreactivity in the visual cortex of Old World monkeys and humans. *Journal of Comparative Neurology*, 301, 417–432.

Brodmann, K. (1909). *Vergleichende Lokalisationslehre der Grosshirnrhinde*. Leipzig: Barth.

Brodmann, K. (1912). Neue Ergibnisse über die vergleichende histologische Lokalisation der Grosshirnrinde mit besonderer Berücksichtigung des Stirnhirns. *Anatomischer Anzeiger*, 41, 157–216.

Brückner, G., Seeger, G., Brauer, K., Härtig, W., Kacza, J. & Bigl, V. (1994). Cortical areas are revealed by distribution patterns of proteoglycan components and parvalbumin in the Mongolian gerbil and rat. *Brain Research*, 658, 67–86.

Bugbee, N. M. & Goldman-Rakic, P. S. (1983). Columnar organization of corticocortical projections in squirrel and rhesus monkeys: Similarity of column width in species differing in cortical volume. *Journal of Comparative Neurology*, 220, 355–364.

Campbell, M. & Morrison, J. (1989). Monoclonal antibody to neurofilament protein (SMI-32) labels a subpopulation of pyramidal neurons in the human and monkey neocortex. *Journal of Comparative Neurology*, 282, 191–205.

Casagrande, V. A. & Kaas, J. H. (1994). The afferent, intrinsic, and efferent connections of primary visual cortex in primates. In *Cerebral Cortex, Volume 10: Primary Visual Cortex in Primates*, eds. A. Peters & K. Rockland, pp. 201–259. New York: Plenum Press.

Celio, M. (1990). Calbindin D-28k and parvalbumin in the rat nervous system. *Neuroscience*, 35, 375–475.

Churchland, P. S. & Sejnowski, T. J. (1992). *The Computational Brain*. Cambridge, MA: MIT Press.

Condé, F., Maire-Lepoivre, E., Audinat, E. & Crépel, F. (1995). Afferent connections of the medial frontal cortex of the rat. II. Cortical and subcortical afferents. *Journal of Comparative Neurology*, 352, 567–593.

Creutzfeldt, O. D. (1977). Generality of functional structure of the neocortex. *Naturwissenschaften*, 64, 507–517.

Creutzfeldt, O. (1978). The neocortical link: Thoughts on the generality of structure and function in the neocortex. In *Architectonics of the Cerebral Cortex*, eds. M. Brazier & H. Ptesche, pp. 367–384. New York: Raen Press.

Crick, F. & Jones, E. G. (1993). Backwardness of human neuroanatomy. *Nature*, 361, 109–110.

Darwin, C. (1871). *The Descent of Man, and Selection in Relation to Sex*. London: John Murray [Facsimile edition: Princeton, NJ: Princeton University Press, 1981].

del Río, M. R. & DeFelipe, J. (1997). Colocalization of parvalbumin and calbindin D-28k in neurons including chandelier cells of the human temporal neocortex. *Journal of Chemical Neuroanatomy*, **12**, 165–173.

Dinopoulos, A. (1994). Reciprocal connections of the motor neocortical area with the contralateral thalamus in the hedgehog (*Erinaceus europaeus*) brain. *European Journal of Neuroscience*, **6**, 374–380.

Douglas, R. J. & Martin, K. A. C. (1998). Neocortex. In *Synaptic Organization of the Brain. Fourth edition*, ed. G. M. Shepherd, pp. 389–438. New York: Oxford University Press.

Dreher, B. (1986). Thalamocortical and corticocortical interconnections in the cat visual system: Relation to the mechanisms of information processing. In *Visual Neuroscience*, ed. J. D. Pettigrew, pp. 290–314. Cambridge: Cambridge University Press.

Dupouy, V., Puget, A., Eschalier, A. & Zajac, J. M. (1996). Species differences in the localization of neuropeptide FF receptors in rodent and lagomorph brain and spinal cord. *Peptides*, **17**, 399–405.

Eccles, J. C. (1984). The cerebral neocortex: A theory of its operation. In *Cerebral Cortex. Vol. 2: Functional Properties of Cortical Cells*, eds. E. G. Jones & A. Peters, pp. 1–36. New York: Plenum.

Elliot Smith, G. (1924). *The Evolution of Man. Essays*. London: Oxford University Press.

Felleman, D. J. & Van Essen, D. C. (1991). Distributed hierarchical processing in the primate cerebral cortex. *Cerebral Cortex*, **1**, 1–47.

Finlay, B. L. & Darlington, R. B. (1995). Linked regularities in the development and evolution of mammalian brains. *Science*, **268**, 1578–1584.

Frackowiak, R. S. J., Friston, K. J., Frith, C. D., Dolan, R. J. & Mazziotta, J. C. (1997). *Human Brain Function*. San Diego: Academic Press.

Funk, A. P. & Rosa, M. G. (1998). Visual responses of neurones in the second visual area of flying foxes (*Pteropus poliocephalus*) after lesions of striate cortex. *Journal*, **513**, 507–519.

Garey, L. J. & Leuba, G. (1986). A quantitative study of neuronal and glial numerical density in the visual cortex of the bottle-nosed-dolphin – Evidence for a specialized subarea and changes with age. *Journal of Comparative Neurology*, **247**, 491–496.

Garey, L. J., Winkelmann, E. & Brauer, K. (1985). Golgi and Nissl studies of the visual cortex of the bottlenose dolphin. *Journal of Comparative Neurology*, **240**, 305–321.

Gaspar, P., Berger, P., Febvret, A., Vigny, A. & Henry, J. P. (1989). Catecholamine innervation of the human cerebral cortex as revealed by comparative immunohistochemistry of tyrosine hydroxylase and dopamine-beta-hydroxylase. *Journal of Comparative Neurology*, **221**, 169–184.

Gebhard, R., Zilles, K., Schleicher, A., Everitt, B. J., Robbins, T. W. & Divac, I. (1995). Parcellation of the frontal cortex of the New World monkey *Callithrix jacchus* by eight neurotransmitter-binding sites. *Anatomy and Embryology (Berlin)*, **191**, 509–517.

Glezer, I. I., Hof, P. R., Leranth, C. & Morgane, P. J. (1992). Morphological and histochemical features of odontocete visual neocortex: Immunocytochemical analysis of pyramidal and nonpyramidal populations of neurons. In *Marine Mammal Sensory Systems*, eds. J.A. Thomas, R.A. Kastelein & A.Y. Supin, pp. 1–38. New York: Plenum Press.

Glezer, I.I., Hof, P.R., Leranth, C. & Morgane, P.J. (1993). Calcium-binding protein-containing neuronal populations in mammalian visual cortex: A comparative study in whales, insectivores, bats, rodents, and primates. *Cerebral Cortex*, **3**, 249–272.

Glezer, I.I., Jacobs, M.S. & Morgane, P.J. (1988). The 'initial brain' concept and its implications for brain evolution in Cetacea. *Behavioral and Brain Sciences*, **11**, 75–116.

Goldman, P.S. & Nauta, W.J. (1977). Columnar distribution of cortico-cortical fibers in the frontal association, limbic, and motor cortex of the developing rhesus monkey. *Brain Research*, **122**, 393–413.

Haug, H. (1987). Brain sizes, surfaces, and neuronal sizes of the cortex cerebri: A stereological investigation of man and his variability and a comparison with some mammals (primates, whales, marsupials, insectivores, and one elephant). *American Journal of Anatomy*, **180**, 126–142.

Hendry, S.H. & Carder, R.K. (1993). Neurochemical compartmentation of monkey and human visual cortex: Similarities and variations in calbindin immunoreactivity across species. *Visual Neuroscience*, **10**, 1109–1120.

Hendry, S.H.C. (1996). The anatomy of the cerebral cortex: Aspects of neuronal morphology and organization. In *Excitatory Amino Acids and the Cerebral Cortex*, eds. F. Conti & T.P. Hicks, pp. 3–20. Cambridge, MA: MIT Press.

Hof, P.R., Glezer, I.I., Archin, N., Janssen, W.G., Morgane, P.J. & Morrison, J.H. (1992). The primary auditory cortex in cetacean and human brain: A comparative analysis of neurofilament protein-containing pyramidal neurons. *Neuroscience Letters*, **146**, 91–95.

Hof, P.R., Glezer, I.I., Revishchin, A.V., Bouras, C., Charnay, Y. & Morgane, P.J. (1995). Distribution of dopaminergic fibers and neurons in visual and auditory cortices of the harbor porpoise and pilot whale. *Brain Research Bulletin*, **36**, 275–284.

Holloway, R.L., Jr. (1966a). Cranial capacity and neuron number: A critique and proposal. *American Journal of Physical Anthropology*, **25**, 305–314.

Holloway, R.L., Jr. (1966b). Cranial capacity, neural reorganization, and hominid evolution: A search for more suitable parameters. *American Anthropologist*, **68**, 103–121.

Horton, J.C. (1984). Cytochrome oxidase patches: A new cytoarchitectonic feature of monkey visual cortex. *Philosophical Transactions of the Royal Society of London*, B**304**, 199–253.

Horton, J.C. & Hedley-Whyte, E.T. (1984). Mapping of cytochrome oxidase patches and ocular dominance columns in human visual cortex. *Philosophical Transactions of the Royal Society of London*, B**304**, 255–272.

Hubel, D.H. (1975). An autoradiographic study of the retino-cortical projections in the tree shrew (*Tupaia glis*). *Brain Research*, **96**, 41–50.

Hubel, D.H. & Wiesel, T.N. (1977). Ferrier lecture. Functional architecture of macaque monkey visual cortex. *Proceedings of the Royal Society of London*, B**198**, 1–59.

Huxley, T.H. (1863). *Evidence as to Man's Place in Nature*. London: Williams and Norgate [1959, Ann Arbor, University of Michigan].

Jerison, H. J. (1961). Quantitative analysis of evolution of the brain in mammals. *Science*, **133**, 1012–1024.

Jerison, H. J. (1973). *Evolution of the Brain and Intelligence*. New York: Academic Press.

Kaas, J. H. (1987). The organization and evolution of neocortex. In *Higher Brain Function: Recent Explorations of the Brain's Emergent Properties*, ed. S. P. Wise, pp. 347–378. New York: John Wiley.

Kaas, J. H. (1995). The evolution of isocortex. *Brain, Behavior and Evolution*, **46**, 187–196.

Killackey, H. P. (1995). Evolution of the human brain: A neuroanatomical perspective. In *The Cognitive Neurosciences*, ed. M. S. Gazzaniga, pp. 1243–1253. Cambridge, MA: MIT Press.

Kosofsky, B. E., Molliver, M. E., Morrison, J. H. & Foote, S. L. (1984). The serotonin and norepinephrine innervation of primary visual cortex in the cynomolgus monkey (*Macaca fascicularis*). *Journal of Comparative Neurology*, **230**, 168–178.

Kritzer, M. F., Cowey, A. & Somogyi, P. (1992). Patterns of inter- and intralaminar GABAergic connections distinguish striate (V1) and extrastriate (V2, V4) visual cortices and their functionally specialized subdivisions in the rhesus monkey. *Journal of Neuroscience*, **12**, 4545–4564.

Kritzer, M. F. & Goldman-Rakic, P. S. (1995). Intrinsic circuit organization of the major layers and sublayers of the dorsolateral prefrontal cortex in the rhesus monkey. *Journal of Comparative Neurology*, **359**, 131–143.

Künzle, H. (1995). Crossed thalamocortical connections in the Madagascan hedgehog tenrec: Dissimilarities to erinaceous hedgehog, similarities to mammals with more differentiated brains. *Neuroscience Letters*, **189**, 89–92.

LaChica, E. A., Beck, P. D. & Casagrande, V. A. (1993). Intrinsic connections of layer III of striate cortex in squirrel monkey and bush baby: Correlations with patterns of cytochrome oxidase. *Journal of Comparative Neurology*, **329**, 163–187.

Le Gros Clark, W. E. (1959). *The Antecedents of Man*. Edinburgh: Edinburgh University Press.

Matano, S. & Hirasaki, E. (1997). Volumetric comparisons in the cerebellar complex of anthropoids, with special reference to locomotor types. *American Journal of Physical Anthropology*, **103**, 173–183.

McGurk, H. & MacDonald, J. (1976). Hearing lips and seeing voices. *Nature*, **264**, 746–748.

McNeill, D. (1992). *Hand and Mind*. Chicago: University of Chicago Press.

Miller, M.W. & Vogt, B. A. (1984). Direct connections of rat visual cortex with sensory, motor, and association cortices. *Journal of Comparative Neurology*, **226**, 184–202.

Morgane, P. J., Glezer, I. I. & Jacobs, M. S. (1988). Visual cortex of the dolphin: An image-analysis study. *Journal of Comparative Neurology*, **273**, 3–25.

Morgane, P. J., Jacobs, M. S. & Galaburda, A. (1985). Conservative features of neocortical evolution in dolphin brain. *Brain, Behavior and Evolution*, **26**, 176–184.

Mountcastle, V. B. (1978). An organizing principle for cerebral function: The unit module and the distributed system. In *The Mindful Brain: Cortical Organization and the Group-Selective Theory of Higher Brain Function*, eds. G. M. Edelman & V. B. Mountcastle, pp. 7–51. Cambridge, MA: MIT Press.

Nishikawa, K. C. (1997). Emergence of novel functions during brain evolution. *BioScience*, **47**, 341–354.

Nudo, R. J. & Masterton, R. B. (1990). Descending pathways to the spinal cord, III: Sites of origin of the corticospinal tract. *Journal of Comparative Neurology*, **296**, 559–583.

Paperna, T. & Malach, R. (1991). Pattern of sensory intermodality relationships in the cerebral cortex of the rat. *Journal of Comparative Neurology*, **308**, 432–456.

Peters, A. & Sethares, C. (1991). Organization of pyramidal neurons in area 17 of monkey visual cortex. *Journal of Comparative Neurology*, **306**, 1–23.

Peters, A. & Yilmaz, E. (1993). Neuronal organization in area 17 of cat visual cortex. *Cerebral Cortex*, **3**, 49–68.

Preuss, T.M. (1993). The role of the neurosciences in primate evolutionary biology: Historical commentary and prospectus. In *Primates and their Relatives in Phylogenetic Perspective*, ed. R.D.E. MacPhee, pp. 333–362. New York: Plenum Press.

Preuss, T.M. (1995a). The argument from animals to humans in cognitive neuroscience. In *The Cognitive Neurosciences*, ed. M.S. Gazzaniga, pp. 1227–1241. Cambridge, MA: MIT Press.

Preuss, T.M. (1995b). Do rats have prefrontal cortex? The Rose–Woolsey–Akert program reconsidered. *Journal of Cognitive Neuroscience*, **7**, 1–24.

Preuss, T.M. (2000). What's human about the human brain? In *The New Cognitive Neurosciences – 2nd Edition*, ed. M.S. Gazzaniga, pp. 1219–1234. Cambridge, MA: MIT Press.

Preuss, T.M. & Goldman-Rakic, P.S. (1991). Architectonics of the parietal and temporal association cortex in the strepsirhine primate *Galago* compared to the anthropoid primate *Macaca*. *Journal of Comparative Neurology*, **310**, 475–506.

Preuss, T.M. & Kaas, J.H. (1996). Parvalbumin-like immunoreactivity of layer V pyramidal cells in the motor and somatosensory cortex of adult primates. *Brain Research*, **712**, 353–357.

Preuss, T.M. & Kaas, J.H. (1999). Human brain evolution. In *Fundamental Neuroscience*, eds. F.E. Bloom, S.C. Landis, J.L. Robert, L.R. Squire & M.J. Zigmond, pp. 1283–1311. San Diego: Academic Press.

Preuss, T.M., Qi, H.-S. & Kaas, J.H. (1999). Distinctive compartmental organization of human primary visual cortex. *Proceedings of the National Academy of Sciences USA*, **96**, 11601–11606.

Preuss, T.M., Qi, H.-X. & Kaas, J.H. (1998). Chimpanzees and humans share specializations of primary visual cortex. *Society for Neuroscience Abstracts*, **24**, 1125.

Rakic, P. (1988). Specification of cerebral cortical areas. *Science*, **241**, 170–176.

Reep, R.L., Goodwin, G.S. & Corwin, J.V. (1990). Topographic organization in the corticocortical connections of medial agranular cortex in rats. *Journal of Comparative Neurology*, **294**, 262–280.

Regidor, J. & Divac, I. (1992). Bilateral thalamocortical projection in hedgehogs: Evolutionary implications. *Brain, Behavior and Evolution*, **39**, 265–269.

Revishchin, A.V. & Garey, L.J. (1996). Mitochondrial distribution in visual and auditory cerebral cortex of the harbour porpoise. *Brain, Behavior and Evolution*, **47**, 257–266.

Richfield, E.K., Young, A.B. & Penney, J.B. (1989). Comparative distributions of dopamine D-1 and D-2 receptors in the cerebral cortex of rats, cats, and monkeys. *Journal of Comparative Neurology*, **286**, 409–426.

Rilling, J.K. & Insel, T.R. (1998). Evolution of the cerebellum in primates: Differences in relative volume among monkeys, apes and humans. *Brain, Behavior and Evolution*, **52**, 308–314.

Rockel, A.J., Hiorns, R.W. & Powell, T.P.S. (1980). The basic uniformity of structure of the neocortex. *Brain*, **103**, 221–224.

Roland, P.E. (1993). *Brain Activation*. New York: Wiley-Liss.

Sacher, G.A. (1982). The role of brain maturation in the evolution of the primates. In *Primate Brain Evolution*, eds. D. Falk & E. Armstrong, pp. 97–112. New York: Plenum Press.

Sanides, F. (1970). Functional architecture of motor and sensory cortices in primates in the light of a new concept of neocortex evolution. In *The Primate Brain*, eds. C.R. Noback & W. Montagna, pp. 137–208. New York: Appleton-Century-Crofts.

Sanides, F. & Sanides, D. (1972). The 'extraverted' neurons of the mammalian cerebral cortex. *Z. Anat. Entwickl. Gesch.*, **136**, 272–293.

Semendeferi, K., Armstrong, E., Schleicher, A., Zilles, K. & Van Hoesen, G.W. (1998). Limbic frontal cortex in hominoids: A comparative study of area 13. *American Journal of Physical Anthropology*, **106**, 129–155.

Semendeferi, K., Damasio, H., Frank, R. & Van Hoesen, G.W. (1997). The evolution of the frontal lobes: A volumetric analysis based on three-dimensional reconstructions of magnetic resonance image scans of human and ape brains. *Journal of Human Evolution*, **32**, 375–388.

Shepherd, G.M. (1988). A basic circuit for cortical organization. In *Perspectives on Memory Research*, ed. M. Gazzaniga, pp. 93–134. Cambridge, MA: MIT Press.

Shepherd, G.M. (1994). *Neurobiology. Third Edition*. New York: Oxford University Press.

Skoglund, T., Pascher, R. & Berthold, C.H. (1996a). Aspects of the quantitative analysis of neurons in the cerebral cortex. *Journal of Neuroscience Methods*, **70**, 201–210.

Skoglund, T.S., Pascher, R. & Berthold, C.H. (1996b). Heterogeneity in the columnar number of neurons in different neocortical areas in the rat. *Neuroscience Letters*, **208**, 97–100.

Stephan, H., Baron, G. & Frahm, H.D. (1988). Comparative size of brains and brain components. In *Comparative Primate Biology, Vol. 4: Neurosciences*, eds. H.D. Steklis & J. Erwin, pp. 1–38. New York: Liss.

Stephan, H., Frahm, H. & Baron, G. (1981). New and revised data on volumes of brain structures in insectivores and primates. *Folia Primatologia*, **35**, 1–29.

Sukekawa, K. (1988). Interconnections of the visual cortex with the frontal cortex in the rat. *Journal für Hirnforschung*, **29**, 83–93.

Szentágothai, J. (1975). The 'module-concept' in cerebral cortex architecture. *Brain Research*, **95**, 475–496.

Szentágothai, J. (1978). The neuron network of the cerebral cortex: A functional interpretation. *Proceedings of the Royal Society of London*, B**201**, 219–248.

Tootell, R.B., Mendola, J.D., Hadjikhani, N.K., Ledden, P.J., Liu, A.K., Reppas, J.B., Sereno, M.I. & Dale, A.M. (1997). Functional analysis of V3A and related areas in human visual cortex. *Journal of Neuroscience*, **17**, 7060–7078.

Tootell, R.B. & Taylor, J.B. (1995). Anatomical evidence for MT and additional cortical visual areas in humans. *Cerebral Cortex*, **5**, 39–55.

Tyler, C.J., Dunlop, S.A., Lund, R.D., Harman, A.M., Dann, J.F., Beazley, L.D. & Lund, J.S. (1998). Anatomical comparison of the macaque and marsupial visual cortex: Common features that may reflect retention of essential cortical elements. *Journal of Comparative Neurology*, **400**, 449–468.

Valverde, F. (1983). A comparative approach to neocortical organization based on the study of the brain of the hedgehog, *Erinaceus europaeus*. In *Ramon y Cajal: Contributions to Neuroscience*, eds. S. Grisolia, C. Guerri, F. Sampson, S. Norton & F. Reinoso-Suarez, pp. 149–170. Amsterdam: Elsevier.

Valverde, F. (1986). Intrinsic neocortical organization: Some comparative aspects. *Neuroscience*, 18, 1–23.

van Eden, C.G., Lamme, V.A.F. & Uylings, H.B.M. (1992). Heterotopic cortical afferents to the medial prefrontal cortex in the rat. A combined retrograde and anterograde tracer study. *European Journal of Neuroscience*, 4, 77–97.

Vogt, B.A. & Miller, M.W. (1983). Cortical connections between rat cingulate cortex and visual, motor, and postsubicular cortices. *Journal of Comparative Neurology*, 216, 192–210.

Wang, Z., Young, L.J., Liu, Y. & Insel, T.R. (1997). Species differences in vasopressin receptor binding are evident early in development: Comparative anatomic studies in prairie and montane voles. *Journal of Comparative Neurology*, 378, 535–546.

White, E.L. (1988). *Cortical Circuits*. Boston: Birhaüser.

Williams, S.M. & Goldman-Rakic, P.S. (1998). Widespread origin of the primate mesofrontal dopamine system. *Cerebral Cortex*, 8, 321–345.

Wong-Riley, M.T.T., Hevner, R.F., Cutlan, R., Earnest, M., Egan, R., Frost, J. & Nguyen, T. (1993). Cytochrome oxidase in the human visual cortex: Distribution in the developing and the adult brain. *Visual Neuroscience*, 10, 41–58.

Zilles, K., Armstrong, E., Schlaug, G. & Schleicher, A. (1986). Quantitative cytoarchitectonics of the posterior cingulate cortex in primates. *Journal of Comparative Neurology*, 253, 514–524.

Zilles, K., Qu, M. & Schleicher, A. (1993). Regional distribution and heterogeneity of alpha-adrenoceptors in the rat and human central nervous system. *Journal für Hirnforschung*, 34, 123–132.

Zilles, K. & Wree, A. (1985). Cortex: Areal and laminar structure. In *The Rat Nervous System. Volume 1. Forebrain and Midbrain*, ed. G. Paxinos, pp. 375–415. Sydney: Academic Press.

8
_____

Pheromonal communication and socialization

Throughout the lives of most mammalian species, the sense of smell plays an important role in response to chemical messengers that are involved in many different behavioral activities. Pheromones are the most important compounds for olfactory communication. The term pheromone was invented by Karlson & Lüscher in 1959. Pheromones are chemical substances that, when emitted from one animal, cause behavioral or physiological responses in other animals of the same species. Pheromones are secreted by specific organs that are widely scattered on the bodies of different animals. Released pheromones stimulate rapid behavioral changes in the neuroendocrine system and subsequently produce a physiological and behavioral change in the receiving individual. Pheromones also indicate an animal's identity and territory. Pheromones in mammals convey specific information concerning species, gender, physiological phases and identities of animals, thus triggering stereotyped behavioral and neuroendocrine responses. Such responses ensure breeding and hierarchical order in the animal group.

Olfactory communications between conspecific mammals facilitate reproductive processes. Pheromones produced by males and females influence their sexual behavior and hormone activity (Marchlewska-Koj, 1984). In most species, males can distinguish between females in estrus or anestrus phases by their scents. Females, too, are able to identify sexually active males by odor. Production of such olfactory stimulants is controlled by gonadal hormones, mainly testosterone. Pheromones produced by males can accelerate puberty in juvenile females, induce estrus in anestrus females and block pregnancy in recently inseminated females. This acceleration of sexual maturation and stimulation of ovulation in mammalian adults has been described in many species including rodents, rabbits, cow, pigs and a few species of primates.

Pregnancy termination by male olfactory signals has been observed in rodents (Marchlewska-Koj, 1983) that require a high level of progesterone for *in utero* blastocyst implantation. Progesterone is released by the corpora lutea, a structure where hormonal activity is stimulated by prolactin that is released from the pituitary gland. It is well documented that male pheromones in these rodents stimulate the neurohormonal systems of females and thus inhibit secretion of prolactin from their hypophyses. Consequently, the level of progesterone decreases and blastocyst implantation does not occur. Implantation failure is followed by estrus and possible copulation. This phenomenon is observed only when recently inseminated females are exposed to a male that is different than the one with which she copulated. Such blockage of pregnancy, described for mice and other species of rodents, may lead to reduction of reproduction and suppression of growth in high-density populations where females repeatedly meet strange males and experience interrupted pregnancies. The same phenomenon may also prevent inbreeding in populations. This form of pregnancy blockage may also represent a form of intermale competition, as has been hypothesized for infanticide of unrelated young by males of some primates, lions, and a few species of rodents. Usually females cannot be fertilized during lactation. When males kill infants, lactation is interrupted, estrus ensues, and females become receptive and may mate with and conceive the offspring of the males that killed their infants.

Male mice not only are able to discriminate females in estrus and diestrus but also between females from congenic strains that have identical genotypes in all but one small chromosomal region. The typical example is a male that distinguishes from the odor of their urine between females that differ at the major histocompatibility complex (MHC), which is named the H-2 gene (Yamazaki *et al.*, 1988). This complex is involved in a number of important immunological functions including graft rejections, cell–cell interactions, and reactions to infections. The H-2 complex is composed of a series of fractions and subfractions. Genes H-2K and H-2D are extremely mutable and are consequently represented by many alleles. Males are able to distinguish between females that differ only at the H-2K and H-2D loci and always prefer to copulate with females that differ from themselves, e.g., an H-2D male selects females with H-2K loci. The ability to discriminate at a single locus helps to develop heterogenic populations of animals with very important complexes of genes that control many immunological functions.

The capacity to recognize conspecifics by their pheromones, and to mark territories with pheromonal secretions is well known in prosimians. The most important studies on primates were conducted by Keverne (1983) and by Michael and colleagues (Michael & Keverne, 1968; Michael et al., 1971, 1974) who demonstrated the existence and the importance of pheromones in these animals, which are considered functionally to be non-microsmatic. An extensive review of the chemoreceptive senses of smell and taste in primates has been presented by Scalfari (1994) and by Natoli (1994). Although the sexual function of pheromones as messages of continuous sexual receptivity has been reduced in women compared to females of some other primates, pheromones appear to play an important role in impulses related to their likes and dislikes. The extent to which this is true for nonhuman primates remains to be determined.

The pheromone's physiochemical function

Animals have evolved chemosensory systems that both discriminate between a large array of natural scents as well as translate olfactory stimuli into complex sensory information (i.e. the presence of food, the anticipation of a danger, and the approach of a mate). Independent collections of chemosensory neurons and neuronal networks process two basic modalities of smell in terrestrial vertebrates: (1) independent discrimination of odorant molecules, and (2) pheromone perception. Pheromones are molecules of fatty acids or steroids that consist of few atoms of carbon (15 on average) and have molecular weights between 180 and 300. Pheromones that interact with sexual behavior have larger molecular weights; those that interact in alarm communication and aggression are relatively less complex and have smaller molecular weights. The most interesting of these are the species-specific pheromones that regulate basic functions such as mating, the timing of estrus cycles and aggressiveness.

In mammals, odorants are detected in the olfactory epithelium of the nose and are processed in the cortical and neocortical centers of the brain that generate cognitive and behavioral responses as either 'adversive' or 'pleasurable.' Unlike odorants, mammals detect pheromones through receptors found in a specialized structure called the vomeronasal organ (VNO). This small tubular structure lies close to the nasal cavity and is lined with receptor cells. Pheromones bind to receptors on the neuron surface of the receptor cells. This action, in turn, triggers signals that travel through non-olfactory pathways via the accessory olfactory bulb. Pheromone signals by-pass higher cognitive centers and go instead to the amygdala, the bed nucleus of the stria terminalis, and to specific nuclei of the ventro-medial hypothalamus. These brain structures govern emotional and neuroendocrine responses that are related to reproductive physiology and aggressive behavior (Bartoshuk & Beauchamp, 1994). This VNO-to-brain pathway constitutes the accessory olfactory system, and it is distinct from the main olfactory system. Thus, while odor discrimination is processed by the main olfactory epithelium, pheromone perception is processed by the vomeronasal system and, in contrast, results in behavioral and endocrine responses that do not involve higher cognitive centers in the brain.

The human VNO was considered to be atrophied in adults until only a few years ago. A clearly identifiable VNO, however, was found near the base of the nasal septum in adults (Monti-Bloch *et al.*, 1994). Initial studies that applied chemical products obtained from adult humans to the VNO showed changes in the autonomic nervous system, as well as in the periodicity of follicle-stimulating and luteinizing hormones from the pituitary gland (Berliner *et al.*, 1996). These results indicate that a potentially functional VNO–hypothalamic–pituitary–gonadal axis exists in humans. But can humans actually use this system to process and respond to chemical signals that are emitted by other humans?

The molecular–genetic data

Recent molecular advances have demonstrated that both the main olfactory epithelium (MOE) and the vomeronasal organ (VNO) sensory neurons utilize unrelated sets of genes to translate the olfactory information into electrical stimuli (Dulac & Axel, 1995; Liman, 1996). This suggests that, despite a common location in the nose and a common embryonic origin in the olfactory placade, the two chemosensory systems may have evolved from independent ancestral sensory systems. In fact, a family of 100 genes that encode pheromone receptors in the VNO recently has been identified and analyzed in mice (Matsunami & Buck, 1997) and in rats (Herrada & Dulac, 1997; Ryba & Tirindelli, 1997). This family of genes joins two others already known to receive olfactory signals – one family that perceives garden-variety odorants in the olfactory epithelium

(Buck & Axel, 1991) and another family that encodes vomeronasal receptors (Dulac & Axel, 1995) and is likely to be additionally responsible for the perception of pheromones. Like the genes for the olfactory receptors, both pheromone receptor families encode proteins with seven transmembrane domains that convey their signals via heterotrimeric GTP-binding proteins (G proteins).

Is the molecular evidence for mice and rats, however, homologous to the molecular evidence for humans? Or has the evolutionary adaptation to tree life for primates, which is associated with reduced olfactory abilities in favor of improvements in the visual sense, also influenced pheromonal perception? Whatever the answer to this question, arboreal primates should, in fact, retain some dependence on pheromones as vestiges of their terrestrial past.

Pheromones in humans

Before discussing chemical communication and its role in social interactions, one must first determine whether the animal under consideration can perceive, identify and translate the incoming chemosensory signals in addition to being able to generate and transmit the same kinds of signals. Humans lack well-differentiated specialized scent glands (although the axillae often are characterized as having specialized scent glands) (Spielman et al., 1995). Instead, the odor of exocrine substances that are enhanced by the enzymatic actions of resident bacteria in addition to several simple products resulting from bacterial degradation have been proposed as putative semichemicals (e.g., a series of aliphatic acids of vaginal origin and androstenol–androstenone of mainly axillary origin). The local quality and quantity of exocrine substrates, the composition and density of resident microorganisms, and the microecological conditions (i.e. hair, pH, temperature etc.) generate a highly distinctive scent in different regions of the human body. Therefore, it can be concluded that *Homo sapiens* are efficient receivers and senders of chemical signals like all species possessing an active olfactory communication system (Stoddart, 1988).

The secretion of semichemicals in virtually any part of the body is dependent basically upon endocrine activity. Endocrine activity, in turn, can be strongly affected by psychological–social events and may be influenced by the environment in which the person lives (Schaal & Porter, 1991). Some of these olfactory signals are perceived consciously and are processed through the main olfactory system. Others (i.e. pheromones) may be processed unconsciously and through the accessory olfactory system.

A central question remains. How do humans use pheromonal communication? Experiments have shown (Schaal *et al.*, 1980) that a mother can identify and discriminate the odor of her newborn infant from that of another child of the same age by smelling garments previously worn by the children. In addition, infants normally prefer axillary pads worn by their own mothers over pads worn by unfamiliar mothers. Therefore, body odors can provide humans with important information about the identity of individuals (Porter & Moore, 1981; Porter *et al.*, 1983, 1985; Russel *et al.*, 1983). Experiments also have demonstrated that adults can recognize gender (73%) and individuality (34%) of non-related children (Ligabue Stricker, 1991).

But can one human's chemical signals be detected by another who does not consciously experience it as an odor? Can excreted chemicals have an immediate or delayed effect upon the neuroendocrinological reproductive system of other humans (Weller & Weller, 1993)? Tests on adults demonstrate that both males and females are able to identify gender, self odor, and partner odor simply by smelling t-shirts that have been worn for some hours without the use of any deodorants or perfumes. Male odor is often described as 'musky,' and female odor is described as 'sweet' (Russel, 1976; Hold & Schleidt, 1977). Moreover, compounds similar to copulin, which have been detected in primates, have been found in women (Michael *et al.*, 1971, 1974). Copulin is a blend of aliphatic acids (e.g., acetic, propionic, butyric, isovaleric and isocaproic) that is usually present in vaginal fluids of healthy women. These acids are under hormonal control and their fluctuations during the menstrual cycle communicate the ovulatory period (McClintock, 1971, 1983). As in other primates, the concentration of these acids in women is higher near the middle of the menstrual cycle. The use of hormonal contraceptives reduces the production of copulin and its fluctuations.

The 'musky' odor of men (Kloek, 1961), is due to metabolites of androstenone (5-androst-16-en-3-one) and androstenol (5-androst-16-en-3-ol), pheromonal substances typically produced by the testes and present in high concentrations in urine, saliva, and axillary sweat. The effect of androstenone and androstenol on social interactions is more constant and stronger than copulin's (Kirk-Smith *et al.*, 1978). The greater intensity of male odor in comparison to female odor is due to greater amounts of skin secretion and concomitantly more odorogenic microflora.

In regard to perception, women are more capable of recognizing biological odors than men, especially during ovulatory periods (e.g., exalto-
lide, synthetic lattone of 15-idrossipentadecanoic acid). This capability
induces a correlation between olfactory and reproductive systems and the
existence of pheromonal communication in humans (LeMagnen, 1952).

And what about the perception of odors related to age? Olfactory tests
conducted on a group of babies using pheromone-like substances demonstrated that, from 3 to 6 years of age, male and female responses to pirro-
line isovalerianate butyrate (which has a female-like odor) were mostly
identical and described as pleasant (69%). On the other hand, strong sex
differences were observed in response to androstenol derivative (which
has a male-like odor) (Ligabue Stricker & Tua, 1993). The ability of both
sexes to recognize the female synthetic pheromone would presumably
facilitate recognition of mothers by very young children. On the other
hand, 62% of males recognized and found pleasant the male synthetic
pheromone in contrast with 69% of females who described it as unpleas-
ant. Subsequent research by the same group at the Department of Animal
and Human Biology at the University of Turin demonstrated that the
ability to distinguish pheromone-like substances as either of male or
female origin varied with age and developed with the physiological stages
of life (Ligabue Stricker & Chiarelli, 1992).

Olfaction tests were conducted on a group of 1318 school children (aged
6 to 14) using the same biologically relevant substances that were used on
infants. Younger males and females showed the same responses to pirro-
line isovalerianate butyrate and to androstenol in a high percentage of
cases (56% at age 6, 37% at age 9). Variability in responses increased gradually with age. Moreover, in females, female pheromones were judged to
be pleasant in frequencies that decreased linearly between age 6 (69%) to
age 13 (12%), concomitant with increased positive responses to male pheromones (23% at age 6, 63% at age 13). Males prior to the age of 13, on the
other hand, did not show any significant differences in the perceptions of
the two smells and, compared to females, showed only a slightly lower
acceptance of the male-like-pheromone and a slightly higher acceptance
of the female-like pheromone.

These results are consistent with the hypothesis that sensitivity to biological smells correlates positively with the emission of pheromones or,
even more, with the hormone development with which they are associated. Before puberty both sexes secrete similar amounts of eccrine
sweat, comparable to that secreted by adult females (Rees & Shuster, 1981).

It is very difficult to distinguish between the scent of boys and girls who have not reached puberty (Schleidt & Hold, 1982), even for adult females who normally perform superiorly on odor discrimination tasks (Doty, 1981). The acquisition of a distinctive odor profile goes hand in hand, not only with the pubertal activation of the elementary semichemical mechanisms of the skin, but probably also with some pubertal enabling of odor perception. Thus the ability of females to distinguish pheromonally active odors at earlier ages than males is probably due to the fact that, in a high percentage of females, the prepuberal hormone mechanisms start considerably earlier than is the case for males.

The correlation between human physiological and olfactory development is paralleled by a correlation between pheromone olfactory sensitivity and hormonal development. Ligabue Stricker & Mazzone (1996) analyzed pheromone perception of 160 subjects with hormonal problems related to reproduction (i.e. impotence, sterility, amenorrhoea, etc.). The olfactory responses of these individuals, who were characterized by abnormal variations in haematic concentrations of gonadotropins and sexual hormones, were compared with those of healthy adults. The results showed that males with pathological hormonal levels manifested changes in pheromone perception, with the positive response to female odors (6.7%) reaching a minimum value not found in healthy people of any age. Interestingly, and in contrast to healthy control subjects, a very high percentage of persons with hormonal and sexual disorders were anosmic for pheromone-like substances.

The above research confirms the strong interactions between olfactory, endocrine, and reproductive systems. This interactive physiological relationship is also suggested by the pathological condition known as Kallman's syndrome (Kallmann et al., 1944) or hypogonadic hypogonadim, which is associated with anosmy due to a genetic defect (Sparkes et al., 1968). Once the relationship between olfactory and hormonal systems is accepted, it is easier to understand and recognize the interactive role of social phenomena on reproductive physiology. For example, McClintock (1971) showed that the menstrual cycles of women who are roommates or close friends tend to converge over time. Some factor must therefore exist that is related to social closeness and interaction, and that shifts the timing of the biological clock in the brain thus causing a change in ovulation and cycling (Stern & McClintock, 1998). It seems, then, that the potential for chemical communication involving sexual function has been preserved during the course of human evolution. What about the pheromonal interaction of stable partners? Interestingly, administration of a synthetic pheromone to stable partners for four months demonstrated that balanced pheromonal overloads do not affect their relationships, unlike the situation when the chemical compound is given to only one of the partners (Ligabue Stricker, 1994). One may therefore conclude that happy paired couples are pheromonally balanced.

The last question is whether histocompatibility antigens can act as olfactory markers that facilitate recognition of suitable partners in humans as is the case for mice (Beauchamp *et al.*, 1985; Lenington, 1994; Potts, 1991; Yamazaki *et al.*, 1981). Selection of a companion who bears antigens that differ from those of an individual mouse is likely to lead to offspring that are mostly heterozygous and that show a wider immune response, giving them a significant advantage in the selection process. Ligabue Stricker and her team demonstrated that some relationship exists between histocompatibility antigens and olfactory perception in humans. In order to evaluate whether or not there are biological factors in our species that influence, to some extent, the choice of partners, studies were conducted on pairs with proven good fitness. Firstly, antigenic differences between single and coupled people were analyzed by comparing the frequency of class I HLA antigens found in 1454 coupled persons (727 pairs) against a control population of 133 singles (Ligabue Stricker *et al.*, 1995). The analysis showed that, in addition to a different antigenic frequency, single and paired people have a different appreciation of pheromone substances, and that this difference is even more evident in pairs whose components have different HLA antigens. In order to produce heterozygous offspring, partners that have different HLA antigens have to be selected in humans as they are in mice. It therefore seems reasonable to assume that such choices are influenced by a pheromone communication system that facilitates the olfactory recognition of genetically suitable mates.

The finding that humans appear to communicate by pheromones opens many possibilities for future basic and applied research. With respect to the latter, the active components of body odor (when clearly identified) may be developed as natural alternative substances for controlling the time of ovulation, and thus as an aid in contraception. As outlined above, other aspects of human behavior and physiology are affected by covert olfactory messages from others during social interactions. Because odors have well-known influences on emotions, human pheromones appear to complement (and add emotional valence to) other sources of interpersonal information.

Acknowledgments

I am obliged for the kind cooperation of Arthur Sansone in revising the text and to my colleague Franca Ligabue Stricker for integrating several bibliographical sources.

References

Bartoshuk, L.M. & Beauchamp, G.K. (1994). Chemical senses. *Annual Review of Psychology*, **45**, 419–449.

Beauchamp, G., Boyse, E. & Yamazaki, K. (1985). Il riconoscimento olfattivo dell' individualita genetica. *Le Scienze*, **10**, 91–97.

Berliner, D.L., Monti-Bloch, L., Jennings-White, C. & Diaz-Sanchez, V.J. (1996). The functionality of the human vomeronasal organ (VNO) evidence for steroid receptors. *Journal of Steroid Biochemistry and Molecular Biology*, **58**, 259–265.

Buck, L. & Axel, R.L. (1991). A novel multigene family may encode odorant receptors: a molecular basis for odor recognition. *Cell*, **65**, 175–187.

Doty, R.L. (1981). Olfactory communication in human. *Chemical Senses*, **6**, 351–376.

Dulac, C. & Axel, R. (1995). A novel family of genes encoding putative pheromone receptor in mammals. *Cell*, **83**, 195–206.

Herrada, G. & Dulac, C. (1997). A novel family of putative pheromone receptors in mammals with a topographically organized and sexually dimorphic distribution. *Cell*, **90**, 763–773.

Hold, B. & Schleidt, M. (1977). The importance of human odour in non-verbal communication. *Zeitschrift fur Tierpsychologie*, **43**, 225–238.

Kallmann, F.J., Schoenfeld, W.A. & Barrera, S.E. (1944). The genetic aspects of primary eunuchoidism. *American Journal of Mental Deficiency*, **48**, 203–236.

Karlson, P. & Lüscher, M. (1959). Pheromones: a new term for a class of biologically active substances. *Nature*, **183**, 55–56.

Keverne, E.B. (1983). Pheromonal influences on the endocrine regulation of reproduction. *Trends in Neuroscience*, **6**, 381–384.

Kirk-Smith, M., Booth, D., Carrol, D. & Davies, P. (1978). Human sexual attitudes affected by androstenol. *Research Communications in Psychology, Psychiatry and Behavior*, **3**, 379–384.

Kloek, J. (1961). The smell of some steroid sex hormones and their metabolites: Reflections and experiments concerning the significance of smell for the mutual relation of the sexes. *Psichiatria, Neurologia, Neurochirurgia*, **64**, 309–344.

LeMagnen, J. (1952). Les phenomenes olfacto-sexuels chez l'homme. *Archives of Science and Physics*, **6**, 125–160.

Lenington, F. (1994). Of Mais, Men and the MHC. *Trends in Ecology and Evolution*, **9**, 455–456.

Ligabue Stricker, F. (1991). I feromoni: conoscenze attuali e brevi cenni sugli esperimenti in corso. *Antropologia Contemporanea*, **14**, 305–314.

Ligabue Stricker, F. (1994). La comunicazione feromonale nell'uomo. *Antropologia Contemporanea*, **17**, 281–192.

Ligabue Stricker, F., Amoroso, A. & Cerutti, N. (1995). Antigeni di istocompatibilita' e percezione olfattiva nell'uomo. *Antropologia Contemporanea*, **18**, 79–86.

Ligabue Stricker, F. & Chiarelli, B. (1992). Research on olfactory perception of biologically relevant substances in a sample of school-children, aged from 6 to 14. VIIIth Congress Europ. Anthrop. Ass. Madrid. *International Journal of Anthropology*, **7**, 67–72.

Ligabue Stricker, F. & Mazzone, M. (1996). Perception of biologically significant substances and gonadotropin, PRL, gonodatropic hormone levels in man. Relata Technica. *International Journal on Dermopharmaceutical Research, Dermopharmaceutical Technology*, **28**, 6–10.

Ligabue Stricker, F. & Tua, N. (1993). Indagine sulle capacità olfattive e l'odore personale di un campione di bambini di età prescolare. Atti IX Congr. Antropol. Ital. *Antropologia contemporanea*, **16**, 181–186.

Liman, E. R. (1996). Pheromone transduction in the vomeronasal organ. *Neurobiology*, **6**, 487–493.

Marchlewska-Koj, A. (1983). Pregnancy blocking by pheromones. In *Pheromones and Reproduction in Mammals*, ed. J. G. Vanderbergh, pp. 151–174. New York: Academic Press.

Marchlewska-Koj, A. (1984). Pheromones in mammalian reproduction. *Oxford Reviews of Reproductive Biology*, **6**, 226–302.

Matsunami, H. & Buck, L. B. (1997). A multigene family encoding a diverse array of putative pheromone receptors in mammals. *Cell*, **90**, 775–784.

McClintock, M. K. (1971). Menstrual synchrony and suppression. *Nature*, **229**, 244–245.

McClintock, M. K. (1983). *Pheromones and Reproduction in Mammals*, ed. J. G. Vandenbergh, pp. 113–149. New York: Academic Press.

Michael, R. P. & Keverne, E. B. (1968). Pheromones in the communication of sexual status in primates. *Nature*, **218**, 746–749.

Michael, R. P., Keverne, E. B. & Bonsall, R. W. (1971). Isolation of male sex attractants from a female primate. *Science*, **172**, 964–966.

Michael, R. P., Bonsall, R. W. & Warner, P. (1974). Human vaginal secretions: volatile fatty acid content. *Science*, **186**, 1217–1219.

Monti-Bloch, L., Jennings-White, C., Dolberg, D. S. & Berliner, D. L. (1994). The human vomeronasal system. *Psychoneuroendocrinology*, **19**, 673–686.

Natoli, E. (1994). La comunicazione chimica nei Primati non umani. *Antropologia Contemporanea*, **17**, 263–272.

Porter, R., Cernoch, J. & Balogh, R. (1985). Odour signatures and kin recognition. *Physiology and Behavior*, **34**, 445–448.

Porter, R., Cernoch, J. & McLaughin, F. (1983). Maternal recognition of neonates through olfactory cues. *Physiology and Behavior*, **30**, 151–154.

Porter, R. & Moore, J. D. (1981). Human kin recognition by olfactory cues. *Psychology and Behaviour*, **27**, 493–495.

Potts, W. K. (1991). Genotype influences mating pattern in seminatural population of mouse. *Nature*, **352**, 619–621.

Rees, J. & Shuster, S. (1981). Pubertal induction of sweat gland activity. *Clinical Science*, **60**, 689–692.

Russel, M. (1976). Human olfactory communication. *Nature*, **260**, 520–522.

Russel, M., Mendelsson, T. & Peeke, H. (1983). Mother's identification of their infant's odors. *Ethology and Sociobiology*, **4**, 29–31.

Ryba, N. J. P. & Tirindelli, R. (1997). A new multigenic family of putative pheromone receptors. *Neuron*, **19**, 371–379.

Scalfari, F. (1994). Il gusto e l'olfatto nei Primati non umani. *Antropologia Contemporanea*, **17**, 253–261.

Schaal, B., Montagner, H., Hertling, E., Bolzoni, D., Moyse, R. & Quichon, R. (1980). Les stimulations olfactives dans les relations entre l'enfant et la mere. *Reproduction, Nutrition, Development*, **20**, 843–858.

Schaal, B. & Porter, R.H. (1991). In *Advances in the Study of Behaviour*, 20, eds. P.J.B. Slater, C. Beer & M. Milinski, pp. 135–199, New York: Academic Press.

Schleidt, M. & Hold, B. (1982). Human odour and identity. In *Olfaction and Endocrine Regulation*, ed. W. Breipohl, pp. 181–194. London: IRL Press.

Sparkes, R.S., Simpson, R.W. & Paulsen, C.A. (1968). Familial hypogonadotropic hypogonadism with anosmia. *Archives of Internal Medicine*, **121**, 534–538.

Spielman, A.I., Zeng, X.N., Leyden, J.J. & Preti, G. (1995). Proteinaceous precursor of human axillary odor: isolation of two novel odor-binding proteins. *Experientia*, **51**, 40–47.

Stern, K. & McClintock, M.K. (1998). Regulation of ovulation by human pheromones. *Nature*, **392**, 177–179.

Stoddart, D.M. (1988). Human odor culture: a zoological perspective. In *Perfumery: The Psychology and Biology of Fragrance*, eds. S. Van Toller & G.H. Dodd, pp. 3–17. London: Chapman & Hall.

Weller, L. & Weller, A. (1993). Human menstrual synchrony: a critical assessment. *Neuroscience and Behavioral Reviews*, **17**, 427–439.

Yamazaki, K., Yamaguchi, M., Beauchamp, G.K., Bard, J., Boyse, E.A. & Thomas, L. (1981). Chemosensation: An aspect of the uniqueness of the individual. In *Biochemistry of Taste and Olfaction*, eds. H.R. Cagan & M.R. Kare. New York: Academic Press.

Yamazaki, K., Beauchamp, G.K., Krupinski, D., Bard, J., Thomas, L. & Boyse, E.A. (1988). Familiar imprinting determines II-2 selective mating preferences. *Science*, **240**, 1331–1332.

RALPH L. HOLLOWAY, DOUGLAS C. BROADFIELD &
MICHAEL S. YUAN

9

Revisiting australopithecine visual striate cortex: newer data from chimpanzee and human brains suggest it could have been reduced during australopithecine times

Although this author's (R.L.H.) disagreements with Harry Jerison are legion (e.g. Holloway, 1966, 1974, 1979), I have always found his ideas stimulating and thus of great value to my own work regarding human brain evolution. I believe we best honor Harry Jerison by taking his ideas seriously, whether or not we agree with them.

There do not appear to be any serious disagreements that the brain became reorganized as well as enlarged during hominid evolution, but there is considerable controversy as to when reorganization, particularly that relating to the reduction of primary visual striate cortex, Brodmann's area 17, had taken place. (Reviews of these questions can be found in Holloway, 1995, 1996.) Since the only way we will ever know for absolutely certain when this process occurred requires travel with a time machine and some histological sectioning of australopithecine brains, one might wonder why we are writing this paper. It is already apparent from the literature on early hominid brain evolution that a major controversy exists regarding the fossil australopithecine endocasts and their interpretation regarding that infamous landmark, the lunate sulcus. Falk (1983, 1985,1986) interprets the paleoneurological evidence from the Taung and Hadar (AL 162–28) endocasts as indicating that the lunate sulcus was in an anterior pongid-like position. Holloway (1981, 1983, 1984) interprets the evidence as suggesting a posterior, more modern-human like position. Basically, the question is when in the course of hominid evolution did reorganization, specifically of the amount of primary visual striate of the cerebral cortex, take place and what is that relationship to the well-documented evidence regarding brain size enlargement during hominid evolution?

[177]

Two other views are those of Armstrong *et al.* (1991) and the scientist we now fête, Harry Jerison. Armstrong *et al.* are of the opinion that the hominid brain first had to enlarge before cortical reorganization involving a reduction of area 17 could have occurred, arguing from modern developmental evidence (see Holloway, 1992, for a critique). Jerison, on the other hand, disagrees with an early reorganization of the lateral extent of area 17, because he believes that reducing the lateral extent of area 17 would have involved an addition of area 17 along the calcarine fissure of the midline, which, without overall brain enlargement would have seriously deformed the midline structures such as the corpus callosum. As Jerison notes, since the medial cortex is involved, fossil endocasts will never be of any use in settling this controversy. It is worth quoting him in full here (Jerison, 1984, pp. 288–289).

> Holloway believes that the lunate sulcus in *Australopithecus africanus* was displaced posteriorly relative to its position in chimpanzees . . . Language systems homologous to those of living humans could then have appeared in *Australopithecus* anteriorly to the sulcus in the vicinity of the angular gyrus. Falk . . . interprets the "lunate" differently, and would have the hominid and chimpanzee *Affenspalte* in similar positions. I have argued still another position, based not on detailed morphology but rather the morphometric consequences of packing primary visual cortex into a primate brain with a posteriorly displaced lunate . . . The anterior border of area 17 is near the lunate, which limits the extent of visual cortex on the lateral surface of the brain. If Holloway's interpretation is correct, I argued, and if hominids and chimpanzees required similar amounts of primary visual cortex to process visual information, the representation of vision in *medial* [emphasis Jerison's] neocortex would have been much greater in early hominids than in living chimpanzees. Packing this additional tissue medially would have required major changes in the medial profile of the brain, especially around the calcarine fissure and the splenium of the corpus callosum, which are among the more major landmarks in mammalian brains.
>
> My argument was uniformitarian . . .: Since the medial callosal region of the brain in placental mammals is similar in appearance in different species, this region in *Australopithecus* should have looked like that of 'good' placental mammals, and visual cortex should have been packed normally. Falk's analysis is consistent with uniformitarianism; Holloway's is not. But the medial surface of the brain is not visible in endocasts, and this controversy cannot be resolved by the fossil evidence alone.

Here, we must seriously disagree with Jerison, as the fossil evidence can certainly provide some evidence regarding the lateral extent of primary visual cortex, and this datum, whether controversial or not, should not be ignored.

The matter of how much striate cortex is (or was) needed to process visual information is unanswerable, and in fact there is considerable variation in amounts of primary visual striate cortex, both in humans and chimpanzees, with no apparent indication of any causal relationship to variation in visual acuity, or processing of visual information. If it can be shown that such morphometric variation of primary visual striate cortex does exist currently in extant species, it certainly allows for the possibility that it existed in the past using the same uniformitarian framework that Jersion championed above. In other words, the neurogenetic bases for expanded and reduced volumes of primary visual striate cortex may be very similar (if not totally homologous) between chimpanzee and modern human. Given a pongid–hominid split of perhaps 5–7 million years ago, such a neurogenetic basis could have been operating in *Australopithecus*, and other early hominids. From the data of Stephan *et al.* (1981), it is clear that the volume of primary visual striate cortex is some 121% less than would be expected for a primate of our brain size, corroborated by the additional fact that our lateral geniculate nucleus is about 140% less than expected (Holloway, 1995, 1996). Passingham & Ettlinger (1973) had shown such a diminution back in 1969, but chose not to stress it (see Holloway, 1979, for a review). We mention this because at least the comparative evidence is unambiguous on whether or not human primary visual striate cortex is less than expected when allometry is considered.

We will show here that indeed, both in modern humans and chimpanzees, there is considerable variability regarding volume of primary visual striate cortex, and that the brain endocasts of the Hadar 162-28 specimen, using Falk's (1983) placement of the lunate, shows a reduction toward the human case.

Newer observations

Variation of primary visual striate cortex in modern humans

Gilissen & Zilles (1995, 1996) and Gilissen *et al.* (1995) have studied the relationships between the following variables: striate cortex volume, depth and area of the calcarine fissure. These variables can be quantified using

MRI scans. Their findings suggest a very high degree of variability of striate cortical volume with coefficients of variation (CV) twice that associated with total brain volume. Striate cortex showed CVs of 18.7 and 19.3%, while total brain volume CV was 9.0–10.6 %, based on two human samples of N = 20 and N = 9. In the Gilissen *et al.* (1995) paper, they found that the projection area of the medial surface (as measured by calcarine length and depth) had CVs of 20–23%, and occipital surface area had a CV of 18.4 %, while cortical surface area (total and non-occipital) had CVs around 9.5%. They conclude that occipital surface area correlates significantly with calcarine length, while the calcarine surface varies independently from the rest of the variables (p. 454). There is no evidence of deformation of the medial surface, splenium of the corpus callosum, or poor visual information processing in these healthy modern humans. (There is a large literature on this question of variation of volume of striate area 17 cortex, and the reader is advised to peruse the references in these authors' papers, as well as the various chapters in Peters & Rockland (eds.), 1994.)

An additional interesting indication of a neurogenetic basis for considerable variability in striate cortical volume comes from the work of Klekamp and his colleagues. Klekamp *et al.* (1994) have shown that the Australian Aborigine's visual striate cortical volume is significantly larger (both absolutely and relatively) than in the German Caucasian sample they measured. There is no evidence of any environmental factors affecting this size difference, and the authors' conclude that some neurogenetic factor in ontogenetic development is most likely the explanation for this difference.

Variation in visual striate cortical volume in chimpanzee brains

That the lunate sulcus in chimpanzee is placed well anterior to where it occasionally exists in modern humans has long been appreciated (see Holloway, 1985, for a review). We know that the lunate is roughly the anterior boundary of primary visual cortex, and this anterior placement is the usual configuration of all apes, and indeed the Old World monkeys as well.

Recently, two very interesting departures from the normal morphometric position of the lunate sulcus have appeared in two common chimpanzees (*Pan troglodytes*) whose brains have been sent to my laboratory for study from Yerkes. 'Frank' and 'Chuck', two male chimpanzees from Yerkes show a fascinating composite of features of the lunate sulcus.

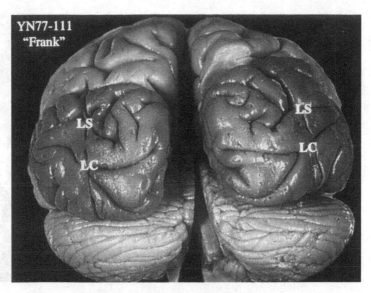

Fig. 9.1. An occipital view of the brain of 'Frank'. LS is the lunate sulcus, and LC is the lateral calcarine fissure. The darker shading is the result of preliminary staining, and the most anterior part of the staining is approximately where the lunate sulcus is usually found in *Pan troglodytes*. These sulci on 'Frank' are in the same position as on the right hemisphere of 'Chuck' in Fig. 9.2.

'Frank' (see Fig. 9.1), shows a pattern that departs significantly from all the other chimpanzee brains these authors have ever seen. The lunate sulcus is clearly in a more posterior position than found in most other chimpanzee hemispheres that we have measured.

'Chuck' is even more surprising, in that the left hemisphere shows a typical anterior pongid position for the lunate sulcus, while the right hemisphere shows a more posterior position (see Fig. 9.2). The medial surface surrounding the calcarine fissure is normal in both brains, and there are no behavioral observations that would indicate that these two chimpanzees had anything but normal vision and information processing. The histological staining we have done thus far indicates that the stripe of Gennari (layer 4c) is visible up to the limit of the lunate sulcus in both chimpanzees, and particularly so in the case of 'Chuck'. Clearly, the neurogenetic bases for variability regarding reduction in the posterior placement of the lunate sulcus is present in modern chimpanzee and modern human. Applying Jerison's penchant for 'uniformitarianism', these observations suggest that similar, if not identical neurogenetic processes obtain in the ontogenetic development of primary visual striate

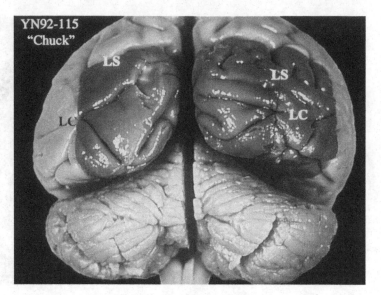

Fig. 9.2. An occipital view of the brain of 'Chuck'. Notice that the left hemispheric position of the lunate is considerably more anterior than on the right side.

cortex. Why should these processes have skipped the Australopithecines? We don't believe they have.

Statistical analysis of the position of the lunate sulcus in *Pan* and *Australopithecus*

Published measurements in Holloway (1983, 1988, 1995) and Holloway & Kimbel (1986) which showed that if Holloway and Falk (1986) do agree on the position of the intraparietal sulcus on the Hadar 162-28 *Australopithecus afarensis* specimen, the modern chimpanzee position of the lunate sulcus is roughly twice as great as the distance for the Hadar specimen, even though many of the chimpanzee hemispheres measured were of smaller brain size than that of the Hadar specimen (i.e. 385–400 cm³).

Our mixed-sex sample of chimpanzee hemispheres has now increased to 39 without 'Frank' and 'Chuck', and measurements of the distance from occipital pole (OP) to lunate sulcus (LS) provide a mean OP–LS distance of 31.55 mm, and a standard deviation (SD) of 4.6 mm, and an average brain weight of 137.8 g for each hemisphere, SD = 32.3 g. The OP–LS distance in 'Frank' is 22 mm (left) and 20 mm (right). In the case of

'Chuck', the right OP–LS distance is 20 mm, while the left OP–LS distance is 35 mm, a value most often seen on chimpanzee brains. If 'Frank' and 'Chuck' are included, the mean OP–LS distance is 30.87 mm, and the SD is 5.24 mm. The mean brain weight is 141.3 g, SD = 32.7 g.

Given an OP–LS distance of 15.5 on the Hadar 162-28 *A. afarensis* endocast, this is 3.49 SD posterior to the mean chimpanzee value. When the two unusual chimpanzees are included, the Hadar specimen's OP–LS distance is 2.93 SD posterior to the chimpanzee mean. Earlier and smaller samples were indicating SDs of approximately 5. As the sample increases so does the variability, and the SD also becomes lower. Such SDs as currently available from these samples indicate a very statistically significant difference between the chimpanzee and *A. afarensis* positioning of the lunate sulcus, if indeed the lunate can be unambiguously determined on the australopithecine brain endocasts.

Summary

Our studies on the variability of morphogenetic characters in both modern humans' and chimpanzees' brains suggest that neurogenetic processes underlying reduction of the volume of primary visual striate cortex, area 17 of Brodmann, are both expressed in these two species. Given that this variability is shared between *Homo* and *Pan*, it would appear possible that some of the australopithecine ancestors of *Homo* could have expressed these variations also, given a pongid–hominid divergence of 5–7 MYA. While the data on these variations cannot prove such a contention, they are supportive of our claims, and the paleoneurological evidence, despite its controversial nature, supports our claims of a diminution of the lateral extent of primary visual cortex by *A. afarensis* times.

Hopes and predictions on the state of brain studies in the year 2010

Hopes are surely easy to pronounce; predictions are another matter, but here goes, anyway. We would hope for far more quantitative information about primate brains, much of it along the lines provided by Stephan and his associates, but which would include within-species variation. That is, we would have the most accurate volumetric data for all neural nuclei as well as fiber tracts for each species of primate with a sample of at least 10 each. We would hope that the scientific community could begin to show a strong interest in within-species variation of brain structure and behavior, so that we might have a better understanding of what are the units of structure and behavior that become targeted by evolutionary processes, and of course, their neurogenetic underpinnings and ontogenetic development. We would hope that scientists interested in human brain evolution (or any other creature's) would finally come to realize that size alone, whether allometrically scaled or not, will not be sufficient to inform us about brain evolution, as the brain's organization must be a critical component of species-specific behavior and evolutionary processes. Of course, this includes the hope that all of these species will still be around in a non-endangered state by 2010. We would also hope that neuroimaging techniques (noninvasive) develop rapidly to permit accurate assessments of cognitive capacities in other animals (particularly *Pan*), such as are becoming available through fMRI and PET on humans. Next, a cure for Alzheimer's so that we can all read about it by 2010!

Needless to say, paleoneurologists can only hope and pray that we will find *the* perfect australopithecine brain endocast, lunate sulcus unambiguously in place, either anterior or posterior, or for that matter completely lacking. We would also keep our hopes high for a frozen complete Neandertal brain, fully intact within its brow-ridged cranium.

We predict that none of the above will come to pass by 2010. Instead, we expect a dozen or so more fossil hominid partial crania to be discovered which will provide limitless opportunities for controversy regarding their brain sizes and organizations. If the frontal lobe is the issue, the requisite fossils will only have the posterior part of the brain present, while if the lunate sulcus is what matters, only the frontal portions of the crania will be preserved. We predict that cranial capacities will continue to be determined using a multitude of techniques, including seed, shot, water displacement, computer imaging and CT-scanning, water dowsers, Tarot Cards, not to forget crystal balls. We finally predict that Harry Jerison's 1973 book will still be a classic in the field, and required reading for all evolutionary neuropaleontologists.

Acknowledgments

The authors are grateful to the editors for including us in the opportunity to fête Harry Jerison. We would like to thank Harold McClure, Dan Anderson, Tom Insel, Jeremey Dahl and Jim Rilling of Yerkes Regional

Primate Center for their cooperation in allowing us access to these many chimpanzee brains, and to Patrick Gannon, Nancy Kheck, and Star Gabriel of Mount Sinai School of Medicine, for their advice and help with sectioning some of the brain tissue. We also wish to thank Sam Marquez, Jill Shapiro, and Chet Sherwood for their comments and suggestions.

References

Armstrong, E., Zilles, K., Curtis, M. & Schleicher, A. (1991). Cortical folding, the lunate sulcus and the evolution of the human brain. *Journal of Human Evolution*, **20**, 341–348.

Falk, D. (1983). The Taung endocast. A reply to Holloway. *American Journal of Physical Anthropology*, **53**, 525–539.

Falk, D. (1985). Hadar AL 162-28 endocast as evidence that brain enlargement preceded cortical reorganization in hominid evolution. *Nature*, **313**, 45–47.

Falk, D. (1986). Reply to Holloway and Kimbel. *Nature*, **321**, 536–537.

Gilissen, E. & Zilles, K. (1995). The relative volume of primary visual cortex and its intersubject variability among humans: a new morphometric study. *Comptes Rendus Academie des Sciences (Paris)* serie II, **t.320**, 897–902.

Gilissen, E. & Zilles, K. (1996). The calcarine sulcus as an estimate of the total volume of the human striate cortex: a morphometric study of reliability and intersubject variability. *Journal of Brain Research*, **37**, 57–66.

Gilissen, E., Iba-Zizen, T., Stievenart, J.-L., Lopez, A., Trad, M., Cabanis, E.A. & Zilles, K. (1995). Is the length of the calcarine sulcus associated with the size of the human visual cortex? A morphometric study with magnetic resonance tomography. *Journal of Brain Research*, **36**, 451–459.

Holloway, R.L. (1966). Cranial capacity and neuron number: critique and proposal. *American Journal of Physical Anthropology*, **52**, 305–314.

Holloway, R.L. (1974). On the meaning of brain size. A review of H.J. Jerison's 1973 *Evolution of the Brain and Intelligence*. *Science*, **184**, 677–679.

Holloway, R.L. (1979). Brain size, allometry, and reorganization: toward a synthesis. In *Development and Evolution of Brain Size: Behavioral Implications*, eds. M.E. Hahn, G. Jensen & B.C. Dudek, pp. 59–88. New York: Academic Press.

Holloway, R.L. (1981). Revisiting the S. African Australopithecine endocasts: results of stereoplotting the lunate sulcus. *American Journal of Physical Anthropology*, **56**, 43–58.

Holloway, R.L. (1983). Cerebral brain endocast pattern of *A. afarensis* hominid. *Nature*, **303**, 420–422.

Holloway, R.L. (1984). The Taung endocast and the lunate sulcus: a rejection of the hypothesis of its anterior placement. *American Journal of Physical Anthropology*, **64**, 285–288.

Holloway, R.L. (1985). The past, present, and future significance of the lunate sulcus in early homind evolution. In *Hominid Evolution: Past, Present, and Future*, ed. P.V. Tobias, pp. 47–62. New York: A.R. Liss.

Holloway, R.L. (1988). 'Robust' Australopithecine brain endocasts: some preliminary observations. In *Evolutionary History of the 'robust' Australopithecines*, ed. F.E. Grine, pp. 97–105. New York: Aldine-deGruyter.

Holloway, R. L. (1992). The failure of the gyrification index (GI) to account for volumetric reorganization in the evolution of the human brain. *Journal of Human Evolution*, **22**, 163–170.

Holloway, R. L. (1995). Toward a synthetic theory of human brain evolution. In *Origins of the Human Brain*, eds. J. P. Changeaux & J. Chavaillon, pp. 42–55. Oxford: Clarendon Press.

Holloway, R. L. (1996). Evolution of the human brain. Chapter 4 in *Handbook of Human Symbolic Evolution*, eds. A. Lock & C. Peters, pp. 74–116. Oxford: Clarendon Press.

Holloway, R. L. & Kimbel, W. H. (1986). Endocast morphology of Hadar AL 162-28. *Nature*, **321**, 538.

Jerison, H. J. (1973). *Evolution of the Brain and Intelligence*. New York: Academic Press.

Jerison, H. J. (1984). Fossil evidence on the evolution of the neocortex. In *Cerebral Cortex. Vol. 8A. Comparative Structure and Evolution of Cerebral Cortex, part I*, eds. E. Jones & A. Peters, pp. 285–309. New York: Plenum.

Klekamp, J., Reidel, A., Harper, C. & Kretschmann, H. J. (1994). Morphometric study on the postnatal growth of the visual cortex of Australian Aborigines and Caucasians. *Journal of Brain Research*, **35**, 541–548.

Passingham, R. & Ettlinger, G. (1973). A comparison of cortical functions in man and other primates. *International Review of Neurobiology*, **16**, 233–299.

Peters, A. & Rockland, K. S. (eds.) (1994). *Cerebral Cortex. Vol. 10. Primary Visual Cortex in Primates*. New York: Plenum.

Stephan, H., Frahm, H. & Baron, G. (1981). New and revised data on volumes of brain structures in insectivores and primates. *Folia Primatologia*, **35**, 1–29.

10

Structural symmetries and asymmetries in human and chimpanzee brains

Humans and chimpanzees share a common prehominid ancestor and, together with gorillas, constitute a group of closely related primates (Falk, 1987a; Ruvolo, 1997; Deinard & Kidd, 1999). Although they have similar body sizes, humans and chimpanzees differ completely in terms of encephalization. The human brain is indeed about three times larger than the chimpanzee's. This dramatic increase in brain size started more than 2 million years ago and characterizes the human lineage. In contrast to the generally acknowledged consensus that brain size relative to body size is a better measure of increased cognitive performance than is absolute brain size, it has recently been suggested that higher cognitive capacity is more closely related to absolute brain size and that absolute brain size more closely reflects the cognitive differences between humans, great apes, and monkeys than encephalization indices (Rumbaugh et al., 1996; Gibson et al., 1998; Gibson et al., Chapter 5, this volume).

Increased brain size is nevertheless also accompanied by decreased interhemispheric transfer speed and thus decreased cognitive processing speed. In order to maintain processing power, the number of elements clustered in one hemisphere is therefore expected to increase. This principle may be at the origin of hemispheric specialization (Ringo et al., 1994). More recently, Anderson (1999) showed by analytical means that if interneural conduction time increases proportionally with interneuronal distance, spatial clustering of interneuronal connections is the only way to increase the number of synaptic events occuring in a given period of time. Empirical evidence tends to support this concept (Aboitiz et al., 1992a,b). It can therefore be expected that large brains will manifest a high degree of structural and functional hemispheric specialization.

When compared with other primates, some aspects of structural brain lateralization in humans indeed appear to represent an extreme situation (Holloway & De La Coste-Lareymondie, 1982; Falk, 1987b) and functional asymmetries show important differences when comparing humans and animals (Lacreuse, 1997). Other aspects of structural asymmetries are, however, shared by humans and chimpanzees (Gannon *et al.*, 1998; Gilissen *et al.*, 1998; Hopkins *et al.*, 1998). It also appears that structural and functional asymmetries exist in numerous vertebrate species (Petersen *et al.*, 1978; Beecher *et al.*, 1979; LeMay *et al.*, 1982; Gilissen, 1992; Glick, 1985; Falk *et al.*, 1990; Fitch *et al.*, 1993; Lewis & Diamond, 1995; Lacreuse, 1997). This raises the question of whether brain size increase is more related to some defined patterns of asymmetries than to others. Certain aspects of structural (a)symmetries in human and chimpanzee brains are reviewed in this chapter.

Cortical shape variability

In any discussion of brain asymmetry, there are three points that must always be considered: (1) the direction of the asymmetry, (2) the degree of the asymmetry, and (3) the variability in the direction of asymmetry at the population level (Galaburda, 1995; Wynn *et al.*, 1996). Because one of the most striking asymmetries of the human brain involves cortical shape (petalias), it is interesting to determine if the variability of cortical shape shows a similar pattern in humans and chimpanzees. Below, the overall cortical shape variability of humans and common chimpanzees (Fig. 10.1) are first compared in order to understand the extent to which the observations of variability of cortical regions observed among humans can be extended to our nearest cousin. Comparison of feature variation in great apes and humans is then used to help clarify the possibilities for early hominids.

Despite the wide range of variation in absolute brain size, intraspecific variability for both male and female adult human brain weight is comparable with that calculated for different samples of male or female nonhuman primates. It is, however, possible that the variability of specific cortical regions can be different when humans are compared with non human primates (i.e. orang-utan, *Cercopithecus* sp.) (Filimonoff, 1933). Intraspecific variability of cortical regions appears to be much larger than that of the whole brain in humans (Gilissen *et al.*, 1995; Gilissen & Zilles, 1996; Kennedy *et al.*, 1998). These observations concerning intraspecific variability of cortical regions can be integrated by studying the locations of maximal variability in overall cortical shape, which can be measured as distances between the external brain surfaces after 3D reconstructions of the brains and after normalization of the different absolute brain volumes (Dabringhaus *et al.*, 1994a,b). The study of cortical shape also appears to be a sensitive method for understanding structure–function relationships (Zilles *et al.*, 1996b, 1998).

MR scans of the brain were carried out on 10 randomly selected healthy right-handed men and on 10 *in situ* formalin-fixed brains of the common chimpanzee *(Pan troglodytes)* that did not show any damage to their surface structure. Although the brain may suffer volumetric changes due to fixation, a more or less uniform and minor change can be assumed for the whole cerebral cortex if no histological processing is involved. Sagittal T1-weighted, 3D gradient-echo (FLASH) images were obtained from humans and from the fixed chimpanzees brains with the use of a 1.5 T superconductive magnet. The scanning parameters were: TR, 40 ms; TE, 5 ms; 1 excitation; 256×256 pixel/image; and 1 mm thick contiguous slices. Images were transferred to an image analyzer where image segmentation procedures were performed in order to extract those portions of the image representing scalp, skull, meninges and the cerebellum, and to separate the two hemispheres on each brain.

A mean brain surface for each of the two MRI data sets was then built up, thereby simultaneously obtaining quantitative information about interindividual variability in shape for each species (Dabringhaus *et al.*, 1994a,b). The study of interindividual variability of brain shape relies on proper alignment (fitting) of each individual brain to a common reference system. For this, we used a fitting procedure that is independent of anatomical landmarks and based on finding the optimal 3D fitting that maximizes the amount of overlap for each pair of brains chosen from a given sample. The fitting is done by linear transformations composed of translations, rotations and isotropic scalings, thus merely changing the position, spatial orientation and size of the individual brain 3D images. The optimal fitting is the one in the set of all possible fittings that minimizes the volume of discordance of two brains, that is, the volume of the region which is occupied by only one of the two brains. After normalization, remaining differences between location of the cortical surfaces of different brains are entirely due to shape, not to size differences.

Three-dimensional images of mean human and chimpanzee cortical surfaces that code the intersubject differences in cortical shape were constructed, using the following procedures (Dabringhaus *et al.*, 1994a,b).

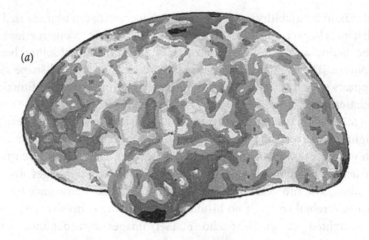

(a)

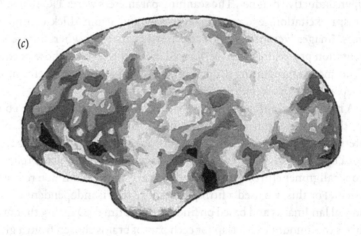

(c)

Fig. 10.1. Lateral views of 'mean' human (a, b) and chimpanzee (c, d) left and right hemispheres. These 'mean' images were obtained from a sample of 10 adult male human brains (right-handers) and brains from 9 adult common chimpanzees (*Pan troglodytes*). After segmentation of the MR scan images, the dimensions and orientations of 3D images of individual left and right hemispheres were standardized with an automatic method. These sets of standardized 3D images were used to create the 3D images of 'mean' human and chimpanzee left and right hemispheres. The intraspecific cortical shape variability is calculated for each voxel from the distances between the external surfaces of individual hemispheres and the 'mean' surfaces. This variability is expressed with a gray scale. White means that the distances between external surfaces of individual hemispheres and the 'mean' surface in a given cortical region are smaller than 1 mm. Light gray means that these distances are between 1 and 1.125 mm. Intermediate gray means that the distances are

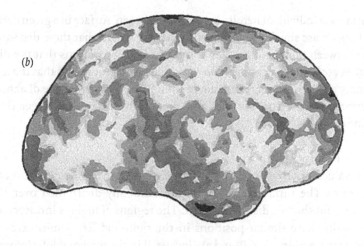

(b)

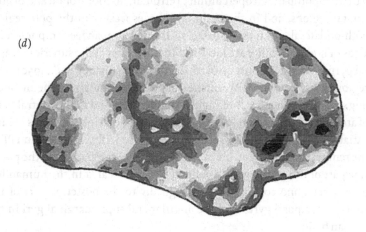

(d)

between 1.125 and 1.375 mm. Dark gray means that the distances are between 1.375 and 2 mm. Black means that the distances between the external surfaces and the 'mean' surface are bigger than 2 mm. Mesial surfaces of the occipital poles (not shown) are also regions of high shape variability.

For each voxel of the mean brain surface, the distance to the nearest voxel of each individual brain surface was determined and a measure of difference in cortical shape was calculated (Raya & Udupa, 1990). The value of this measure was attached to the corresponding starting point on the mean brain surface. The intersubject variability in cortical shape is visualized with a gray scale. White means that the distances between external surfaces of individual hemispheres and the 'mean' surface in a given cortical region are smaller than 1 mm. Light gray means that these distances are between 1 mm and 1.125 mm. Intermediate gray means that the distances are between 1.125 mm and 1.375 mm. Dark gray means that the distances are between 1.375 mm and 2 mm. Black means that the distances between the external surfaces and the 'mean' surface are bigger than 2 mm.

Results

The values for surface variation distance range from 0 mm to 3 mm (mean 1.7 mm). The surface variablity is not randomly distributed over the cortex, but shows a distinct pattern. The regions of highest intraspecific variability have similar positions in the right and left hemispheres of chimpanzees (Fig. 10.1c,d), and are localized in the temporal lobe (central part); temporoparietal operculum; prefrontal, inferior frontal and orbitofrontal regions; and in the occipital lobe (especially in the pole region, both on lateral and mesial surfaces). In the chimpanzee temporal lobe, areas of high variability are localized in the region of the superior temporal gyrus, labeled TA on a cytoarchitectonic map (Bailey et al., 1950). This region partly comprises Wernicke's area in the human left hemisphere (Fig. 10.1a). Another focus of high variability is found in the central parts of areas TE1 and TE2, and in area TG of the temporal lobe. Regions of high variability also cover the posterior part of TA, as well as areas PG and PF in the temporoparietal operculum. These areas are comparable to the posterior part of the more broadly defined Wernicke's area in the human left hemisphere, and correspond topologically to the posterior part of the superior temporal gyrus and the angular and supramarginal gyri in the human brain.

The inferior frontal areas of chimpanzees correspond partly to Broca's area and its homolog in the right hemisphere of humans. This region is called area FCBm in cytoarchitectonic studies (Bailey et al., 1950). The prefrontal and orbitofrontal regions correspond to cytoarchitectonically defined areas FE and FDp. The regions of highest variability in the occipital lobe have positions comparable to those of areas OC, OB and parts of area OA (Bailey et al., 1950).

Regions of high variability are found in the human brain in temporal, inferior frontal and prefrontal areas and are located in positions similar to those described for chimpanzees (Fig. 10.1a,b). Variability of the occipital lobe is more restricted to the pole region, including the mesial surface. Most of the foci of variability in hemispheric shape are thus comparable in the two species.

In human brains, some areas of the cortical surface appear to be more variable than others. Regions of highest variability are localized in the lower parietal lobe, the prefrontal cortex and the temporal lobe, together with Wernicke's area of the left hemisphere and its counterpart in the right hemisphere. These regions are known to have played an important role in the evolution of the human brain, constituting the centers for receptive language and praxic functions on the left side, and for spatial perception and integration of aspects of musical stimuli and tonal aspects of speech on the right side (Bryden, 1982; Perecman, 1983; Schlaug *et al.*, 1995; Witelson & Kigar, 1988). The areas which represent Broca's area, regions of the prefrontal cortex, and the occipital pole show a similarly high intraspecific variability for both hemispheres. With the exception of the occipital pole, these cortical regions were particularly progressive in the evolution of the human brain. The region of the superior part of the pre- and postcentral gyrus (central region) is also high variable among humans.

When compared with that of humans, the high intraspecific variability of the occipital region is more symmetrical in chimpanzees. The chimpanzee brain shows more variability in the inferior frontal, right occipital, and temporal cortices, and less variability in the region of the superior part of the pre- and postcentral gyrus. Nevertheless, the distribution of cortical regions of highest intraspecific shape variability is roughly the same in chimpanzees and humans. The differences in their extent between the two species, as well as the more symmetrical pattern of variability of the occipital region in chimpanzees, may simply be the result of relatively small sample sizes in the present study.

The cortical regions of highest intraspecific variability in both species, such as temporoparietal regions and the occipital pole, are not similarly progressive in primate brain evolution (Armstrong, 1990; Frahm *et al.*, 1984; Deacon, 1988; Gilissen & Zilles, 1995). The present study demonstrates a localized and considerable variability in regions with associative and higher sensory functions. This can be interpreted as a sign of relative instability in structural determination of the cortex. This holds true if we conceptualize brain evolution as an ongoing process, and not as a mechanism leading to endpoints within a simple 'scala naturae' scheme.

Petalias

Petalia is a term commonly used by anatomists (Hadziselimovic & Kus, 1966) to describe the extension of one cerebral hemisphere beyond the other. A larger frontal (rostral) or caudal projection is usually coupled with a larger lateral extent of the more projecting hemisphere relative to the other. In humans, the posterior portion of the left hemisphere and, less strikingly, the anterior portion of the right hemisphere have been found to be commonly wider and to project further more often than their lateral counterparts. The concurrence of right frontal and left occipital petalias is common in most right-handed individuals (LeMay, 1976; LeMay & Kido, 1978).

Zilles *et al.* (1996a) reinvestigated this issue by using 3D reconstructions of 29 human brains (from 15 right-handed males and 14 left-handed males) and nine brains from common chimpanzees. Interactive or computerized procedures were used in order to separate the left and right hemispheres. Mirror images of the right hemisphere 3D reconstructions were created in order to fit the 3D reconstructions of both hemispheres on each other. The dimensions and the orientation of the left and mirrored right 3D reconstructions were normalized by the automated method described earlier in this chapter. For each sample, three 'mean' surfaces were then created. They included a mean left hemisphere surface, a mean right surface, and a mean generic (mixed left + right) surface. The distance of the respective voxels between left and (mirrored) right 3D reconstructions provided a measure of brain surface asymmetry. Statistically significant asymmetry was evaluated for all voxels with *t*-tests.

Results

The study of Zilles *et al.* (1996a) revealed left–right petalia patterns in humans. The directions of the petalia patterns observed in right-handed males were expected from previous studies (LeMay, 1976, 1977; LeMay & Kido, 1978; LeMay *et al.*, 1982; Falk *et al.*, 1991). A large part of the lateral surface of the left occipital lobe is wider than its right counterpart. The right hemisphere is wider in the frontal lobe on the lateral surface and in the rostral and dorsal parts of the temporal lobe. In the region of the upper motor and premotor cortex as well as in the parietal lobe, the lateral surface of the right hemisphere shows small patchy-like protrusions. The brains of right-handed men therefore show a set of localized asymmetries that comprise petalias as well as patchy protrusions located on the mesial and lateral cortical surfaces of the hemispheres.

It is the extrastriate visual cortex that shows the largest difference between the two hemispheres. In this region, the left hemisphere is wider than the right. The asymmetries are statistically significant on the mesial and lateral surfaces in the visual cortex (i.e. leftward asymmetries in striate and extrastriate areas), in regions of the prefrontal cortex (i.e. rightward asymmetries in areas 46 and 10), and in premotor cortex (rightward asymmetry in area 44). Asymmetries of the prefrontal cortex appear to be related to cognitive lateralization and handedness (for a review, see Zilles *et al.*, 1996a). Functional correlates of occipital cortex asymmetries require further investigation. The overall pattern of cortical shape asymmetries tends to be less pronounced in left-handed males. For instance, the occurence of frontal petalia in favor of the right hemisphere is significant in right-handed but not in left-handed males.

Compared with humans, the hemispheres of the chimpanzee brain appear to be relatively symmetrical. In pioneering studies, LeMay *et al.* (1982) suggested that asymmetries of ape brain shape tended to resemble those observed in humans. However, according to findings based on analysis of 135 great ape endocasts by Holloway & De la Coste-Lareymondie (1982), common chimpanzees tend to show very little brain shape asymmetries. Among great apes, only gorillas show clear asymmetries favoring left occipital, but not right frontal petalia patterns. The torque pattern (i.e. the combination of a left occipital and right frontal petalia) seems to be confined to *Homo*. Nevertheless, the study by Zilles *et al.* (1996a) in humans clearly shows that the left occipital petalia is a far more striking feature than the right frontal petalia (see also Fig. 10.2). In the more symmetric brains of left-handed individuals, it is the frontal petalia that vanishes. The situation regarding petalia patterns in gorillas therefore seems to be in continuity with the human situation.

Visualization by Zilles *et al.* (1996a) of the petalia pattern in humans, especially that of right-handers, contrasts to some extent with the classical definition (Le May & Kido, 1978, p. 471):

> (a) the left occipital pole is frequently wider and protrudes further posteriorly than the right; (b) the right frontal area often measures wider than the left, and the right frontal pole usually protrudes either as far forward as the left or extends beyond the left.

Zilles *et al.* (1996a) identified wider regions on the lateral and mesial surface of the hemispheres, but no clear rostral or caudal projection of the hemispheres beyond their lateral counterpart. Figure 10.2 illustrates these results based on the sample of 9 common chimpanzees used by Zilles *et al.* (1996a) and a sample from 32 right-handed men. The purpose of this Fig. is to offer a better visualization of the human petalia pattern in right-handed males. The left occipital petalia appears to be far more important than the right frontal one. In addition, most of the mesial surface of the left occipital lobe distorts the midline and protrudes into the right side, a situation that is commonly observed in human brains (Galaburda *et al.*, 1978a).

Planum temporale

In the classical anatomical nomenclature, the planum temporale (PT) refers to the plane area of the temporal bone (Toldt, 1921), but since the work of Geschwind & Levitsky (1968) this term widely refers to an area on the posterior superior temporal gyrus. This region is of particular interest for the study of structural correlates of cerebral functional asymmetries in humans. The planum temporale comprises higher-order auditory association cortex and constitutes the major part of classical 'Wernicke's language area' in the left hemisphere. In a majority of cases, the left PT is larger than the right. Geschwind & Levitsky (1968) examined the outside border of the planum temporale and found that 65 of the 100 randomly selected brains they examined had a larger left planum, 11 had the reverse asymmetry, and 24 had no bias. Studies on normal subjects support the assumption that PT (a)symmetry is related to functional lateralization (Steinmetz & Galaburda, 1991). The positive significant correlation between the degree of surface asymmetry of the planum temporale and the degree of volume asymmetry of the temporoparietal area Tpt (Galaburda *et al.*, 1978b) and angular gyrus area PG (Eidelberg & Galaburda, 1984) suggests linked asymmetries in language areas. Other results, however, suggest that the PT is likely to be involved in auditory processing more than in specifically linguistic functions (Binder *et al.*, 1996). Even so, processing of auditory features in the PT is probably highly elaborate, as witnessed by the exaggerated leftward PT asymmetry displayed by musicians with perfect pitch (Schlaug *et al.*, 1995).

Numerous other studies (see Geschwind, 1974; Galaburda, 1995; Galaburda *et al.*, 1990; Steinmetz, 1996; Shapleske *et al.*, 1999, for reviews) have confirmed that the left planum temporale is larger than the right in the majority of human brains, particularly in right-handed individuals.

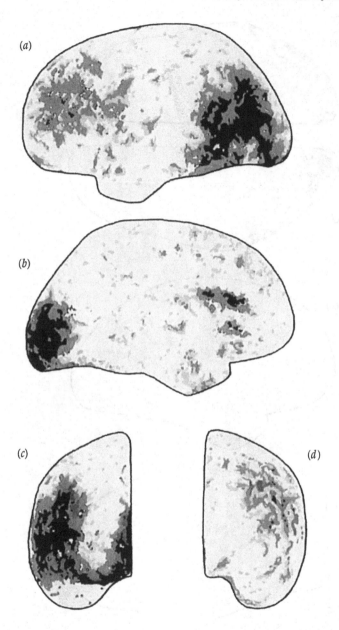

Fig. 10.2. Three-dimensional images of a mixed left and right hemisphere for humans (N = 32, a–f) and chimpanzees (N = 9, g–i). Different views of cortical shape asymmetries between left and right hemispheres are represented for male right-handed humans and chimpanzees: (a, g) lateral, (b, h) mesial, (c, i) caudal, (d, j) frontal, (e, k) dorsal and (f, l) ventral views. The brains were

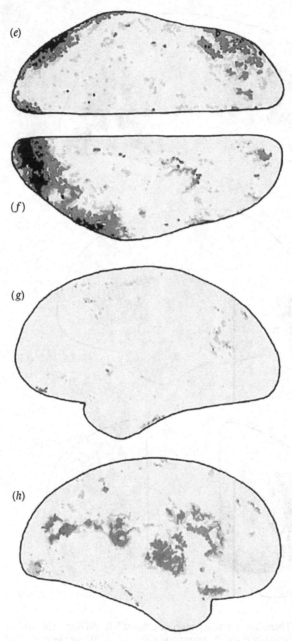

Fig. 10.2 (*cont.*)
reconstructed from T1-weighted images after MR scans. The differences in
patchy or confluent (petalia) local protrusions are displayed with a *t*-test
expressed with a 4 gray level code. White, *p*-value = 0.5 or more; light gray,

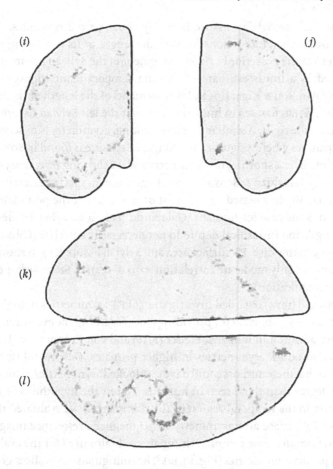

(i) *(j)* *(k)* *(l)*

p-value between 0.1 and 0.05; dark gray, p-value between 0.05 and 0.002; black, p-value = 0.001 or smaller. Significant cortical shape asymmetry between the two hemispheres is illustrated in dark gray and black. (The distance between the external brain surfaces of left and right hemispheres is approximately 0.75–2.50 mm.) The frontal (patchy) protrusions are in favor of the right hemisphere (frontal petalia), the parietal and occipital protrusions are in favor of the left hemisphere (occipital petalia). Note that the left occipital petalia appears to be far more striking than the right frontal petalia. Rostral or caudal projections of one hemisphere relative to the other are not clear features on these images. In addition, most of the mesial surface of the left occipital lobe is wider and protrudes into the right side. The petalia pattern is absent in chimpanzees.

The depth of the Sylvian fissure is nearly equal on the two sides. PT surface area is therefore proportional to the length of its outer margin. The length of the posterior horizontal segment of the Sylvian fissure has been used as a linear estimate of planum temporale anteroposterior extent by Witelson & Kigar (1992). Measurements of the length of the left and right Sylvian fissures in humans show that the left Sylvian fissure is longer than the right. A similar, but less striking, asymmetry is observed in chimpanzees where a significantly longer left fissure is found in 80% of the specimens, 12% showing no asymmetry and 8% showing reverse asymmetry (Yeni-Komshian & Benson, 1976). In nonhuman species, lateralization is generally less biased to the right or to the left at the population level than is the case for humans (Galaburda et al., 1990). Nevertheless, sulcal length and intrasulcal depth do not necessarily correlate (Gilissen et al., 1995). In this case, PT surface area and Sylvian fissure length show a significant but only moderate correlation ($r = 0.6$–0.7) (H. Steinmetz, personal communication).

Geschwind (1974) regarded investigation of PT asymmetries in higher primates as very important for providing clues regarding the evolution of brain lateralization in humans. Pfeifer (1936) and von Economo & Horn (1930) found no PT asymmetries in higher primates. Geschwind (1974) suggested that these authors could have overlooked asymmetries of much smaller degree than those seen in humans. To test the hypothesis of an asymmetry in the temporal region of the chimpanzee, we evaluated the degree of PT surface area asymmetry in 3D magnetic resonance images obtained from the same common chimpanzees brains used for the evaluation of petalia asymmetries (Fig. 10.3a). The contiguous brain slices generated using fast low-angle shot (FLASH) sequences show excellent gray matter–white matter contrast and are devoid of important distortion (see Steinmetz & Galaburda, 1991, for a review).

The anterior border of the PT is classically defined as Heschl's sulcus, which is the transverse sulcus caudal to Heschl's convolution. This definition of the anterior border of the PT is reliable between observers. As compared with monkeys, Heschl's convolution is a prominent structure in great apes and humans (Fig. 10.3a,b) (Geschwind, 1974; Gannon et al., 1998; Hopkins et al., 1998). The posterior border of the PT is defined as the posterior end of the horizontal segment of the Sylvian fissure. When present, the cortex buried in the posterior (terminal) ascending ramus of the Sylvian fissure is excluded from the measurements (Steinmetz, 1996). At least in humans, this definition of the PT posterior border is favored by

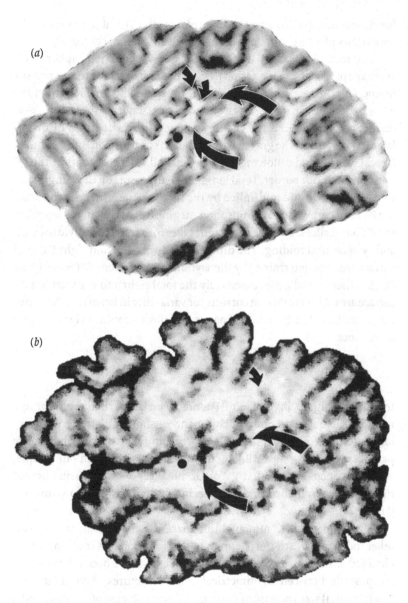

Fig. 10.3. Morphometry of the intrasylvian temporoparietal cortex on parasagittal magnetic resonance images of the right hemisphere of (a) common chimpanzee and (b) human. The anterior part of the brain is at the left; dot, the anterior (first) transverse gyrus of Heschl (H1); large arrows, the anterior and posterior borders of the planum temporale (PT); small arrows, the lower and upper end of the planum parietale (PP). Courtesy of Professor E.A. Cabanis (CHNO XV–XX, Paris).

functional data (Steinmetz & Galaburda, 1991). Critical appraisal of the boundaries of PT in humans is discussed by Shapleske *et al.* (1999).

Total surface area of PT was measured on each brain hemisphere with an image processing workstation ($N = 10$; five females, four males, one sex unknown) (Gilissen *et al.*, 1998). For this purpose, the total length of the PT was determined on a series of subsequent sagittal slices. On 14–16 images per hemisphere, the cursor was traced manually from medial to lateral slices within the gray matter of the PT, starting from the bottom of Heschl's sulcus and following all the gyral and sulcal contours of the PT until the posterior border. Total length measurements on each single slice were summed up and multiplied by the slice thickness in order to obtain the PT total surface area. PT morphometry measured the curved length of the PT on all slices. This measurement takes into account individual variability of cortical folding. The difference between left and right PT total surface area was determined by the asymmetry coefficient $dPT = (R - L)/0.5 (R + L)$, where R and L are respectively the total right and the total left PT surface area. This coefficient corrects for variability in brain size. Negative values indicate left PT predominance and positive values right PT predominance.

Results

In humans (Fig. 10.4*a*), the left PT tends to be larger than the right in a majority of subjects. Common chimpanzees showed a strong tendency for a left-larger-than-right PT approaching statistical significance (sample mean, −0.206; *t* Value, −1.690; *p* (1-tail), 0.062). In our sample, seven specimens showed left PT predominance, two specimens showed right PT predominance, and one specimen was very close to symmetry (Fig. 10.4*b*).

PT asymmetry in common chimpanzees has been evaluated in two other independent studies (Gannon *et al.*, 1998; Hopkins *et al.*, 1998) that obtained similar results (left-larger-than-right PT). Three relationships are possible between asymmetrical brain structures. Asymmetry can result from (1) size increase of one side, (2) size decrease of the other side, or (3) a combination of both (1) and (2). Based on 100 human cadaver brains, Galaburda *et al.* (1987) concluded that structural changes away from symmetry involved size decrease of one side (right PT) rather than size increase of the other (left PT). In this case, asymmetry would correspond to a reduced state compared to symmetry and would imply a

(a)

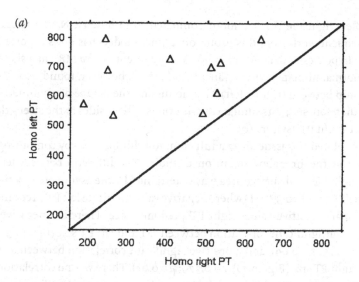

(b)

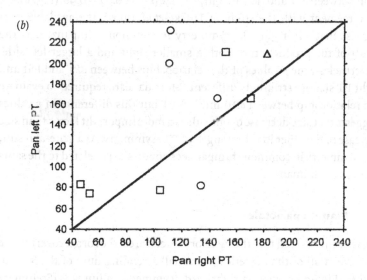

Fig. 10.4. (a) Surface area (mm²) of the left planum temporale (PT) plotted against the right PT for 10 randomly selected adult human cadaver brains (data from Steinmetz *et al.*, 1990). The diagonal represents equal left and right PT surface areas. The left PT is statistically significantly larger than the right one (asymmetry coefficient sample mean, −0.540; *t* value, −4.559; *p* (1-tail), 0.0007). (b) Surface area (mm²) of the left planum temporale (PT) plotted against the right PT for 10 adult common chimpanzee cadaver brains. The diagonal represents equal left and right PT surface areas. Circles, males; squares, females; triangle, unknown sex (asymmetry coefficient sample mean, −0.206; *t* value, −1.690; *p* (1-tail), 0.062).

smaller (right + left) PT amount compared to symmetry. Nevertheless, subsequent work from this group on animal models has not supported their hypothesis (Galaburda, 1994). A more recent *in vivo* MR analysis of 221 normal human subjects (Jäncke *et al.*, 1997), however, found no relationship between (right + left) PT amount and the degree of asymmetry and therefore suggests similar contributions of both sides to the strength of left–right PT asymmetry.

I explored this issue on 37 adult common chimpanzees by combining data from the three above-mentioned studies. The difference between left and right PT total surface area was determined by the asymmetry coefficient $dPT = (R-L)/0.5(R+L)$ where negative values indicate left PT predominance and positive values right PT predominance. There is a negative, albeit nonsignificant correlation between dPT and left PT size (Fig. 10.5*a*) ($r = -0.275$; $p = 0.09$), and a positive significant correlation between dPT and right PT size (Fig. 10.5*b*) ($r = 0.379$; $p = 0.02$). There was no correlation at all between dPT and (left + right) PT size ($r = 0.004$; $p = 0.98$) (Fig. 10.5*c*). In agreement with the study of Jäncke *et al.* (1997), the available data suggest that left–right PT asymmetry in common chimpanzees is the result of the production of both a smaller right and a larger left side. Nevertheless, the p values of the relationships between dPT and left and right PT size are strikingly different. More data are required to evaluate the relationship between dPT and left PT but this difference in p values suggests that size decrease of one side is a more important factor than size increase of the other in the strength of PT asymmetry. As a general result, PT asymmetry in common chimpanzees appears to be related to the same factors as in humans.

Planum parietale

It has been observed that the inferior parietal area, the cortex covering the posterior wall of the posterior (terminal) ascending limb of the Sylvian fissure (Fig. 10.3), shows a rightward asymmetry in humans (Steinmetz *et al.*, 1990; Jäncke *et al.*, 1994) (Fig. 10.6a). This region involves functions lateralized to the right hemisphere, such as attention or visual abilities. Measurements of the surface area of this region in common chimpanzees were realized on the same sample (Gilissen *et al.*, 1998) with the same method as for the PT surface area. When measurable, the planum parietale (PP) surface area was symmetrical in two chimpanzees, three chimpanzees showed a slight left PP predominance and four showed a right PP

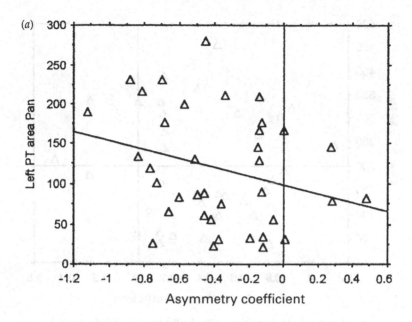

(a)

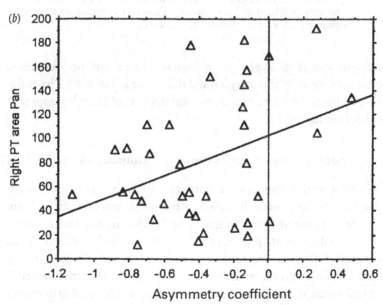

(b)

Fig. 10.5. (a) Relationship between left PT surface area and asymmetry coefficient (dPT) ($r = -0.275$; $p = 0.09$) (data from Gannon *et al.*, 1998; Hopkins *et al.*, 1998; and E.G. unpublished data). (b) Relationship between right PT surface area and asymmetry coefficient (dPT) ($r = 0.379$; $p = 0.02$) (data from Gannon *et al.*, 1998; Hopkins *et al.*, 1998; and E.G. unpublished data).

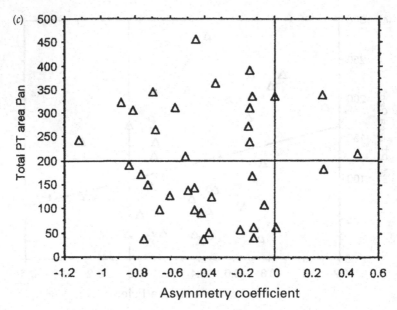

Fig. 10.5. (*cont.*) (*c*) Relationship between left + right PT surface area and asymmetry coefficient (*dPT*) (*r* = 0.004; *p* = 0.98) (data from Gannon *et al.*, 1998, Hopkins *et al.*, 1998; and E.G. unpublished data).

predominance (Fig. 10.6*b*). As in humans, there was no correlation between asymmetry of this region and that of the adjacent PT. The evolutionary histories of these two anatomical markers of laterality appear to be clearly independent.

A note on handedness in common chimpanzees

Brain structural asymmetries in humans are clearly related to handedness. Can this parameter be taken into account when studying brain structural asymmetries in chimpanzees? Results suggest that asymmetries in handedness are present in great apes, but further investigations are required that account for the over representation of some types of handedness measures in most studies. Moreover, the cognitive demands of a task influence the pattern of hand preference. The need to develop a common protocol that can be used to measure hand preferences across species is therefore a crucial requirement of this research (Hopkins & Morris, 1993). In a study of 30 common chimpanzees, Finch (1941) observed 800 reaches each performed on four different tasks. With a

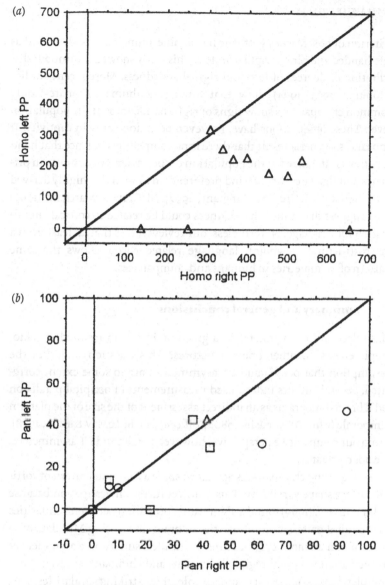

Fig. 10.6. (*a*) Surface area (mm²) of the left planum parietale (PP) plotted against the right PP for 10 randomly selected adult human cadaver brains (data from Steinmetz *et al.*, 1990). The diagonal represents equal left and right PP surface areas, three specimens have no left PP (asymmetry coefficient sample mean, 0.988; *t* value, 4.123; *p* (1-tail), 0.001). (*b*) Surface area (mm²) of the left planum parietale (PP) plotted against the right PP for 10 adult common chimpanzee cadaver brains. The diagonal represents equal left and right PT surface areas. Circles, males; squares, females; triangle, unknown sex; one specimen has no left nor right PP and one specimen has no left PP (asymmetry coefficient sample mean, 0.127; *t* value, 0.420; *p* (1-tail), 0.342).

criterion of 90% reaches with one hand, nine animals can be described as left-handed and nine as right-handed. This study shows a continuous distribution of degrees of left- and right-handedness. More recent studies (Hopkins, 1993, 1994) show that among nonhuman primates, only common chimpanzees show signs of right-handedness at the population level. These observations have, however, been done only in captivity. It appears as a general result that there is no compelling evidence that hand function is lateralized at the population or species level in nonhuman primates and that laterality of hand preference in humans is a highly derived characteristic (McGrew & Marchant, 1997). McGrew & Marchant (1997) then suggest that human handedness could be related to cortical lateralization for language. Nevertheless, our review shows that, at least from a macrostructural viewpoint, language related cortex shows the same pattern of asymmetries in humans and chimpanzees.

Summary and general conclusions

Has selection for asymmetry in a given brain region resulted in pleiotropic effects on other brain structures? This question underlies the assumption that petalia and PT asymmetries are to some extent correlated. Several authors indeed used measurements of occipital petalia on axial brain tomograms as an indirect assessment of the size of the planum temporale (Chui & Damasio, 1980; Koff et al., 1986; LeMay & Kido, 1978). From our comparative perspective, however, petalia and PT asymmetries are not correlated.

Humans and chimpanzees appear to share a common pattern of cortical surface shape variability. This requires further investigation because Lohmann et al. (1999) found a significant correlation between similarities in the sulcal pattern and similarities in brain shape using MRI data of 19 pairs of human monozygotic twins. Intrasulcal surface area asymmetries in the parietotemporal region in humans and chimpanzees, even if not completely similar at least in our sample, show striking similarities. This characteristic doesn't deserve to be considered as an epiphenomenon because in normal development, gyri formation serves largely to accomodate cortical connectivity (Dehay et al., 1996). Nevertheless, asymmetries of cortical shape, determined by 3D fitting of left and right hemispheres in humans and chimpanzees, show that the typical human pattern of fronto-occipital petalia is absent in chimpanzees. Moreover, if it is the degree of asymmetries which is the most biologically relevant variable, as has often been suggested (see, for instance, Schlaug *et al.*, 1995; Steinmetz, 1996), the intrasulcal asymmetries in the parietotemporal region in humans and chimpanzees show, at least in our sample, striking differences (but see Gannon *et al.*, 1998; Hopkins *et al.*, 1998). The tendency of common chimpanzees to show humanlike PT and PP asymmetries suggests, in any case, that the onset of morphological asymmetry of language areas is part of an evolutionary process that has not been limited to humans (see also Gannon *et al.*, 1998; Hopkins *et al.*, 1998).

The combination of a left occipital and right frontal petalia appears to remain the only human specific pattern of asymmetry. In contrast with humans, right frontal petalia seems to be a more striking structural asymmetry than left occipital petalia in macaques (Falk *et al.*, 1990; Cheverud *et al.*, 1990). In gorillas, Holloway & De La Coste-Lareymondie (1982) identified clear asymmetries favoring the left occipital, but not the right frontal petalial pattern. The petalial pattern in gorillas seems to be in continuity with the human situation where a left occipital petalia is a far more striking feature than a right frontal petalia (Zilles *et al.*, 1996a; Fig. 10.2). The absence of petalia in chimpanzees may therefore represent another species-specific characteristic, the functional significance of which remains to be elucidated. It seems, at least, to be possible to conclude tentatively from this comparative review that patterns of asymmetries are not intercorrelated and that humans show an extreme stage of 'mosaic' structural asymmetries, when compared with chimpanzees and probably with gorillas.

Are brains built economically? This paraphrase of Ewald R. Weibel (1998) leads to the question of whether brain asymmetries represent an example of optimization of biological design. Brain structural asymmetries subserve functions and it can be argued that structures should be matched to functional requirements (Schmidt-Nielsen, 1998). It is, however, impossible to quantify the optimized relationship between a given structure and a given function because a structure can subserve several functions, and a function can be related to several structural substrates. It is therefore essential to establish the dominant function of a given structure. Asymmetries in the parietotemporal region provide an example of a structural feature that seems likely to have evolved in the common ancestor of chimpanzees and humans about 8 million years ago (Gannon *et al.*, 1998). However, a cross-species definition of the functions subserved by brain structural asymmetries still eludes our understanding. Moreover, species-specific behaviors may have arisen from very small changes in neuronal circuits (Katz & Harris-Warrick, 1999). At least a further step could be reached by addressing the question of gender differences with respect to brain organization in general (see Falk, Chapter 5, this volume) and to brain lateralization in particular (Amunts *et al.*, 2000) in great apes brains.

Acknowledgments

The author thanks K. Zilles, A. Dabringhaus, K. Amunts, A. Schleicher, T. Schormann (C.&O. Vogt-Institute of Brain Research, Düsseldorf, Germany), G. Schlaug (Department of Neurology, Beth Israel Deaconess Hospital, Boston), J. Rademacher, E. Rädisch (Department of Neurology, University of Düsseldorf), H. Steinmetz (Department of Neurology, University of Frankfurt am Main), E.A. Cabanis (Centre Hospitalier National d'Ophtalmologie des XV-XX, Paris), M. Mann (University of Nebraska Medical Center, Omaha, Nebraska), J.M. Allman (California Institute of Technology), J. Maina, J.C. Allan, and M. Broekman (University of the Witwatersrand Medical School) for their help and support in various parts of this work. MR scans were carried out by G. Schlaug, E. Rädisch, H. Steinmetz, and E.A. Cabanis. Image processing was realized by A. Dabringhaus. All the topics presented in this review were developed during postdoctoral stages in the Centre Hospitalier National d'Ophtalmologie des XV-XX, in the C.&O. Vogt-Institute of Brain Research, and in the California Institute of Technology. I especially express my deepest gratitude to Professor Emmanuel A. Cabanis and to Professor Karl Zilles. I started to work on brain structure variability with Professor Cabanis and became aware of the importance of brain shape as a structural parameter with Professor Zilles, who encouraged me to work on comparative aspects of brain structure. However, all weaknesses of this review are entirely my own responsibility.

References

Aboitiz, F., Scheibel, A.B. & Zaidel, E. (1992a). Morphometry of the sylvian fissure and the corpus callosum, with emphasis on sex differences. *Brain*, 115, 1521–1541.

Aboitiz, F., Scheibel, A.B., Fisher, R.S. & Zaidel, E. (1992b). Individual differences in brain asymmetries and fiber composition in the human corpus callosum. *Brain Research*, 598, 154–161.

Amunts, K., Jäncke, L., Mohlberg, H., Steinmetz, H. & Zilles, K. (2000). Interhemispheric asymmetry of the human motor cortex related to handedness and gender. *Neuropsychologia*, 38, 304–312.

Anderson, B. (1999). Commentary – Ringo, Doty, Demeter and Simard, *Cerebral Cortex* 1994; 4: 331–343: A proof of the need for the spatial clustering of interneuronal connections to enhance cortical computation. *Cerebral Cortex*, **9**, 2–3.

Armstrong, E. (1990). Evolution of the brain. In *The Human Nervous System*, ed. G. Paxinos, pp. 1–16. New York: Academic Press.

Bailey, P., von Bonin, G. & McCulloch, W. (1950). *The Isocortex of the Chimpanzee*. Urbana: The University of Illinois Press.

Beecher, M.D., Petersen, M.R., Zoloth, S.R., Moody, D.B. & Stebbins, W.C. (1979). Perception of conspecific vocalizations by japanese macaques. Evidence for selective attention and neural lateralization. *Brain Behavior and Evolution*, **16**, 443–460.

Binder, J.R., Frost, J.A., Hammeke, T.A., Rao, S.M. & Cox, R.W. (1996). Function of the left planum temporale in auditory and linguistic processing. *Brain*, **119**, 1239–1247.

Bryden, M.P. (1982). *Laterality, Functional Asymmetry in the Intact Brain*. New York: Academic Press.

Cheverud, J., Falk, D., Hildebolt, C., Moore, A.J., Helmkamp, R.C. & Vannier, M. (1990). Heritability and association of cortical petalias in rhesus macaques (*Macaca mulatta*). *Brain, Behavior, and Evolution*, **35**, 368–372.

Chui, H.C. & Damasio, A.R. (1980). Human cerebral asymmetries evaluated by computed tomography. *Journal of Neurology, Neurosurgery, and Psychiatry*, **43**, 873–878.

Dabringhaus, A., Schormann, T., Schleicher, A., Zilles, K., Schlaug, G. & Steinmetz, H. (1994a). Interindividuelle Variabilität des menschlichen Gehirns: Cortexoberfläche, Corpus callosum und CA-CP-Linie. *Annals of Anatomy*, **176** (Suppl.), 285.

Dabringhaus, A., Schormann, T., Schlaug, G., Steinmetz, H. & Zilles, K. (1994b). Variabilität der Cortexoberfläche beim Menschen in Abhängigkeit von Geschlecht und genetischer Konkordanz. *Annals of Anatomy*, **176** (Suppl.), 61.

Deacon, T.W. (1988). Human brain evolution: II. Embryology and brain allometry. In *Intelligence and Evolutionary Biology*, eds. H.J. Jerison & I. Jerison, pp. 383–416. Berlin: Springer Verlag.

Dehay, C., Giroud, P., Berland, M., Killackey, H. & Kennedy, H. (1996). Contribution of thalamic input to the specification of cytoarchitectonic cortical fields in the primate: effects of bilateral enucleation in the fetal monkey on the boundaries, dimensions, and gyrification of striate and extrastriate cortex. *The Journal of Comparative Neurology*, **67**, 70–89.

Deinard, A. & Kidd, K. (1999). Evolution of a HOXB6 intergenic region within the great apes and humans. *Journal of Human Evolution*, **36**, 687–703.

Eidelberg, D. & Galaburda, A.M. (1984). Inferior parietal lobule. Divergent architectonic asymmetries in the human brain. *Archives of Neurology*, **41**, 843–852.

Falk, D. (1987a). Hominid paleoneurology. *Annual Review of Anthropology*, **16**, 13–30.

Falk, D. (1987b). Brain lateralization in primates and its evolution in hominids. *Yearbook of Physical Anthropology*, **30**, 107–125.

Falk, D., Hildebolt, C., Cheverud, J., Vannier, M., Helmkamp, R.C. & Konigsberg, L. (1990). Cortical asymmetries in frontal lobes of rhesus monkeys (*Macaca mulatta*). *Brain Research*, **512**, 40–45.

Falk, D., Hildebolt, C., Cheverud, J., Kohn, L.A.P., Figiel, G. & Vannier, M. (1991).

Human cortical asymmetries determined with 3D MR technology. *Journal of Neuroscience Methods*, **39**, 185–191.

Filimonoff, I.N. (1933). Über die Variabilität der Grosshirnrindenstruktur. Mitteilung III: Regio occipitalis bei den höheren und niederen Affen. *Journal für Psychologie und Neurologie*, **45**, 69–137.

Finch, G. (1941). Chimpanzee handedness. *Science*, **94**, 117–118.

Fitch, R.H., Brown, C.P., O'Connor, K. & Tallal, P. (1993). Functional lateralization for auditory temporal processing in male and female rats. *Behavioral Neuroscience*, **107**, 844–850.

Frahm, H., Stephan, H. & Baron, G. (1984). Comparison of brain structure volumes in Insectivora and Primates. V. Area striata (AS). *Journal für Hirnforschung*, **25**, 537–557.

Galaburda, A.M. (1994). Developmental dyslexia and animal studies: at interface between cognition and neurology. *Cognition*, **50**, 133–149.

Galaburda, A.M. (1995). Anatomic basis of dominance. In *Brain Asymmetry*, eds. R.J. Davidson & K. Hugdahl, pp. 51–73. Cambridge, Massachussets: MIT Press.

Galaburda, A.M., LeMay, M., Kemper, T.L. & Geschwind, N. (1978a). Right-left asymmetries in the brain. *Science*, **199**, 852–856.

Galaburda, A.M., Sanides, F. & Geschwind, N. (1978b). Human brain. Cytoarchitectonic left–right asymmetries in the temporal speech region. *Archives of Neurology*, **35**, 812–817.

Galaburda, A.M., Corsiglia, J., Rosen, G.D. & Sherman, G.F. (1987). Planum Temporale asymmetry, reappraisal since Geschwind and Levitsky. *Neuropsychologia*, **25**, 853–868.

Galaburda, A.M., Rosen, G.D. & Sherman, G.F. (1990). Individual variability in cortical organization: its relationship to brain laterality and implications to function. *Neuropsychologia*, **28**, 529–546.

Gannon, P.J., Holloway, R.L., Broadfield, D.C. & Braun, A.R. (1998). Asymmetry of chimpanzee Planum Temporale: humanlike pattern of Wernicke's brain language area homolog. *Science*, **279**, 220–222.

Geschwind, N. (1974). The anatomical basis of hemispheric differentiation. In *Hemisphere Function in the Human Brain*, eds. S.J. Diamond & J.G. Beaumont, pp. 7–24. London: Elek Science.

Geschwind, N. & Levitsky, W. (1968). Human brain: left–right asymmetries in temporal speech region. *Science*, **161**, 186–187.

Gibson, K.R., Rumbaugh, D. & Byrne, R. (1998). Bigger is better: primate brain size in relationship to cognition. *American Journal of Physical Anthropology Supplement*, **26**, 101.

Gilissen, E. (1992). The neocortical sulci of the capuchin monkey (*Cebus*): evidence for asymmetry in the sylvian sulcus and comparison with other primates. *Comptes Rendus de l'Académie des Sciences Paris, Série III*, **314**, 165–170.

Gilissen, E., Iba-Zizen, M.-T., Stievenart, J.-L., Lopez, A., Trad, M., Cabanis, E.A. & Zilles, K. (1995). Is the length of the calcarine sulcus associated with the size of the human visual cortex? A morphometric study with magnetic resonance tomography. *Journal of Brain Research*, **36**, 451–459.

Gilissen, E. & Zilles, K. (1995). The relative volume of the primary visual cortex and its intersubject variability among humans: a new morphometric study. *Comptes Rendus de l'Académie des Sciences Paris, Série 2a*, **320**, 897–902.

Gilissen, E. & Zilles, K. (1996). The calcarine sulcus as an estimate of the total volume of the human striate cortex: A morphometric study of reliability and intersubject variability. *Journal of Brain Research*, **37**, 57–66.

Gilissen, E., Amunts, K., Schlaug, G. & Zilles, K. (1998). Left-right asymmetries in the temporoparietal intrasylvian cortex of common chimpanzees. *American Journal of Physical Anthropology Supplement*, **26**, 86.

Glick, S. D. (1985). *Cerebral Lateralization in Nonhuman Species*. New York: Academic Press.

Hadziselimovic, H. & Cus, M. (1966). The appearance of internal structures of the brain in relation to configuration of the human skull. *Acta Anatomica*, **63**, 289–299.

Holloway, R. L. & De La Coste-Lareymondie, M.-C. (1982). Brain endocast asymmetry in pongids and hominids: some preliminary findings on the paleontology of cerebral dominance. *American Journal of Physical Anthropology*, **58**, 101–110.

Hopkins, W. D. (1993). Posture and reaching in chimpanzees (*Pan troglodytes*) and orangutans (*Pongo pygmaeus*). *Journal of Comparative Psychology*, **107**, 162–168.

Hopkins, W. D. (1994). Hand preferences for bimanual feeding in 140 captive chimpanzees (*Pan troglodytes*): rearing and ontogenetic determinants. *Developmental Psychology*, **27**, 395–407.

Hopkins, W. D. & Morris, R. D. (1993). Handedness in great apes: a review of findings. *International Journal of Primatology*, **14**, 1–25.

Hopkins, W. D., Marino, L., Rilling, J. K. & MacGregor, L. A. (1998). Planum Temporale asymmetries in great apes as revealed by MRI. *Neuroreport*, **9**, 2913–2918.

Jäncke, L., Schlaug, G., Huang, Y. & Steinmetz, H. (1994). Asymmetry of the Planum Parietale. *NeuroReport*, **5**, 1161–1163.

Jäncke, L., Preis, S., Huang, Y. & Steinmetz, H. (1997). Relationship between size and asymmetry of right vs. left Planum Temporale. *Society for Neuroscience Abstracts*, **23**, 1059.

Katz, P. S. & Harris-Warrick, R. M. (1999). The evolution of neuronal circuits underlying species-specific behavior. *Current Opinion in Neurobiology*, **9**, 628–633.

Kennedy, D. N., Lange, N., Makris, N., Bates, J., Meyer, J. & Caviness, Jr, V. S. (1998). Gyri of the human neocortex: an MRI-based analysis of volume and variance. *Cerebral Cortex*, **8**, 372–384.

Koff, E., Naeser, M. A., Pieniadz, J. M., Foundas, A. L. & Levine, H. L. (1986). Computed tomographic scan hemispheric asymmetries in right- and left-handed male and female subjects. *Archives of Neurology*, **43**, 487–491.

Lacreuse, A. (1997). Latéralité chez l'animal. *Annales de la Fondation Fyssen*, **12**, 41–51.

LeMay, M. (1976). Morphological cerebral asymmetries of modern man, fossil man, and nonhuman primates. *Annals of the New York Academy of Sciences*, **280**, 349–366.

LeMay, M. (1977). Asymmetries of the skull and handedness. Phrenology revisited. *Journal of the Neurological Sciences*, **32**, 243–253.

LeMay, M. & Kido, D. K. (1978). Asymmetries of the cerebral hemispheres on computed tomograms. *Journal of Computer Assisted Tomography*, **2**, 471–476.

LeMay, M., Billig, M. S. & Geschwind, N. (1982). Asymmetries of the brain and skulls of nonhuman primates. In *Primate Brain Evolution*, eds. E. Armstrong & D. Falk, pp. 263–277. New York and London, Plenum Press.

Lewis, D. W. & Diamond, M. C. (1995). The influence of gonadal steroids on the asymmetry of the cerebral cortex. In *Brain Asymmetry*, eds. R. J. Davidson & K. Hugdahl, pp. 31–50. Cambridge, Massachussets: MIT Press.

Lohmann, G., von Cramon, D. Y. & Steinmetz, H. (1999) Sulcal variability of twins. *Cerebral Cortex*, **9**, 754–763.

McGrew, W.C. & Marchant, L.F. (1997). On the other hand: current issues in and meta-analysis of the behavioral laterality of hand function in nonhuman primates. *Yearbook of Physical Anthropology*, **40**, 201–232.

Perecman, E. (1983). *Cognitive Processing in the Right Hemisphere.* Toronto: Academic Press.

Petersen, M.R., Beecher, M.D., Zoloth, S.R., Moody, D.B. & Stebbins, W.C. (1978). Neural lateralization of species-specific vocalizations by japanese macaques (*Macaca fuscata*). *Science*, **202**, 324–327.

Pfeifer, R.A. (1936). Pathologie der Hörstrahlung und der corticalen Hörsphäre. In *Handbuch der Neurologie, Vol. VI*, eds. O. Bumke & O. Foerster. Berlin: Springer.

Raya, S.P. & Udupa, J.K. (1990). Shape-based interpolation of multidimensional objects. *IEEE Transactions of Medical Imaging*, **9**, 32–42.

Ringo, J.L., Doty, R.W., Demeter, S. & Simard, P.Y. (1994). Time is of the essence: a conjecture that hemispheric specialization arises from interhemispheric conduction delay. *Cerebral Cortex*, **4**, 331–343.

Ruvolo, M. (1997). Molecular phylogeny of the hominoids: inferences from multiple independent DNA data sets. *Molecular Biology and Evolution*, **14**, 248–265.

Rumbaugh, D.M., Savage-Rumbaugh, S. & Washburn, D.A. (1996). Toward a new outlook on primate learning and behavior: complex learning and emergent processes in comparative perspective. *Japanese Psychological Research*, **38**, 113–125.

Schlaug, G., Jäncke, L., Huang, Y. & Steinmetz, H. (1995). In vivo evidence of structural brain asymmetry in musicians. *Science*, **267**, 699–701.

Schmidt-Nielsen, K. (1998). How much structure is enough? In *Principles of Animal Design. The Optimization and Symmorphosis Debate*, eds. E.R. Weibel, C.R. Taylor & L. Bolis, pp. 11–12. Cambridge: Cambridge University Press.

Shapleske, J., Rossell, S.L., Woodruff, P.W.R. & David, A.S. (1999). The planum temporale: a systematic, quantitative review of its structural, functional and clinical significance. *Brain Research Reviews*, **29**, 26–49.

Steinmetz, H. (1996). Structure, function and cerebral asymmetry: in vivo morphometry of the planum temporale. *Neuroscience and Biobehavioral Reviews*, **20**, 587–591.

Steinmetz, H. & Galaburda, A.M. (1991). Planum Temporale asymmetry: in-vivo morphometry affords a new perspective for neuro-behavioral research. *Reading and Writing: An Interdisciplinary Journal*, **3**, 331–343.

Steinmetz, H., Rademacher, J., Jäncke, L., Huang, Y., Thron, A. & Zilles, K. (1990). Total surface of temporoparietal intrasylvian cortex: diverging left–right asymmetries. *Brain and Language*, **39**, 357–372.

Toldt, C. (1921). *Anatomischer Atlas für Studierende und Ärzte.* Berlin: Urban & Schwarzenberg.

von Economo, C. & Horn, L. (1930). Über Windungsrelief, Masse, und Rindenarchitektonik der Supratemporalfläche. *Zeitschrift der Gesellschaft für Neurologie und Psychiatrie*, **130**, 678–757.

Weibel, E.R. (1998). Symmorphosis and optimization of biological design: introduction and questions. In *Principles of Animal Design. The Optimization and Symmorphosis Debate*, eds. E.R. Weibel, C.R. Taylor & L. Bolis, pp. 1–10. Cambridge: Cambridge University Press.

Witelson, S.F. & Kigar, D.L. (1988). Asymmetry in brain function follows asymmetry in anatomical form: gross, microscopic, postmortem and imaging studies. In

Handbook of Neuropsychology, vol. 1, eds. F. Boller & J. Grafman, pp. 111–142. Amsterdam: Elsevier.

Witelson, S.F. & Kigar, D.L. (1992). Sylvian fissure morphology and asymmetry in men and women: bilateral differences in relation to handedness in men. *Journal of Comparative Neurology*, **323**, 326–340.

Wynn, T.G., Tierson, F.D. & Palmer, C.T. (1996). Evolution of sex differences in spatial cognition. *Yearbook of Physical Anthropology*, **39**, 11–42.

Yeni-Komshian, G.H. & Benson, D.A. (1976). Anatomical study of cerebral asymmetry in the temporal lobe of humans, chimpanzees, and rhesus monkeys. *Science*, **192**, 387–389.

Zilles, K., Dabringhaus, A., Geyer, S., Amunts, K., Qü, M., Schleicher, A., Gilissen, E., Schlaug, G. & Steinmetz, H. (1996a). Structural asymmetries in the human forebrain and the forebrain of non-human primates and rats. *Neuroscience and Biobehavioral Reviews*, **20**, 593–605.

Zilles, K., Falkai, P., Schormann, T., Steinmetz, H. & Palomero-Gallagher, N. (1996b). Cortical surface in schizophrenic patients and controls: MRI, 3-D reconstruction and *in vivo* morphometry. *Neuroimage*, **3**, S525.

Zilles, K., Schormann, T., Steinmetz, H. & Falkai, P. (1998). Shape of cortical surface in schizophrenics. *European Journal of Neuroscience*, **10**, Suppl. 10, 328.

11
_____

Language areas of the hominoid brain: a dynamic communicative shift on the upper east side planum

Recently it was demonstrated that brains of chimpanzees (*Pan troglodytes*) show a humanlike differentially enlarged left planum temporale, an area that in humans is part of the receptive 'language' region of the cerebral cortex (Gannon *et al.*, 1998b). This new finding addressed a highly controversial issue within the disciplines of neurology, neurobiology, evolutionary biology, anthropology, linguistics and psychology, to name but a few. Prior to this finding it had been widely accepted that pronounced hemispheric asymmetry of this brain language region was unique to humans and, as such, could readily have been included as a component within the pervasive 'human language organ' (linguistics-based) concept formulated by Noam Chomsky (Chomsky, 1972). Not surprisingly, this prospective paradigm shift gave rise to many new questions and criticisms. For example, it is not clear whether this left hemisphere-lateralized language region is as remarkable in other closely related primates, particularly other great apes, but also lesser apes and even Old World monkeys. Based upon a century of human studies, it would appear reasonable to hypothesize that the markedly asymmetric planum temporale is involved with ape 'language' or other species specific, interindividual communication modalities. However, although this region is markedly anatomically lateralized to the left hemisphere in apes, it may not be functionally analogous. Further, as recent studies (Binder *et al.*, 1996) have suggested, the planum temporale may not be involved with high-level receptive language processing in humans but may simply represent an early stage relay station. Perhaps this feature shared by humans and apes is not as remarkable as we have proposed. Future studies should address this comparative functionality issue.

Gross anatomic evidence of hemispheric lateralization of the planum temporale homolog, area Tpt in more distantly related primates such as Old World monkeys, has not been clearly demonstrated (Galaburda *et al.*, 1978b). However, this may be due to the limitations of methods and approaches that were utilized. It is entirely possible that the planum temporale/Tpt and other language region homologs might be functionally lateralized for semantic-level communication at the cognitive level of other species. As such, anatomic, behavioral, functional or other comparative evidence, within an inclusive multidisciplinary approach, should be used to discern where and at what level, such functionally pertinent cortical asymmetries originated.

The common ancestor of chimpanzees, bonobos and modern humans that lived within the *'East Side Story'*, a New York City characterization of the East African Rift Valley (Coppens, 1994) may have utilized this brain region for language/communication. Subsequently, environmental influences might have catalyzed a rapid differentiation of the unique form of human language. Here we portray the planum temporale, located on the upper east side of the temporal lobe superior surface, as the result of synchronous temporal events that took place on the Rift Valley five to eight million years ago. Within this evolutionary context, it would be important to investigate whether human brain language areas are 'hard wired' within the vocal/auditory (speaking/hearing) mode of communication or are modality equipotential and demonstrate plasticity in combination with the gestural/visual modality. As discussed below, studies of congenitally deaf, sign language (gestural/visual) using humans indicate that such plasticity may be inherent to the human condition. Further investigation of factors and repercussions related to brain language area evolution would represent a novel and productive endeavor. Provocative issues such as these may offer further insight into both the functional plasticity and evolution of human brain language areas and the underlying suite of modules and mechanisms that may be even more broadly based within primates than previously thought.

Anatomy, function and plasticity of receptive language areas in humans

Human brain receptive language regions were originally characterized in the wake of nineteenth century phrenologic principles, but were clearly more scientifically based on the array of neurological, communicative

deficits that arose from traumatic or cerebrovascular lesions of the cerebral cortex. At that time lesion sites and magnitude were documented
postmortem, often a long time after they occurred. As such, the discipline
of aphasiology emerged and the often inclusive term 'Wernicke's aphasia'
was inaugurated by one of the earliest workers, Carl Wernicke, in his
landmark work '*Der Aphasische Symptomenkomplex*' (Wernicke, 1874). The
peak of aphasiology was in the twentieth century, but use of this powerful, natural lesion-based approach continues, often in conjunction with
new technologies such as anatomic and functional imaging (Damasio,
1992). It is important to note that aphasias still represent the earliest
neurological manifestation of impaired language functions and as such
are a key initial component used to localize lesions prior to utilization of
modern diagnostic techniques such as computerized tomography (Porta-
Etessam *et al.*, 1997).

Subsequently, around the mid-twentieth century, as delineated com-
prehensively in a classic monograph '*Speech and Brain Mechanisms*' (Penfield
& Roberts, 1959), intraoperative electrocortical stimulation mapping
(IESM) techniques were used. This ground breaking new approach
involved micro electrical stimulation of exposed cortical surface areas in
awake, alert individuals that were undergoing brain surgery to remove
lesions adjacent to brain language areas. Temporary language deficits
that arose upon stimulation of specific left hemisphere cortical areas provided detailed information related both to the potential for surgical
sparing of these regions as well their precise regional localization and
variation. This method was developed in the 1980s and became incorporated into broader approaches (Howard *et al.*, 2000; Simos *et al.*, 1999b).
More recently, imaging techniques such as positron emission tomography (PET) and functional magnetic resonance imaging (fMRI) have been
used extensively and have further expanded, refined and altered our
understanding of these brain regions (Damasio, 1997; Fitch *et al.*, 1997;
Karbe *et al.*, 1995; Paus *et al.*, 1996; Semrud-Clikeman, 1997; Tallal *et al.*,
1998; Tzourio *et al.*, 1998; Zatorre *et al.*, 1996, 1998). However, comparisons
of techniques such as fMRI and IESM may or may not produce similar
results and thus reflect technical differences between these approaches
(Modayur *et al.*, 1997; Roux *et al.*, 1999; Schlosser *et al.*, 1999; Simos *et al.*,
1999a).

Left hemisphere predominance of the planum temporale is more pronounced than any other example of human brain interhemispheric asymmetry. An early landmark study of planum temporale anatomic

asymmetry in humans (Geschwind & Levitsky, 1968) subsequently gave rise to a large number of studies on this region of the cerebral cortex (Barta *et al.*, 1995; Foundas *et al.*, 1994; Galaburda, 1993; Galaburda *et al.*, 1978b; Jancke *et al.*, 1994; Jancke & Steinmetz, 1993; Preis *et al.*, 1999; Shapleske *et al.*, 1999; Shenton *et al.*, 1995; Steinmetz, 1996; Steinmetz *et al.*, 1989, 1991; Takami *et al.*, 1993; Westbury *et al.*, 1999; Yamadori *et al.*, 1982; Zatorre *et al.*, 1998). It is still widely accepted that asymmetry of this brain region is unique to humans and human language (e.g., Anderson *et al.*, 1999; Preis *et al.*, 1999; Shapleske *et al.*, 1999; Tzourio *et al.*, 1998). The planum temporale, a component of auditory association cortex in direct association with the primary auditory cortex located within Heschl's gyrus on the left hemisphere, represents an important initial site within Wernicke's posterior receptive language area. In essence, planum temporale may be the first down-line integrator and executor of mosaic (vocal-auditory and/or gestural-visual) communicative information that is distributed among complex cognitive associative components within discrete elements of the temporal, parietal and frontal lobe association cortices. As discussed below, although planum temporale is the major component of auditory association cortex, it may be equipotential with regard to its role in production and comprehension of both spoken and signed human languages and perhaps gestural components in both modalities.

Because it has now been demonstrated that left hemisphere predominance of planum temporale is also present in chimpanzees and other great apes, the evolutionary and functional significance of this purported key language area in humans should be reappraised (Gannon *et al.*, 1998a,b; Hopkins *et al.*, 1998b). However, there are a series of outstanding questions with regard to the precise role of planum temporale within the current inclusive concept of Wernicke's receptive language area. For example, even in speaking/hearing humans it is not clear to what degree planum temporale is involved with processing reception or even production of language (Barta *et al.*, 1995). Unfortunately, one of the confounding variables associated with designation of specific functions to language area subregions such as planum temporale may be the complex, dynamic and potentially intangible nature of regional interactions. Aphasia-producing lesions are rarely, if ever, limited to a subregion such as the planum temporale and the nature of tasks for functional imaging studies may be either too specific or global and range from single words to whole sentences (e.g., Muller *et al.*, 1999; Price *et al.*, 1996). However, after more than a century of aphasiology and the application of techniques such as electrophysiology and functional imaging, it is generally well accepted that there is considerable intercommunication both within and between language production and reception sites (Romanski *et al.*, 1999). Further, human 'language' is modally independent, and as such may be spoken/heard, signed/seen, written/seen, brailled/touched or transmitted/received in an almost limitless diversity of ways as witnessed recently during a digital technology-driven special lecture at the White House (Hawkin, 1998; http://www.intel.com/intel/community/hawkins.htm). It has yet to be determined, however, whether the same brain language areas used to communicate via this wide diversity of modalities in humans are used for species-specific communicative tasks in nonhuman primates such as chimpanzees and bonobos.

In addition to compelling questions regarding the specific role of planum temporale in human and chimpanzee 'languages', there are a number of other outstanding issues. For example, even though it has been proposed (Binder *et al.*, 1996) that the planum temporale is likely only involved in early auditory processing, while specifically linguistic functions are mediated by polymodal association areas distributed elsewhere in the left hemisphere, is the planum temporale used for such (lower level) language functions in the deaf-from-birth, sign language using population? In fact, are Heschl's gyrus and the planum temporale developed to the same degree, and if so, does the planum temporale demonstrate left hemisphere predominant asymmetry in deaf individuals? Although a recent sign language aphasia study did not address directly the role of the planum temporale, it was concluded that left hemisphere dominance for language is not driven by physical characteristics of the linguistic signal or motor aspects of its production, but rather stem from higher-order properties of the system (Hickok *et al.*, 1996). Similarly, another sign language study concluded there are strong biological constraints that render these particular brain areas well designed to process linguistic information independently of the linguistic structure or the modality of language (Neville *et al.*, 1998). These authors also reported that American sign language users and English speakers activate classic left hemisphere language areas with some right hemisphere region homotype activation in signers. Interestingly, in a recent lecture, Neville also reported a preliminary finding that primary auditory cortex in the left hemisphere was activated during American sign language perception in deaf from birth individuals (Neville, 1998). Although concurrent activation of the planum temporale was not reported or addressed, participation of this adjacent auditory association site was implied.

In support of this compelling concept of regional polymodal equipotential, many studies have indicated a role for the visual modality in 'language' tasks. For example, it has been shown that (visual) reading and sentence processing takes place in the perisylvian association cortex (Just *et al.*, 1996). Similarly, it was demonstrated that (visual) lip-reading both augmented speech perception and independently activated auditory cortex (Calvert *et al.*, 1997). A subsequent study demonstrated that speech perception, via the vocal auditory channel, was significantly enhanced when the speaker's face was visible even though the listener was not a proficient lip reader (Calvert *et al.*, 1999). Similarly, it was noted that regions in the superior temporal sulcus were activated by viewing eye and mouth movements which, it was suggested, may be functionally related to nearby regions involved with lip-reading and perception of hand and body movement (Puce *et al.*, 1998). Further, a recent PET study demonstrated left planum temporale involvement in processing unvoiced/whispered (masked – thus inaudible) speech (Paus *et al.*, 1996). Other examples of non-auditory, potentially polymodal activation of brain language areas include demonstration of cortical activity which underlies 'inner voices' or auditory hallucinations that have no discernible motor or audible components, located in Broca's area or auditory association areas (Suzuki *et al.*, 1993). Similarly, within the occipital lobe, visual cortex was activated in blind individuals via Braille-somatosensory stimulation (Cohen *et al.*, 1997; Sadato *et al.*, 1996). Interestingly, a recent review concluded that current evidence supported the notion that cross-modal reorganization did not occur only in individuals that were deaf or blind from birth and that such neural plasticity may take place in the adult human brain (Kujala *et al.*, 2000).

These studies of auditory and visual cortices indicate an inherent cross-modal plasticity that may have broad evolutionary implications. The specific role that is played by planum temporale within the complex functional mosaic of Wernicke's language area in humans or other primates using the speaking/hearing or gestural/visual modalities is not as yet fully elucidated. However, we consider that the evidence for a polymodal role of the planum temporale is compelling, particularly within the context of non-auditory based communicative modalities such as human sign language and normal polymodal communication with use of gesture (Goldin-Meadow, 1998, 1999; Iverson & Goldin-Meadow, 1998).

Further, the fact that chimpanzees and other primates may use primarily, species-specific forms of a gestural–visual 'language' that may include both manual, facial and whole body components, is supportive (Hopkins & Leavens, 1998; Steklis & Harnad, 1976). Within this global framework, it is proposed that speech and gestures arose from a common neural, psychological and evolutionary substrate of semantic, syntactic and conceptual representation (Call, 1980; Glosser *et al.*, 1986; Greenfield & Savage-Rumbaugh, 1993; Steklis & Harnad, 1976).

Asymmetry of planum temporale homolog in nonhuman primates

Sylvian fissure length as an indicator of planum temporale asymmetry

The length and course of the Sylvian fissure on the left and right hemispheres of humans has served as a brain surface indicator of L > R hemispheric asymmetric expression of the more deeply located planum temporale and primary auditory cortex, Heschl's gyrus (Foundas *et al.*, 1999; LeMay, 1976; Musiek & Reeves, 1990; Rubens *et al.*, 1976; Seidenwurm *et al.*, 1985; Steinmetz *et al.*, 1990; Witelson & Kigar, 1992). On the left hemisphere the Sylvian fissure is longer, extends more posteriorly and is situated lower than the right Sylvian fissure, which terminates more anteriorly and ascends superiorly. Prior to our detailed anatomic description of Heschl's gyrus and planum temporale with L > R asymmetry in chimpanzees, previous studies had utilized Sylvian fissure measures to infer left hemisphere predominance of planum temporale in newborn and adult humans, fossil humans, great apes and even New World and Old World monkeys (Falk, 1978; Falk *et al.*, 1986; Galaburda *et al.*, 1978a; LeMay, 1976; LeMay & Geschwind, 1975) (Fig. 11.1). For example, an extensive study of Sylvian fissure length in humans, chimpanzees and macaques showed that chimpanzees were similar to humans (Sylvian fissure being L > R) but that macaques were symmetric (Yeni-Komshian & Benson, 1976). An earlier study demonstrated that only great apes showed Sylvian fissure asymmetries, that of *Pongo* being most pronounced, the chimpanzee intermediate and that of *Gorilla* least discernible (LeMay & Geschwind, 1975). Apparently the magnitude of this finding inspired the authors to write in a brief abstract that 'Studies in the orangutan might be more likely to help in understanding the evolution of handedness or language than studies in chimpanzees' (LeMay & Geschwind, 1975, p. 48).

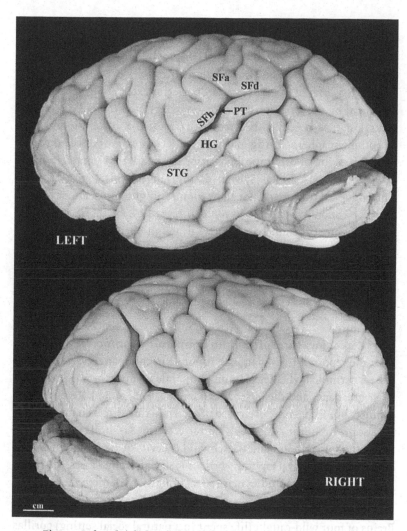

Fig. 11.1. Left and right hemispheres of an adult, captivity-reared, female chimpanzee (*Pan troglodytes*). Abbreviations: STG, superior temporal gyrus; SFh, SFa, and SFd, horizontal, ascending and descending limbs of the Sylvian fissure; PT, planum temporale; HG, Heschl's gyrus.

However, our preliminary data in great apes do not support this contention.

In an endocast study of Old World monkeys, Falk reported L>R Sylvian fissure asymmetry (Falk, 1978). A subsequent study of post-mortem immersion fixed brains of Old World and New World monkeys showed similar findings of L > R Sylvian fissure asymmetry (Heilbroner & Holloway, 1988). Conversely, other studies on a large sample ($n = 32$, perfusion-fixed *Macaca fascicularis* and *M. mulatta* brains) demonstrated that not only was the Sylvian fissure symmetric ($p = 0.97$) but there was a marked masking of the *Sylvian point* (posterior extent of Sylvian fissure; Fig. 11.2a) by the adjacent posterior boundary of the middle temporal gyrus (Fig. 11.2b) on either the left or right side in 62% of hemispheres and on both hemispheres contiguously in 37% (Gannon, 1995). Because differential masking of this critical posterior landmark represented in many cases up to 15% of total Sylvian fissure length, this highly variable morphological trait would not allow for meaningful use of either natural or other endocasts, at least in *Macaca*, regardless of the fact that the Sylvian fissure is symmetric. Clearly, although our preliminary studies have demonstrated that the planum temporale homolog (area Tpt) in macaques is markedly L > R asymmetric at the cytoarchitectonic volumetric level, this character is not manifest at the macroanatomic level (Gannon et al., 1999; Preuss & Goldman-Rakic, 1991).

Direct measures of planum temporale asymmetry

After the report of L > R planum temporale in chimpanzees, it remained to be determined whether planum temporale asymmetry was present in other great apes and the lesser apes (Gannon et al., 1998b). Recently, two distinct approaches have been used to ascertain this; direct anatomic visualization with linear measures (Gannon et al., 1998a) similar to the original method used in humans (Geschwind & Levitsky, 1968), and magnetic resonance imaging (Hopkins et al., 1998b). In some cases, different findings of these two studies may reflect limitations of methods used.

Gorilla Heschl's gyrus and planum temporale

Brains of four wild-caught (life spent in a natural social setting) gorillas *Gorilla gorilla gorilla* from the Smithsonian Institution were studied. In three brains, Heschl's gyrus was prominent bilaterally and the boundaries of planum temporale were readily identifiable (Fig. 11.3). In one brain, although Heschl's gyrus was prominent, the boundaries of planum temporale were ambiguous. Linear caliper measures of the lateral margin of planum temporale on three specimens showed that it was significantly ($P < 0.005$) larger on the left hemisphere. This brain language region in gorillas may be similar in anatomy and hemispheric asymmetry to that of humans and chimpanzees (Gannon et al., 1998a).

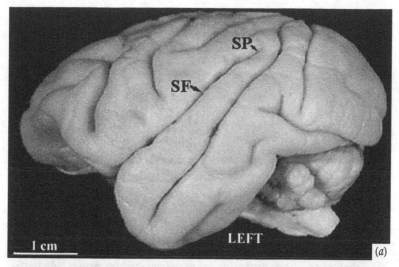

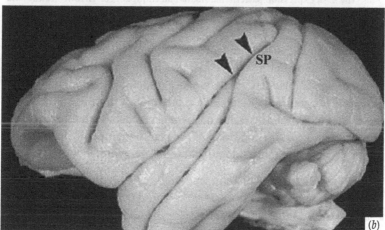

Fig. 11.2. Two left hemispheres of *Macaca fascicularis* brains. (*a*) Determination of Sylvian fissure (SF) length from endocasts or cortical surface measures requires a fully exposed Sylvian point (SP). (*b*) Arrows indicate an operculated Sylvian point and the length of SF hidden deep to the brain surface. This represents the most common SF morphology (62%) observed in our sample (*n* = 32).

Orangutan Heschl's gyrus and planum temporale

Five wild-caught orangutan brains (*Pongo pygmaeus*) were studied at the Smithsonian Institution. A high degree of variation was present in expression of Heschl's gyrus and the planum temporale compared to chimpanzees and gorillas (Fig. 11.4). Linear measures of lateral planum

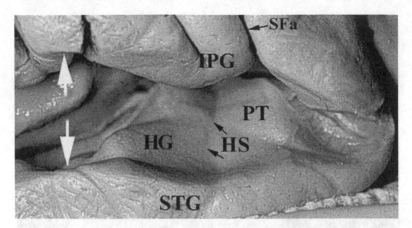

Fig. 11.3. The left superior temporal plane of a wild-caught, adult male gorilla (*Gorilla gorilla*) brain. In four gorilla brains, Heschl's gyrus (HG) and planum temporale (PT) showed a left hemisphere (L>R) predominance, comparable to the L>R expression pattern in humans and chimpanzees. Arrows indicate the Sylvian fissure. Abbreviations: IPG, inferior parietal gyrus; HS, Heschl's sulcus.

temporale showed that it was 53 ± 46% larger on the left in three brains, symmetric in one brain, and 32% larger on the right in one brain. The apparent left hemisphere predominance of planum temporale was not statistically significant (P = 0.3). Our preliminary findings differ from those of LeMay and Geschwind who considered that orangutans expressed a humanlike condition of the planum temporale by inference from Sylvian fissure morphology (LeMay & Geschwind, 1975).

Heschl's gyrus and planum temporale in hylobatids

The morphology of Heschl's gyrus and planum temporale was studied in a sample of the lesser ape family (Hylobatidae) brains, which included representation of two genera: gibbons (*Hylobates*) and siamangs (*Symphalangus*). Hylobatids are thought to have separated from the primate lineage leading to great apes and humans as early as 20 million years ago (Fleagle, 1988) and are the earliest living hominoid representatives, situated at the base of differentiation of this group.

In brains of three wild caught gibbons (*Hylobates lar*) from the Smithsonian Institution collection, Heschl's gyrus was prominently represented bilaterally in two (Fig. 11.5) and one showed a flat superior temporal plane. Surprisingly, it has been reported that Heschl's gyrus was not apparent or well developed in *Hylobates lar* and, for this reason, the authors did not include this species in their study (Hopkins *et al.*, 1998a).

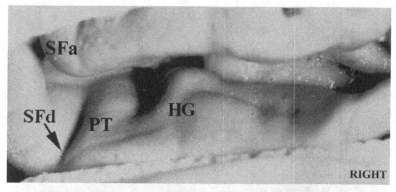

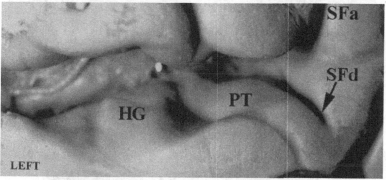

Fig. 11.4. Left and right hemispheres of a wild-caught, adult male orangutan (*Pongo pygmaeus*) brain. Lateral view inside the SF onto the planar surfaces of the superior temporal gyri. Within our sample (*n* = 5), a high degree of variation was characteristic of planum temporale (PT) and Heschl's gyrus (HG) expression. Although HG was as pronounced as in chimpanzees and gorillas, a less robust L > R PT pattern was present. See legend to Fig. 11.1 for abbreviations.

Perhaps the method used, anatomic magnetic resonance imaging, did not capture gross anatomic subtleties that are clearly evident upon direct observation (Fig. 11.5). Either way, since the morphology of the posterior Sylvian fissure differs from great apes and humans (i.e. does not bifurcate) and posterior anatomic landmarks of planum temporale (or Tpt) are ambiguous, we considered it inappropriate to quantify its extent. Determination of the posterior boundary of area Tpt, to be at the level of the Sylvian point, would allow a realistic analysis of asymmetry to be conducted.

We hypothesized that siamangs would show prominent morphology of the Heschl's gyrus/planum temporale complex since their body (and

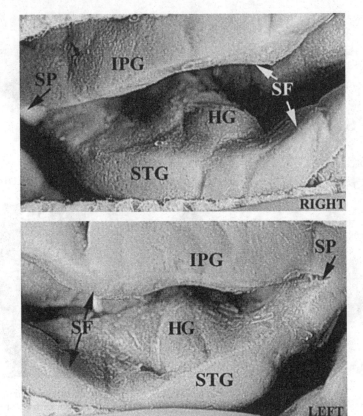

Fig. 11.5. Left and right hemispheres of a wild-caught gibbon (*Hylobates lar*) brain. In three specimens, HG was prominent. However, since the morphology of the posterior Sylvian fissure differs from that of great apes (does not bifurcate), the gross anatomic landmarks of PT were vague and not quantifiable. See legends to Figs. 11.1–11.3 for abbreviations.

brain) size is considerably larger than gibbons. However, unlike gibbons, in brains of three wild caught siamangs (*Symphalangus syndactylus*) only one showed a weakly represented Heschl's gyrus and the other two essentially showed a featureless superior temporal plane similar to macaques (Fig. 11.6).

Heschl's gyrus and planum temporale morphology in macaques

The morphology of Heschl's gyrus and the planum temporale was studied in four female and four male perfusion fixed brains of macaques (*Macaca*

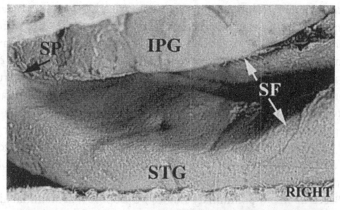

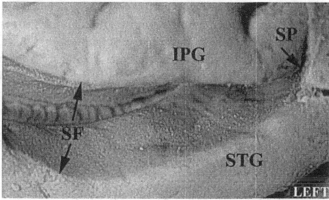

Fig. 11.6. The left and right hemispheres of a wild-caught siamang (*Symphalangus syndactylus*) brain. In the sample of three siamangs, HG was weakly represented unilaterally in one brain, and the remainder showed a flat superior temporal plane. As with the gibbons, since the landmarks of HG were indistinct it was not possible to quantify PT. See legends to Figs. 11.1–11.3 for abbreviations.

fascicularis). In all specimens, there was no gross anatomic evidence for the presence of Heschl's gyrus and, similar to siamangs, the posterior–most superior temporal plane was flat and there was no posterior bifurcation of the Sylvian fissure (Fig. 11.2a).

Overview of Heschl's gyrus/planum temporale anatomy in nonhuman primates

It appears that the morphological expression of these key brain receptive 'language' areas followed a progressive evolutionary trajectory during recent primate evolution: (1) in macaques, Heschl's gyrus and planum temporale (and Sylvian fissure) asymmetry (Gannon et al., 1998a) are not expressed at the gross anatomic level. However, pronounced volumetric asymmetries at the cytoarchitectonic level are evident (Gannon et al., 1999); (2) in lesser apes, particularly in gibbons, Heschl's gyrus is expressed more overtly although planum temporale may not be asymmetric. This may represent a key period during hominoid brain 'language' area evolution when these basal areas underwent modification and elaboration; (3) in great apes, Heschl's gyrus is robustly expressed and planum temporale is predominantly lateralized to the left hemisphere, particularly in chimpanzees and gorillas.

Based upon our preliminary studies we propose that an initial distinguishable suite of human-like receptive language area anatomic traits appeared in our common ancestor with early hominoids around 20 million years ago (although functional asymmetries may have been present prior to this). This differs from the interpretation of Hopkins and co-workers who placed this event around 15 million years ago after divergence from lesser apes (Hopkins et al., 1998a). Subsequently, these traits were gradually elaborated until they became anatomically expressed more prominently, likely within our common ancestor with orangutans around 14 million years ago, and arriving at the human condition in our common ancestor with gorillas around 10 million years ago.

Potential functional significance of brain language areas in nonhuman primates

We have demonstrated that great apes possess a lateralized gross anatomical neural substrate that is comparable to that of modern humans, for whom the area appears to be involved in the perception of language and/or communication. These gross features are manifest to a minor degree in lesser apes but not in Old World monkeys. In fact, it appears that there may be a graded expression of this feature that complements the evolutionary distance between the common ancestors of living hominoids. A comparable finding of neural gradation was recently shown in the expression of cellular morphological specializations of the anterior cingulate cortex, a region that plays a major role in the regulation of many aspects of cognitive processes such as self awareness, emotionality and vocalization (Nimchinsky et al., 1999). Interestingly, this study showed that bonobos closely resembled humans, whereas chimpanzees and gorillas were intermediate, and orangutans rarely displayed the trait. Gibbons and other primates did not express it. Similar to the planum temporale, this finding suggests that the anterior cingulate cortex may have been a region that experienced strong adaptive pressure during the past 16 million years of primate evolution.

These findings lead us to the key question of what might the behavioral correlate of a derived human-like anatomical trait, such as the planum temporale, be in chimpanzees or bonobos? Clearly, members of the genus *Pan* do not have a recognizable interindividual communication system as diversified as that of humans, but they do have a relatively sophisticated polymodal system that subserves adequately their communicative needs and perhaps beyond. Recently, there has been a growing interest in chimpanzee cognitive and communicative abilities. There is considerable evidence, albeit anecdotal in many cases, indicating that chimpanzees and bonobos are highly advanced cognitively compared to other primates and possess a complex communicative repertoire which humans have yet to decipher. For example, it is generally well accepted that chimpanzees possess a *sense of self,* which represents a cognitive milestone; i.e. accretion of the dynamic perspective of self versus others. Chimpanzees and bonobos are thought to possess an array of purportedly derived cognitive traits such as imitation, causality, perception, deception, lying, prediction, forward planning, teaching, compassion, sadness, joking, laughter, tool use, finger pointing, handedness, hunting, nonreproductive social pan-sex, and to be at the equivalent cognitive level of two to three year old humans (Savage-Rumbaugh *et al.*, 1993). Over the past four decades, the extensive body of work conducted on the use of American sign language and arbitrary symbols by chimpanzees has clearly demonstrated that they possess both highly advanced cognitive skills, a proto-linguistic capacity and a marked potential for their ability to communicate with another species, namely humans (Gardner & Gardner, 1969, 1978; Langs *et al.*, 1996; Savage-Rumbaugh, 1990; Savage-Rumbaugh & Rumbaugh, 1978; Savage-Rumbaugh *et al.*, 1985). Many of these studies also indicated that chimpanzees, in a manner similar to human children, are able to cognate considerably more than they can express (Savage-Rumbaugh *et al.*, 1993). It would be interesting and educational to see whether we, as a more cognitively sophisticated species, would be better qualified to comprehend natural chimpanzee 'language' than they are at comprehending ours. In light of this compelling concept, the bonobo Kanzi must represent a great ape prodigy with regard to his remarkable ability to comprehend spoken human language in addition to his personal trans-specific human language communicative speciality, lexigrams (Savage-Rumbaugh & Lewin, 1994). If an individual such as Kanzi can come to understand basic semantic elements of our language, albeit at the level of a two to three year old human child, is it not appropriate that we should come to understand natural ape language, at the very least to the level of a two to three year old bonobo? Other legendary chimpanzees and bonobos such as Washoe, Sherman, Austin, Kanzi's sister Panbanisha and her son Nyota amongst others, may offer new insight into the trans-specific communicative abilities of our closest living relative. Nyota in particular, who is currently being raised at The Language Research Center of Georgia State University, with extensive use of human language almost from birth, may introduce us to new arenas of trans-specific cognitive understanding, since critical periods of development, hitherto not accessed, may be realized (Savage-Rumbaugh, 1998).

Scenario for communicative shifts on the upper east side planum

At around six to eight million years ago, at which time it is generally considered that early humans split off from our common ancestor with living chimpanzees and bonobos, a major adaptive shift occurred; the onset of a bipedal gait. This involved a radical departure, for the first time in primate evolutionary history, away from use of four limbs or forelimbs for locomotion. Bipedal gait represented a rapidly incorporated locomotor complex, which involved inauguration of a biomechanical masterpiece within the foot (Jaffe et al., 1991). This novel ligament-based arch system of the bipedal foot was certainly designed to subserve relatively effortless wide-ranging locomotion, without which it simply would not have been possible to walk great distances.

Clearly, these bipedal early human ancestors had likely already diverged genetically and quite literally moved away, or became isolated from the resource-rich, restricted territorial setting still utilized by modern chimpanzees and bonobos. Such a radical shift away from what may represent a long established basal social system would have turned the communicative repertoire of members within this newly wide-ranging group upside down. Between-group and interindividual communicative interactions within this non-territorial setting without well-defined boundaries, would likely have occurred much more frequently and have been significantly less constrained than previous territorial boundary based interactions with strangers. In turn, these new social demands would have required development of a new suite of cognitive and communicative skills that would have been necessary to provide greater insight into the motives and intent of strangers. Such enhanced abilities would likely have been highly adaptive, thus strongly selected for, as they would have provided for mutually productive communicative outcomes. Such outcomes may have included sharing and wide distribution of knowledge. Knowledge referral would have offered, for example, critical and mutually beneficial information regarding distant dangers and threats, location of widely dispersed food resources, technological advances and skills, and hunting strategies. Such communicative sophistication may also have promoted the potential for rapid gene flow through a large dispersed group of individuals, owing to wider awareness of population dynamics. Further, an ability to provide offspring with detailed survival-related information, and as such, to furnish *referred experience* in advance. Naive young individuals would not have been required to experience a potentially life-threatening situation firsthand. Instead, they would be equipped already with the knowledge and insight required in making critical survival decisions. Wide dispersal of innovative information derived from a larger population would also have allowed for the rapid and wide incorporation of knowledge provided by rarer and more gifted, innovative individuals. In such a non-tethered situation, the application and enhancement of such knowledge and information may have mirrored massive rapid advances in modern day events such as the industrial revolution, computer science and earth and space travel.

As discussed above, at this early time in the development of communicative diversity, the primary modality used was likely gestural/visual (G/V) as in living bonobos and chimpanzees. Why a shift to primacy of the vocal/auditory (V/A) modality took place during early hominid evolution has many possible answers. Clearly, the brain appears to be equipotential for these two input/output modalities as evidenced from the activation of brain language areas in deaf-from-birth signing humans. The brain does not seem to select radically for the modality so long as the information is communication-based and even in a V/A specialized species such as ourselves, is able to accommodate the plasticity of phenotypic outcome the system requires to shift modes when and if it becomes necessary. A great deal of evolutionary insight may be offered by this simple and well-documented fact.

A gestural origin of V/A human language was originally suggested by Gordon Hewes, and although his perspective differed somewhat to that proposed here, it was an early inspirational piece (Hewes, 1973). More recently, Corballis offered another explanation which essentially proposed the change from G/V to V/A language freed the hands for the manufacture of tools and weapons and allowed the V/A channel to be used consecutively for teaching, presumably of tool manufacture and use (Corballis, 1991). Visual demonstration of methodological nuances in tool production would seem to outweigh verbal description or explanation, even in speaking–hearing individuals. In addition, it would seem that there are many situations of tool or weapon use such as close-quarters hunting where silent G/V versus noisy V/A communication would provide a distinct advantage and in fact G/V communication has been used extensively as a language adjunct by modern human groups such as the Khoi San population from South Africa and native North Americans. In contrast, under many other circumstances where multiple individuals are involved in rapid debate of complex issues, other rules would apply. In such an exchange, primary use of the V/A modality would likely be required to mediate the rapid and dynamic shift of individual contributions and interjections. Use of the G/V channel may not have allowed for efficient and productive interchange due to the need to look at each communicator in sequence. Conversely, even during primary use of the V/A mode in living humans, gesture is an integral and important component of our communicative whole, or as elegantly stated by Susan Goldin-Meadow 'for both speakers and listeners, gesture and speech are two aspects of a single process, with each modality contributing its own unique level of representation' (Goldin-Meadow, 1998, p. 29). A recent study showed that congenitally blind speakers gesture despite their lack of a visual model, even when they speak to a blind listener, suggesting that this is an innate behavior that does not require a model or an attentive partner (Iverson & Goldin-Meadow, 1998). In a developmental context, it has been noted that children at the one-word stage produce and perceive gestures along with speech in a manner similar to adults (Goldin-Meadow, 1998). Similarly, it was noted recently by Michael Corballis that in many modern human populations, gesture is used extensively to augment speech and that human spoken language may have evolved primarily from systems of manual gestures, not vocalizations (Corballis, 1999). Although we consider that vocalization may have played some perhaps minor role in evolution of a holistic polymodal, polygestural (not just manual) communicative package, we concur with this position wholeheartedly.

In sum, we propose that the shift from G/V to V/A primacy during hominid evolution represented a progressive series of interconnected events. This long term major adaptive shift was based on the need to expand the efficiency and coordination of cognitive/communicative abilities within the context of behavioral and technological advances. In any case, the neural substrates that underlie these communicative abilities at different levels are designed to subserve species specific tasks that parallel the cognitive capacity of a particular species. Further, a wealth of multi-disciplinary evidence has indicated that the highly plastic, adaptable cerebral cortex does not seem to be affected by the expressive or perceptive modality being utilized by a particular primate species or human group, only that the information being conveyed or conceived is communicative in nature.

Acknowledgments

We thank Richard Thorington and Jeremy Jacobs, for use of the ape brain collection at the Smithsonian Institution, Division of Mammals; Joseph Erwin, for consultation and photos of a chimpanzee brain in his collection; Allen Braun, for consultation; Maria Deftereos, for brain curation, digital graphics and photography; Ralph Holloway, for consultation; Douglas Broadfield, for assistance with the hylobatid brain analysis; and Chester Sherwood, for curation assistance. Thanks especially to the NSF-SBER and NSF-IBN divisions of the National Science Foundation for their support of this work.

References

Anderson, B., Southern, B.D. & Powers, R.E. (1999). Anatomic asymmetries of the posterior superior temporal lobes: a postmortem study. *Neuropsychiatry, Neuropsychology and Behavioral Neurology*, 12, 247–254.

Barta, P.E., Petty, R.G., McGilchrist, I., Lewis, R.W., Jerram, M., Casanova, M.F., Powers, R.E., Brill, L.B. II & Pearlson, G.D. (1995). Asymmetry of the planum temporale: methodological considerations and clinical associations. *Psychiatry Research*, 61, 37–50.

Binder, J.R., Frost, J.A., Hammeke, T.A., Rao, S.M. & Cox, R.W. (1996). Function of the left planum temporale in auditory and linguistic processing. *Brain*, 119, 1239–1247.

Call, J.D. (1980). Some prelinguistic aspects of language development. *Journal of the American Psychoanalytic Association*, 28, 259–289.

Calvert, G.A., Brammer, M.J., Bullmore, E.T., Campbell, R., Iversen, S.D. & David, A.S. (1999). Response amplification in sensory-specific cortices during crossmodal binding. *NeuroReport,* **10**, 2619–2623.

Calvert, G.A., Bullmore, E.T., Brammer, M.J., Campbell, R., Williams, S.C., McGuire, P.K., Woodruff, P.W., Iversen, S.D. & David, A.S. (1997). Activation of auditory cortex during silent lipreading. *Science,* **276**, 593–596.

Chomsky, N. (1972). *Language and Mind.* New York: Harcourt Brace Jovanovich.

Cohen, L.G., Celnik, P., Pascual-Leone, A., Corwell, B., Falz, L., Dambrosia, J., Honda, M., Sadato, N., Gerloff, C., Catala, M.D. & Hallett, M. (1997). Functional relevance of cross-modal plasticity in blind humans. *Nature,* **389**, 180–183.

Coppens, Y. (1994). East side story: the origin of humankind. *Scientific American,* **270**, 88–95.

Corballis, M.C. (1991). *The Lopsided Ape.* New York: Oxford University Press.

Corballis, M.C. (1999). The gestural origins of language. *American Scientist,* **87**, 138–145.

Damasio, A.R. (1992). Aphasia. *New England Journal of Medicine,* **326**, 531–539.

Damasio, A.R. (1997). Brain and language: what a difference a decade makes. *Current Opinion in Neurobiology,* **10**, 177–178.

Falk, D. (1978). Cerebral asymmetry in Old World monkeys. *Acta Anatomica (Basel),* **101**, 334–339.

Falk, D., Cheverud, J., Vannier, M.W. & Conroy, G.C. (1986). Advanced computer graphics technology reveals cortical asymmetry in endocasts of rhesus monkeys. *Folia Primatologica (Basel),* **46**, 98–103.

Fitch, R.H., Miller, S. & Tallal, P. (1997). Neurobiology of speech perception. *Annual Review of Neuroscience,* **20**, 331–353.

Fleagle, J. (1988). *Primate Adaptation and Evolution.* New York: Academic Press.

Foundas, A.L., Faulhaber, J.R., Kulynych, J.J., Browning, C.A. & Weinberger, D.R. (1999). Hemispheric and sex-linked differences in Sylvian fissure morphology: a quantitative approach using volumetric magnetic resonance imaging. *Neuropsychiatry, Neuropsychology and Behavioral Neurology,* **12**, 1–10.

Foundas, A.L., Leonard, C.M., Gilmore, R., Fennell, E. & Heilman, K.M. (1994). Planum temporale asymmetry and language dominance. *Neuropsychologia,* **32**, 1225–1231.

Galaburda, A.M. (1993). The planum temporale. *Archives of Neurology,* **50**, 457.

Galaburda, A.M., LeMay, M., Kemper, T.L. & Geschwind, N. (1978a). Right-left asymmetrics in the brain. *Science,* **199**, 852–856.

Galaburda, A.M., Sanides, F. & Geschwind, N. (1978b). Human brain. Cytoarchitectonic left–right asymmetries in the temporal speech region. *Archives of Neurology,* **35**, 812–817.

Gannon, P. (1995). *Asymmetry in the Cerebral Cortex of Macaca fascicularis: A Basal Substrate for the Evolution of Brain Mechanisms Underlying Language.* City University of New York, New York.

Gannon, P.J., Broadfield, D.C., Kheck, N.M., Hof, P.R., Braun, A.R., Erwin, J.M. & Holloway, R.L. (1998a). Brain language area evolution I: Anatomic expression of Heschl's gyrus and planum temporale asymmetry in great apes, lesser apes and Old World monkeys. *Society for Neuroscience Abstract,* **160**, 64.15

Gannon, P.J., Holloway, R.L., Broadfield, D.C. & Braun, A.R. (1998b). Asymmetry of chimpanzee planum temporale: humanlike pattern of Wernicke's brain language area homolog. *Science,* **279**, 220–222.

Gannon, P.J., Kheck, N.M. & Hof, P.R. (1999). Brain language area evolution III: Left hemisphere predominant asymmetry of cytoarchitectonic, but not gross anatomic, planum temporale homolog in Old World monkeys. *Society for Neuroscience Abstract*, **105**, 47.17.

Gardner, R. A. & Gardner, B. T. (1969). Teaching sign language to a chimpanzee. *Science*, **165**, 664–672.

Gardner, R. A. & Gardner, B. T. (1978). Comparative psychology and language acquisition. *Annals of the New York Academy of Sciences*, **309**, 37–76.

Geschwind, N. & Levitsky, W. (1968). Human brain: left-right asymmetries in temporal speech region. *Science*, **161**, 186–187.

Glosser, G., Wiener, M. & Kaplan, E. (1986). Communicative gestures in aphasia. *Brain and Language*, **27**, 345–359.

Goldin-Meadow, S. (1998). The development of gesture and speech as an integrated system. *New Directions for Child Development*, **79**, 29–42.

Goldin-Meadow, S. (1999). What children contribute to language-learning. *Science Progress*, **82**, 89–102.

Greenfield, P. M. & Savage-Rumbaugh, E. S. (1993). Comparing communicative competence in child and chimp: the pragmatics of repetition. *Journal of Child Language*, **20**, 1–26.

Hawkin, S. (1998). *Imagination and Change: Science in the Next Millenium*. In *Presidential Millenium Evenings*, ed. B. Clinton. White House.

Heilbroner, P. L. & Holloway, R. L. (1988). Anatomical brain asymmetries in New World and Old World monkeys: stages of temporal lobe development in primate evolution [published erratum appears in *American Journal of Physical Anthropology* 1988 Sep; 77(1): 141]. *American Journal of Physical Anthropology*, **76**, 39–48.

Hewes, G. W. (1973). Primate communication and the gestural origins of language. *Current Anthropology*, **14**, 5–24.

Hickok, G., Bellugi, U. & Klima, E. S. (1996). The neurobiology of sign language and its implications for the neural basis of language. *Nature*, **381**, 699–702.

Hopkins, W. D. & Leavens, D. A. (1998). Hand use and gestural communication in chimpanzees (*Pan troglodytes*). *Journal of Comparative Psychology*, **112**, 95–99.

Hopkins, W. D., Marino, L., Rilling, J. K. & MacGregor, L. A. (1998a). Planum temporale asymmetries in great apes as revealed by magnetic resonance imaging (MRI). *Neuroreport*, **9**, 2913–2918.

Hopkins, W. D., Marino, L., Rilling, J. K. & MacGregor, L. A. (1998b). Planum temporale asymmetries in great apes as revealed by magnetic resonance imaging (MRI) [In Process Citation]. *NeuroReport*, **9**, 2913–2918.

Howard, M. A., Volkov, I. O., Mirsky, R., Garell, P. C., Noh, M. D., Granner, M., Damasio, H., Steinschneider, M., Reale, R. A., Hind, J. E. & Brugge, J. F. (2000). Auditory cortex on the human posterior superior temporal gyrus. *Journal of Comparative Neurology*, **416**, 79–92.

Iverson, J. M. & Goldin-Meadow, S. (1998). Why people gesture when they speak. *Nature*, **396**, 228.

Jaffe, W. J., Gannon, P. J. & Laitman, J. T. (1991). Paleontology, embryology, and anatomy of the foot. In *Disorders of the Foot and Ankle: Medical and Surgical Management*, ed. M. J. Jahss. Philadelphia: W. B. Saunders.

Jancke, L., Schlaug, G., Huang, Y. & Steinmetz, H. (1994). Asymmetry of the planum parietale. *NeuroReport*, **5**, 1161–1163.

Jancke, L. & Steinmetz, H. (1993). Auditory lateralization and planum temporale asymmetry. *NeuroReport*, **5**, 169–172.

Just, M. A., Carpenter, P. A., Keller, T. A., Eddy, W. F. & Thulborn, K. R. (1996). Brain activation modulated by sentence comprehension. *Science*, **274**, 114–116.

Karbe, H., Wurker, M., Herholz, K., Ghaemi, M., Pietrzyk, U., Kessler, J. & Heiss, W.D. (1995). Planum temporale and Brodmann's area 22. Magnetic resonance imaging and high-resolution positron emission tomography demonstrate functional left–right asymmetry. *Archives of Neurology*, **52**, 869–874.

Kujala, T., Alho, K. & Naatanen, R. (2000). Cross-modal reorganization of human cortical functions. *Trends in Neurosciences*, **23**, 115–120.

Langs, R., Badalamenti, A.F. & Savage-Rumbaugh, S. (1996). Two mathematically defined expressive language structures in humans and chimpanzees. *Behavioral Science*, **41**, 124–135.

LeMay, M. (1976). Morphological cerebral asymmetries of modern man, fossil man, and nonhuman primate. *Annals of the New York Academy of Sciences*, **280**, 349–366.

LeMay, M., Billig, M. & Geschwind, N. (1982). Asymmetries of the brains and skulls of nonhuman primates. In *Primate Brain Evolution: Methods and Concepts*, eds. E. Armstrong & D. Falk, pp. 263–277. New York: Plenum Press.

LeMay, M. & Geschwind, N. (1975). Hemispheric differences in the brains of great apes. *Brain, Behavior and Evolution (Basel)*, **11**, 48–52.

Modayur, B., Prothero, J., Ojemann, G., Maravilla, K. & Brinkley, J. (1997). Visualization-based mapping of language function in the brain. *Neuroimage*, **6**, 245–258.

Muller, R.A., Behen, M.E., Rothermel, R.D., Muzik, O., Chakraborty, P.K. & Chugani, H.T. (1999). Brain organization for language in children, adolescents, and adults with left hemisphere lesion: a PET study. *Progress in Neuro-psychopharmacology and Biological Psychiatry (Oxford)*, **23**, 657–668.

Musiek, F.E. & Reeves, A.G. (1990). Asymmetries of the auditory areas of the cerebrum. *Journal of the American Academy of Audiology*, **1**, 240–245.

Neville, H.J. (1998). Specificity and plasticity in human brain development: special lecture. *Society for Neuroscience*, **24**, Nov. 9.

Neville, H.J., Bavelier, D., Corina, D., Rauschecker, J., Karni, A., Lalwani, A., Braun, A., Clark, V., Jezzard, P. & Turner, R. (1998). Cerebral organization for language in deaf and hearing subjects: biological constraints and effects of experience. *Proceedings of the National Academy of Sciences, USA*, **95**, 922–929.

Nimchinsky, E.A., Gilissen, E., Allman, J.M., Perl, D.P., Erwin, J.M. & Hof, P.R. (1999). A neuronal morphologic type unique to humans and great apes. *Proceedings of the National Academy of Sciences, USA*, **96**, 5268–5273.

Paus, T., Perry, D.W., Zatorre, R.J., Worsley, K.J. & Evans, A.C. (1996). Modulation of cerebral blood flow in the human auditory cortex during speech: role of motor-to-sensory discharges. *European Journal of Neuroscience*, **8**, 2236–2246.

Penfield, W. & Roberts, L. (1959). *Speech and Brain Mechanisms*. Princeton: Princeton University Press.

Porta-Etessam, J., Nunez-Lopez, R., Balsalobre, J., Lopez, E., Hernandez, A. & Luna, A. (1997). Language and aphasias. *Revue Neurologique*, **25**, 1269–1277.

Preis, S., Jancke, L., Schmitz-Hillebrecht, J. & Steinmetz, H. (1999). Child age and planum temporale asymmetry. *Brain and Cognition*, **40**, 441–452.

Preuss, T.M. & Goldman-Rakic, P.S. (1991). Architectonics of the parietal and temporal association cortex in the strepsirhine primate *Galago* compared to the anthropoid primate *Macaca*. *Journal of Comparative Neurology*, **310**, 475–506.

Price, C.J., Wise, R.J., Warburton, E.A., Moore, C.J., Howard, D., Patterson, K.,

Frackowiak, R.S. & Friston, K.J. (1996). Hearing and saying. The functional neuro-anatomy of auditory word processing. *Brain*, **119**, 919–931.

Puce, A., Allison, T., Bentin, S., Gore, J.C. & McCarthy, G. (1998). Temporal cortex activation in humans viewing eye and mouth movements. *Journal of Neuroscience*, **18**, 2188–2199.

Romanski, L.M., Tian, B., Fritz, J., Mishkin, M., Goldman-Rakic, P.S. & Rauschecker, J.P. (1999). Dual streams of auditory afferents target multiple domains in the primate prefrontal cortex. *Nature Neuroscience*, **2**, 1131–1136.

Roux, F.E., Boulanouar, K., Ibarrola, D., Tremoulet, M., Henry, P., Manelfe, C. & Berry, I. (1999). Importance and limitations of the validation of functional MRI of motor function and language using preoperative cortical stimulation. *Journal of Neuroradiology*, **26**, S82–S88.

Rubens, A.B., Mahowald, M.W. & Hutton, J.T. (1976). Asymmetry of the lateral (Sylvian) fissures in man. *Neurology*, **26**, 620–624.

Sadato, N., Pascual-Leone, A., Grafman, J., Ibanez, V., Deiber, M.P., Dold, G. & Hallett, M. (1996). Activation of the primary visual cortex by Braille reading in blind subjects. *Nature*, **380**, 526–528.

Savage-Rumbaugh, E.S. (1990). Language acquisition in a nonhuman species: implications for the innateness debate. *Developmental Psychobiology*, **23**, 599–620.

Savage-Rumbaugh, E.S., Murphy, J., Sevcik, R.A., Brakke, K.E., Williams, S.L. & Rumbaugh, D.M. (1993). Language comprehension in ape and child. *Monographs of the Society for Research in Child Development*, **58**, 1–222.

Savage-Rumbaugh, E.S. & Rumbaugh, D.M. (1978). Symbolization, language, and chimpanzees: a theoretical reevaluation based on initial language acquisition processes in four young *Pan troglodytes*. *Brain and Language*, **6**, 265–300.

Savage-Rumbaugh, S. (1998). Nyota. http://www.gsu.edu/~wwwlrc/biographies/nyota.html. Language Research Center.

Savage-Rumbaugh, S. & Lewin, R. (1994). *Kanzi: An Ape at the Brink of the Human Mind*. New York: John Wiley & Sons Inc.

Savage-Rumbaugh, S., Rumbaugh, D.M. & McDonald, K. (1985) Language learning in two species of apes. *Neuroscience and Biobehavioral Reviews (Oxford)*, **9**, 653–665.

Schlosser, M.J., Luby, M., Spencer, D.D., Awad, I.A. & McCarthy, G. (1999). Comparative localization of auditory comprehension by using functional magnetic resonance imaging and cortical stimulation. *Journal of Neurosurgery*, **91**, 626–635.

Seidenwurm, D., Bird, C.R., Enzmann, D.R. & Marshall, W.H. (1985). Left–right temporal region asymmetry in infants and children. *American Journal of Neuroradiology*, **6**, 777–779.

Semrud-Clikeman, M. (1997). Evidence from imaging on the relationship between brain structure and developmental language disorders. *Seminars in Pediatric Neurology*, **4**, 117–124.

Shapleske, J., Rossell, S.L., Woodruff, P.W. & David, A.S. (1999). The planum temporale: a systematic, quantitative review of its structural, functional and clinical significance. *Brain Research Reviews*, **29**, 26–49.

Shenton, M.E., McCarley, R.W. & Tamminga, C.A. (1995). Cortex, IX. Heschl's gyrus and the planum temporale. *American Journal of Psychiatry*, **152**, 966.

Simos, P.G., Breier, J.I., Maggio, W.W., Gormley, W.B., Zouridakis, G., Willmore, L.J., Wheless, J.W., Constantinou, J.E. & Papanicolaou, A.C. (1999a). Atypical

240   PATRICK J. GANNON ET AL.

temporal lobe language representation: MEG and intraoperative stimulation mapping correlation. *NeuroReport*, **10**, 139–142.

Simos, P.G., Papanicolaou, A.C., Breier, J.I., Wheless, J.W., Constantinou, J.E., Gormley, W.B. & Maggio, W.W. (1999b). Localization of language-specific cortex by using magnetic source imaging and electrical stimulation mapping. *Journal of Neurosurgery*, **91**, 787–796.

Steinmetz, H. (1996). Structure, functional and cerebral asymmetry: *in vivo* morphometry of the planum temporale. *Neuroscience and Biobehavioral Reviews*, **20**, 587–591.

Steinmetz, H., Ebeling, U., Huang, Y.X. & Kahn, T. (1990). Sulcus topography of the parietal opercular region: an anatomic and MR study. *Brain and Language*, **38**, 515–533.

Steinmetz, H., Rademacher, J., Huang, Y.X., Hefter, H., Zilles, K., Thron, A. & Freund, H.J. (1989). Cerebral asymmetry: MR planimetry of the human planum temporale. *Journal of Computer Assisted Tomography*, **13**, 996–1005.

Steinmetz, H., Volkmann, J., Jancke, L. & Freund, H.J. (1991). Anatomical left-right asymmetry of language-related temporal cortex is different in left- and right-handers. *Annals of Neurology*, **29**, 315–319.

Steklis, H.D. & Harnad, S.R. (1976). From hand to mouth: some critical stages in the evolution of language. *Annals of the New York Academy of Sciences*, **80**, 445–455.

Suzuki, M., Yuasa, S., Minabe, Y., Murata, M. & Kurachi, M. (1993). Left superior temporal blood flow increases in schizophrenic and schizophreniform patients with auditory hallucination: a longitudinal case study using 123I-IMP SPECT. *European Archives of Psychiatry and Clinical Neuroscience*, **24**, 257–261.

Takami, K., Sakurai, A., Mukai, F. & Yamadori, T. (1993). A further study on the left-right asymmetry of the planum temporale. *Okajima Folia Anatomica Japonica*, **70**, 59–61.

Tallal, P., Merzenich, M., Miller, S. & Jenkins, W. (1998). Language learning impairment: integrating research and remediation. *Scandinavian Journal of Psychology*, **39**, 197–199.

Tzourio, N., Nkanga-Ngila, B. & Mazoyer, B. (1998). Left planum temporale surface correlates with functional dominance during story listening. *NeuroReport*, **9**, 829–833.

Wernicke, C. (1874). *Der Aphasische Symptomenkomplex*. Breslau: Cohn & Weigert.

Westbury, C.F., Zatorre, R.J. & Evans, A.C. (1999) Quantifying variability in the planum temporale: a probability map. *Cerebral Cortex*, **9**, 392–405.

Witelson, S.F. & Kigar, D.L. (1992). Sylvian fissure morphology and asymmetry in men and women: bilateral differences in relation to handedness in men. *Journal of Comparative Neurology*, **323**, 326–340.

Yamadori, T., Sukekawa, K., Umetani, T. & Yamadori, A. (1982). A quantitative study on the left-right asymmetry of the planum temporale. *Okajima Folia Anatomica Japonica*, **58**, 627–634.

Yeni-Komshian, G.H. & Benson, D.A. (1976). Anatomical study of cerebral asymmetry in the temporal lobe of humans, chimpanzees, and rhesus monkeys. *Science*, **192**, 387–389.

Zatorre, R.J., Meyer, E., Gjedde, A. & Evans, A.C. (1996). PET studies of phonetic processing of speech: review, replication, and reanalysis. *Cerebral Cortex*, **6**, 21–30.

Zatorre, R.J., Perry, D.W., Beckett, C.A., Westbury, C.F. & Evans, A.C. (1998). Functional anatomy of musical processing in listeners with absolute pitch and relative pitch. *Proceedings of the National Academy of Science, USA*, **95**, 3172–3177.

12

The promise and the peril in hominin brain evolution

There is always a temptation to treat an endocast as if it were a 'fossil brain', no matter how often one repeats the caveat that it is at most an impression of a brain on the skull. It is almost impossible to avoid this identification of an endocast with a brain when one analyzes endocasts for information about the evolution of the brain, but this rarely leads to serious problems in actual work with the endocasts.

HARRY JERISON, 1973

It is just over a quarter of a century since Harry Jerison published the first edition of his seminal work, *Evolution of the Brain and Intelligence* (1973). At the time and in the decades since then, we see it as one of the most significant paleo-neurobiological landmarks which heralded the final quarter of the twentieth century. As we enter the twenty-first century, that work remains ineluctably a signpost for the coming era. It is pleasurable indeed to offer homage to Dr Jerison – who was born one day before me in what seems to have been something of an *annus mirabilis*, 1925 – and to offer him my thanks for his inspiration and his friendship.

When we consider the ancient hominins, one is struck by the fact of how few have yielded good natural endocranial casts (endocasts). In the South African dolomitic limestone cave deposits, conditions seem to have been appropriate for the formation of natural endocasts, at least in those crania whose position in the deposit was upside down, completely or obliquely, so that soft matrix could readily gain access to the calvaria through the upturned foramen magnum. When such an unconsolidated filling became calcified, an endocast was available. We have a small number of such natural endocasts and of them those of the Taung skull and of the Swartkrans specimen SK 1585 are two of the most perfectly formed. When crania end up lying in the cave deposit the right way up in a position approximating to the Frankfurt plane, the result is empty crania or crania containing a small encrustation of calcite, the calvarial cavity constituting a virtual cavern within which mini-stalactites and -stalagmites may grow. Such empty crania are exemplified by Sts 5 ('Mrs Ples') and Stw 505 ('Mr Ples') of Sterkfontein and most of the fossil hominin crania of East Africa. In these, artificial endocasts can be made with plaster of Paris or plastic materials (Tobias, 1971, 1994).

More recently, it has proved possible to use computerized tomographic (CT) X-ray scanning techniques to determine features such as size, shape and surface vasculature of the endocasts, even when these are enclosed within a relatively intact calvaria and even when the investigator is presented with an incomplete calvaria and a partial endocast. Such techniques have recently been applied to several South African specimens, notably the Taung skull, the Makapansgat calvaria and contained endocast MLD 37/38, and the large male cranium of Stw 505, all three of these specimens from three different South African sites being classified as belonging to the species, *Australopithecus africanus*. These studies have added to the available small samples of early hominin endocranial capacity values.

Some results of these recent studies are reviewed here. The data for these early African hominins are examined from several points of view: demography, diet and nutrition, and paleoecology.

The application of computerized X-ray tomography to fossil hominin skulls

In the 1980s, two groups of investigators, one in America and one in Europe, started to apply high resolution computed tomography to fossil hominin skulls. The introduction in the 1970s of computerized tomography or CT scanning (Hounsfield, 1973) offered the opportunity for overcoming the difficulty posed by excessive mineralization (Wind, 1980). The method was first applied in the Netherlands to the study of the internal structure of the temporal bone, which had much of morphological interest to inform the paleoanthropologist (Wind, 1984; Zonneveld & Wind, 1985; Wind & Zonneveld, 1985).

At about the same time, in the USA, Conroy & Vannier (1984, 1985), developed a research strategy using recent advances in high-resolution computed tomography to produce accurate, non-invasive, intracranial capacity measurements of matrix-filled fossil skulls. The advances in computer imaging techniques allowed them to produce geometrically accurate three-dimensional images of fossil crania from two-dimensional CT data. The method was developed by Vannier and his colleagues (1983a, b, c, d, e; 1984) initially for the design of craniofacial surgical repairs and reconstructions. Together, Conroy and Vannier applied the approach to matrix-filled crania. The first such instances were two 30-million year old fossil mammal crania, one of *Stenopsochoerus sp.* and one of *Merycoidodon culbertsonii*. The calvariae were completely filled with a hard sandstone matrix. The two specimens yielded images in which the sandstone matrix was clearly distinguishable from the fossilized bone. Not only did they obtain endocranial capacity values, but the endocranial outlines could be processed through a computer reconstruction algorithm to produce a three-dimensional model of the matrix-filled cranial cavity. Since the brain is unique among the organs of the body in that it fits snugly within a bony box ('braincase'), the model produced in this way may be regarded as a 'virtual endocast'. The method employed is described in detail by Conroy & Vannier (1985).

Conroy assessed the accuracy of their method for the determining of endocranial capacity by applying it to four modern crania, two of humans, one of gorilla and one of baboon. On these crania the capacity was obtained directly by the filling of the empty crania with seed and the determining of the volume of seed required to fill the calvariae. Values derived from the CT scanner all lay within 1–3% of the values directly determined by the seed method (Conroy & Vannier, 1985). They concluded, 'We believe these new non-invasive computer imaging techniques can have important applications in future paleoanthropological investigations by allowing anthropologists to view and analyze fossil primate material in ways never before possible' (Conroy & Vannier, 1985, p. 424).

Application to the Taung skull

Conroy, Vannier and I, assisted by D.E. Ricklan, scanned the Taung skull as a trial run. We were able to obtain a clear picture of the extent of the part of the endocast that remains in position against the posterior surface of the frontal bone and in the anterior cranial fossa. This part of the endocast had been severed from the remainder by the dynamite blast with which the discoverer, a lime miner named M. de Bruyn, had laid the specimen bare in October–November 1924. The chief value of the CT scans of the Taung child was in the revealing of its developing permanent tooth germs. These were visualized far more precisely than could be achieved with straight X-rays: the resulting images were chiefly responsible for the reassessment of the age of the Taung child as about four years, instead of the six years which Dart (1925) had originally estimated on the basis of dental emergence. Up to the present, we have not employed CT scanning to re-estimate the total endocranial capacity of the Taung skull, but this is on the author's program.

Application to an *Australopithecus* fossil from Makapansgat

The first australopithecine cranium to which the new method for the determination of endocranial capacity was applied was specimen MLD 37/38 from Member 4 in the Makapansgat cave system, some 300 km north of Johannesburg (Conroy *et al.*, 1990). This fossil was doubly taxing: not only did it contain a heavily calcified and very solid matrix, but also the anterior part of the calvaria and its contained partial endocast (estimated to be about 12.5% of the total capacity) were missing, having been removed by weathering processes on the surface of the Makapansgat hillside where it was discovered still embedded in Member 4 deposit. Previously the total endocranial capacity of MLD 37/38 had been estimated at 480 cm³ (Dart, 1962) and 435 cm³ (Holloway, 1972).

The scans of the cranium were made in Johannesburg, where the cranium reposes in the Department of Anatomical Sciences of the University of the Witwatersrand. Contiguous, non-overlapping, high-resolution CT scans were taken at a slice thickness of 2 mm with a Siemens DR3 CT scanner in the Department of Radiology, Hillbrow Hospital, Johannesburg. The digital scans and digital radiographs that were used for localization ('topograms') were stored on single-sided, double density floppy disks for transportation to the Mallinckrodt Institute of Radiology at Washington University Medical School, St. Louis, Missouri, where they were analyzed on a Siemens Evaluscope-DR reviewing console. Hard copies of all images were made with a Matrix Instruments MI-10 camera.

In this case, it was necessary to develop a new technique in order to restore missing portions of the calvaria and endocast. A total of 46 continuous transaxial CT slices were used from the foramen magnum inferiorly to the superior plane of the calvaria. A volume was extracted from each slice as follows. The interface between the matrix and the endocranial surface of the calvarial bone was easily determined. An endocranial

'region of interest' (ROI) was created by tracing the contour of the interface with the Evaluscope's built-in digitizer resistor pad and stylus. Once
this ROI was established, the STATISTIC command calculated the area of
the ROI in square centimeters. When this value was multiplied by 0.2 cm
(the thickness of the slices), the endocranial slice volume in cubic centimeters was obtained. The slice volumes for all of the slices were stored.
The sum of the slice volumes gave the total endocranial volume of the
specimen MLD 37/38. The first 23 slices were straightforward. CT slices 24
to 46 traversed both the preserved and the missing portions of the calvaria and endocast. In each of these affected slices, the missing cerebrum
was restored by drawing. The area circumscribed by the tracing was then
rendered opaque on the computer screen so that it formed a symmetrical
fit with the preserved portion of the calvaria and endocast. The volumes
of the preserved and of the reconstructed portions of the endocast were
calculated as described above and recorded: the volumes obtained being
372 cm³ and 53 cm³ respectively. The total value thus obtained is 425 cm³,
which is close to Holloway's (1972) estimate of 435 cm³ from ectocranial
measurements and a revised formula. Both values are appreciably lower
than the 480 cm³ that had been estimated by Dart (1962).

Sterkfontein hominin 505: another kind of problem

A large cranium, Stw 505, was found *in situ* in Sterkfontein Member 4, the
stratum which is the richest source of the species *Australopithecus africanus*.
In this specimen most of the left side of the calvaria is included, extending
up to the midline in places. The calvaria is empty, that is, devoid of an
endocast. Some fracture-distortion of the vault is present. It was necessary therefore first to obtain an undistorted image and then to produce a
computer-generated image of the complete calvaria, on the assumption
that the vault was symmetrical. The repository of this cranium, like that
of the MLD 37/38 cranium, is the fossil laboratory of the Department of
Anatomical Sciences of the University of the Witwatersrand,
Johannesburg. The CT scans were taken on a Siemens Somatom Plus 4 CT
Scanner at Selby Park Medical Centre, Marshalltown, Johannesburg. The
detailed method employed is given in Conroy *et al.* (1998a).

A complete series of high-resolution, 1 mm thick, transaxial CT scans
was made of the calvaria. Even though the cranium is heavily mineral-
ized, the CT scans do not show any noticeable artifacts. From these CT
data the author's collaborators in Vienna, H. Seidler, H. Prossinger, G.W.
Weber, and others, Wolfgang Recheis and D. zur Nedden in Innsbruck,

and the St. Louis group led by G.C. Conroy and including A. Kane and B. Brunsden, produced a geometrically accurate, three-dimensional computer model of the cranium. The model's accuracy was tested by comparisons of its dimensions with those taken on the original cranium. The accuracy was within 0.5%. It was not difficult to determine the mid-sagittal plane of the Stw 505 cranium and thus a complete 3D reconstruction could be made, on the assumption of symmetry.

The program allowed the enclosed endocranial cavity to be rendered into a separate 3D object or a 'virtual endocast', by making the cranium transparent. The volume of the 'virtual endocast' is 513 cm^3. The 'virtual endocast' fits congruously and tightly into the cranium, as imaged. The validity of this method was tested on ten recent *Homo sapiens* crania, whose capacity was determined also by the mustard seed method. The observed error was about 2% of the total capacity.

A second method was used on Stw 505, namely by the calculation of the volume of each 1 mm CT slice (similar to the method used in the case of MLD 37/38). In this instance there were 106 slices and the endocranial volume obtained was 518 cm^3.

In a third approach, we filled the hemi-calvaria with water, after blocking deficiencies and building up the margin to the estimated median sagittal plane. The water was then poured in each case into a glass measuring cylinder. A certain amount of leakage and spillage occurred during this operation, so there is more variability among the series of nine such readings. Thus, the values obtained varied from 482 cm^3 to 536 cm^3 with a mean value of 515 cm^3.

Three different methods thus gave values of 513 cm^3, 518 cm^3 and 515 cm^3 (mean value of water displacement determinations). On this basis, we have proposed 515 cm^3 as an acceptable value for the endocranial capacity of this large cranium of A. *africanus* from Sterkfontein (Conroy *et al.*, 1998a,b).

Resulting new statistics for the capacities of A. *africanus*

Hitherto, the sample range of capacities of A. *africanus* had been 428–485 cm^3 for a sample of six specimens. The previous sample mean had been 441.2 cm^3, with a standard deviation of 19.6 cm^3 and a coefficient of variation (CV) of 4.44% (Tobias, 1987). In contrast, the values of CV for *Homo habilis* were 12.85% and for *Homo erectus* in Asia the values varied between 9.86% and 10.79%. It was clear to me from these values that the previous sample of endocranial capacities of A. *africanus* seriously under-

Table 12.1. *Endocranial capacity estimates for* A. africanus *specimens*

Specimen	Capacity (cm³)	Source
MLD 37/38	425	Conroy *et al.*, 1990
Sts 60	428	Holloway, 1975
Sts 71	428	Holloway, 1975
Sts 19	436	Holloway, 1975
Sts 5	485	Holloway, 1975
Stw 505	515	Conroy *et al.*, 1998a,b
Taung 1	440	Holloway, 1975
Mean	451	This study

represented the variability of capacities in the species. We must have sampled, up to then, only a small proportion of the expected variability of *A. africanus*, with the then available sample of six values. The 95% population limits (rounded off to the nearest cubic centimeter) then stood at 392–490 cm³

The revised estimate for MLD 37/38 obtained by the CT scanning method, and the new value for Stw 505 obtained as described above, have improved these figures somewhat.

The sample range is now 425–515 cm³ (in place of the previous 428–485 cm³). That is, the interval between the smallest and largest values thus far available has increased from 57 cm³ to 90 cm³. It should be remembered that the seven values include data for presumptive males and for presumptive females. Clearly we should expect both smaller and larger values as further specimens become available.

The mean capacity for *A. africanus* now stands at 451 cm³ (in place of the former 441.2 cm³). The standard deviation is now greater at 34.96 cm³ instead of the former 19.6 cm³, whilst the coefficient of variation has risen from the former 4.44% to 7.75%. The 95% population limits (rounded off) now stand at 364–538 cm³.

The new figures show that we are approaching what seems to be a more reasonable estimate of the population variability in the species *A. africanus*. Table 12.1 gives the latest list of individual values for *A. africanus* specimens.

Some other endocranial revelations by CT scanning

The use of CT scanning makes it possible to visualize many other fine details of cranial and endocranial morphology. For example, the anatomy of the bony labyrinth of the inner ear (e.g. Spoor *et al.*, 1994), the pattern of the paranasal sinuses and of the degree and ramifications of cranial pneumatization in general (e.g. Seidler *et al.*, 1997), and the impressions of the cranial venous sinuses on the interior of the calvaria, such as the presence or absence of enlarged occipital and marginal sinuses (Conroy *et al.*, 1990) have all been rendered accessible where conventional X-rays had yielded disappointing results.

In the endocast-filled calvaria of MLD 37/38, for example, serial scans through the posterior cranial fossa have shown the absence of the characteristic grooves which enlarged occipital and marginal sinuses imprint upon the endocranium. Thus, this specimen of *A. africanus* resembles in this respect most of the other crania of *A. africanus* and differs from most of the crania of the robust australopithecines and of those assigned to *A. afarensis*, which agree in possessing the striking occipital and marginal sinus enlargement. It seems that in MLD 37/38 the blood from the surface of the cerebrum drained to the jugular venous system by the lateral route, through the transverse and sigmoid venous sinuses. As testimony of this, the serial scans of MLD 37/38 show clearly a well-developed groove for the sigmoid sinus. Such fine and developmentally and physiologically important traits would not be detectable in endocast-filled crania other than through the use of CT scanning – unless one resorted to the invasive technique of extracting the filling of the calvaria, which might require 'removing part of the braincase to expose the natural fossil endocast' (Radinsky, 1972). Clearly, however, such an invasive method would seriously endanger the calvaria. Custodians of rare and precious specimens would be most unwilling to embark upon such a procedure.

It may be mentioned in passing that the study by CT scans of the fine internal structure of fossil bones is not confined to crania. For example, Macchiarelli *et al.* (1998) have obtained singularly beautiful results by applying CT scanning to the trabecular architecture within the ilium of the os coxae.

Limiting factors in the phylogenetic increase of brain size?

Elsewhere I have shown that both *A. robustus* and *H. habilis* show high risk demographic patterns, *H. habilis* having an appreciably higher risk pattern than that of *A. robustus*. In contrast, the earlier hominin species, *A. africanus*, had a low risk demographic pattern (Tobias, 1968, 1991, 1999). In examining the possible causal factors related to these demographic differences, I found evidence to support the hypothesis that changes in the demographic pattern depended upon alterations in the environment. The less challenging conditions of life when A. africanus lived on the planet, from about 3.2 to 2.6 million years ago, appeared to be correlated with the smaller percentage of A. africanus fossils that represented individuals which had died before the attainment of full anatomical maturity. The well-known deterioration in Africa's climate, largely through tectonic uplift bringing in its wake cooling and drying, from 2.6–2.5 million years onwards, seems to have posed a more serious strain on the chances of survival of the hominins which were living in Africa at that time. This, in turn, reflected itself in higher percentages of anatomically immature individuals of the robust australopithecines and of their contemporary H. habilis and, at Zhoukoudian, among the Asian sample of H. erectus pekinensis.

Both A. robustus and H. habilis shared an equally hostile African environment and it is therefore understandable that both showed high risk demographic patterns. However, one of those two taxa – H. habilis – was at a greater demographic risk than the other. Climate alone does not seem adequate to explain this difference between the two contemporary hominins. I am grateful to S.U. Dani for the suggestion that I explore the possible consequences of marrying the data on absolute and relative brain sizes (i.e. endocranial capacities) to the data on demographic patterns (Tobias, 1996).

Increasing brain size, or encephalization, might be expected to have made extra demands upon the body's nutritional reserves and the population's resource base. This is because, of all the tissues in the body, neural tissue has the greatest nutritional requirements and constitutes a major metabolic burden to the ontogenetically developing organism. (See also Aiello et al., Chapter 3, this volume.) It might therefore be postulated that, at a time of minimal encephalization, a population's demands on the resource base would be minimal; during a phase of greater encephalization, these demands would be enhanced, whilst a population undergoing strong encephalization would be subject to an appreciable increase in its nutritional demands.

First, it is often assumed that a population with larger adult brain sizes would have a larger mean brain size at birth. This is not necessarily so. It is questionable whether the capacity of the pelvis or birth canal of modern human females is three times as great as that of gorillas, chimpanzees or A. africanus although the respective adult brain sizes are on average about 3 to 1. It is instructive to compare the brain size at birth with that in adulthood. In living humans, the brain size at birth is approximately 25% of that in the adult; in gorillas and chimpanzees, the corresponding figure is of the order of 60%. If the small-brained, ancestral australopithecines resembled the living great apes in this respect, it would follow that during the evolution of the genus *Homo* from *Australopithecus* and during the further evolution of some of the species within the genus *Homo*, there must have occurred a series of diminutions in the percentage of the adult brain size which was already present at birth. Thus, it is reasonable to surmise that the percentage dropped from 60% by steps and stages until the modern human value of about 25% was attained. It would follow that, during encephalization, most of the hominins' increase in brain size must have been largely postnatal. If this reasoning is true, most of the trebling in brain size that has occurred in hominins during the last two million years has taken place when the developing fetus was no longer ensconced within the womb.

Secondly, an important implication of this ontogenetic timing of brain enlargement is that the encephalizing processes – or at least a significant proportion of them – took place postnatally in a creature that was subject to the vicissitudes of the environment and fluctuating food resources. In other words, encephalization in the hominins (although not necessarily in monkeys and baboons, nor in the cetaceans) was a highly vulnerable process. Since Loren Eiseley (1958) touched on this subject in *The Immense Journey*, and Epstein (1973) and Tobias (1971) developed it, a number of subsequent studies, such as those of Martin (1980, 1981), Armstrong (1983), and Hofman (1982), have explored the possible metabolic constraints on human brain weight at birth, postnatal growth and brain enlargement.

Thirdly, another aspect of the problem of the vulnerability of the brain is that this factor might be expected to pose a more serious challenge to development and survival at times when hominins were living in more straitened environmental circumstances.

Demographic patterns and brain size

We may test this hypothesis on a relationship of brain size to demographic pattern by reference to the three early hominin species we have been examining.

A. africanus was modestly more encephalized than the chimpanzee, the respective values for Jerison's (1970) Encephalization Quotient (EQ) being

45% and 34% (as percentages of modern *H. sapiens* values) and for Hemmer's (1971) Constant of Cephalization (CC) 36% and 31% (relative to *H. sapiens* values). This small encephalic advantage of *A. africanus* over chimpanzee would have made small extra demands on the resource base. Moreover, the resource base was presumably tolerable to adequate at this mesic period. Only 35% of *A. africanus* individuals died in the 20-and-under age category.

A. robustus was slightly more encephalized than *A. africanus*, the respective values for EQ being 46% and 45% and for CC 42% and 36%. It lived in the cooler, drier and more demanding environment of Africa after 2.6–2.5 million years, so survival was at a premium. The remains of 60.5% of individuals fall into the 20-and-under category.

H. habilis was appreciably more encephalized than *A. africanus*, and had reached or passed the 50% mark in relation to the mean encephalization values of modern humans. The respective values for EQ of *H. habilis* and *A. africanus* are 53% and 45% and for CC 49% and 36%. *H. habilis* lived in the same cooler, more arid conditions as did *A. robustus*, but its greater encephalic nutritional demands must have placed it at a decided disadvantage in the struggle for survival. No fewer than 73% of the age-determinable individuals were 20 years and under at the time of death.

These figures appear to show that the differential demographic patterns among these three early hominin species had two principal determinants. One was the circumambient climate, which could explain part of the differences, namely those between *A. africanus* on the one hand and *A. robustus* and *H. habilis* on the other, but could not distinguish between the two latter synchronic species, the robust australopithecine and *H. habilis*. The second factor was the intensity of encephalizing pressures to which the various taxa were exposed and this appears to account for the differences between the demographic patterns of *A. robustus* and *H. habilis* populations.

It is concluded that, while the increased metabolic burden of larger brains would have been a restrictive handicap under any environmental circumstances, the presence of such encephalizing pressures in the face of a sharply adverse environment, such as beset Africa from 2.6–2.5 million years onwards, would be expected to have made survival even more difficult and would have contributed to a lowering of the average expectation of life. On the other hand, it must be assumed that the change to a high risk demographic pattern went hand in hand with an enhancement or at least the maintenance of the selection pressures favoring encephalization. These evident evolutionary advantages of encephalization (Falk,

1987, 1990) must have more than compensated for the high metabolic and demographic cost of the exercise. This study leads to the conclusion that, controlled by the currently accepted dating framework, the differences among the demographic patterns evinced by several ancient hominin species may be understood as the consequences of changing ecological conditions and of varying evolutionary pressures favoring differing degrees of encephalization.

Water and brain food

The tectonic changes in Africa from 2.6–2.5 million years ago probably had major effects on water resources. A consequence of uplift would be river reversal and other changes of drainage patterns, including the drying up of lakes previously fed with an adequate inflow of water. The availability of fresh water may in itself have had a serious effect on the chances of survival of the hominins (and other animals) living in the vicinity. There is, however, an additional factor that may have influenced the development of the brains of species whose individuals were bigger-brained. This refers to the presence in part of the food chain of a specific chemical considered to be of great importance in the development of brains. Crawford *et al.* (1998) have pointed out that the modern brain, which is 60% lipid, requires docosahexaenoic acid (DHA) for its growth, structure and function. In an analysis of the chemistry of the brains of 42 species of vertebrates, they found that the chemistry of the brain was consistently the same and that the relative brain size (assessed in relation to body size) varied in relation to the DHA supply. They inferred that vertebrates have used DHA in photoreceptors and to optimize the evolution of the brain. The dependence of the visual system and the brain, in general, on DHA has been demonstrated in laboratory experiments and in studies on preterm infant vision and cognitive function. Crawford and his collaborators went further and claimed that the evolution of the large hominin brain depended on the marine (or ?aquatic) food chain with its abundant supply of DHA. Both plants and animals which are adapted to life in the water have a high content of DHA, whereas savanna-dwelling life forms are poor in DHA.

Their claim appears to be supported by the observations of Puech (1992) on the patterns of microwear of the cheek-teeth. These wear patterns suggest that the australopithecine diet included marshland plants, sappy aquatic herbs and grasses, while those of H. *habilis* suggest the inclusion of reeds, sedges, marsh plants, fruits and molluscs in their dietary regimen.

If the claim that DHA is vitally important for the enlargement of the hominin brain is sustained, it would follow that one route by which the deterioration of the African climate and ecology from 2.6–2.5 million years ago affected hominin survival at a time of marked encephalization (as in *H. habilis*) might have been by the decline in DHA resources consequent upon river capture, river reversal, rearrangement of drainage patterns, and drying up of formerly well-filled lakes. Under these conditions, it may be possible for testable causal links to be hypothesized between paleo-ecology, paleo-demography, dependence on the marine and aquatic food chain, and encephalization.

Seen in this light, brain size and its change in hominin evolution become far more than mere characters to be added to the tally of traits available for purposes of hominin systematics. Rather, when placed in the broader contexts considered here, we see brain size change as a marker to climatic and dietary features and changes in them; and it was a probable limiting factor in the survival of populations whose degree of encephalization was burgeoning, at times when the ecology was more exacting.

These correlations and connections are presented here very tentatively. They pose a series of hypotheses, the refinement and testing of which may well occupy the endeavors of some students of brain evolution in the coming century.

Acknowledgments

I am grateful for stimulating and fruitful interaction with G.C. Conroy, M. Vannier, H. Seidler, H. Prossinger, G. Weber, W. Recheis, R. Ziegler, D. zur Nedden and other colleagues at Vienna, Innsbruck, St. Louis and Johannesburg.

My thanks are due to Professor Dean Falk and Professor Kathleen Gibson for their generous invitation to contribute a chapter to this Festschrift, even though I was unable to attend the Symposium in honor of Harry Jerison – and for their patience. This work was made possible through generous grants from the PAST Fund, the National Research Foundation, the University of the Witwatersrand, the Wenner Gren Foundation, the L.S.B. Leakey Foundation and the Ford Foundation.

As always I owe an enormous debt of gratitude to Heather White.

References

Armstrong, E. (1983). A look at relative brain size in mammals. *Neuroscience Letters*, **34**, 101–104.

Conroy, G.C. & Vannier, M.W. (1984). Noninvasive three-dimensional computer imaging of matrix-filled fossil skulls by high-resolution computed tomography. *Science*, **26**, 456–458.

Conroy, G.C. & Vannier, M.W. (1985). Endocranial volume determination of matrix-filled fossil skulls using high-resolution computed tomography. In *Hominid Evolution: Past, Present and Future*, ed. P.V. Tobias, pp. 419–426. New York: Alan R. Liss.

Conroy, G.C., Vannier, M.W. & Tobias, P.V. (1990). Endocranial features of *Australopithecus africanus* revealed by 2- and 3-D computed tomography. *Science*, **247**, 838–841.

Conroy, G.C., Weber, G.W., Seidler, H., Tobias, P.V., Kane, A. & Brunsden, B. (1998a). Endocranial capacity in an early hominid cranium from Sterkfontein, South Africa. *Science*, **280**, 1730–1731.

Conroy, G.C., Kane, A., Seidler, H., Weber, G. & Tobias, P. (1998b). Endocranial capacity of Stw 505 ('Mr. Ples'), a large new hominid cranium from Sterkfontein. *American Journal of Physical Anthropology Supplement.*, **26**, 69–70.

Crawford, M., Bloom, M., Cunnane, S., Broadhurst, L., Harbige, L. & Ghebremeskel, K. (1998). The evolution of the brain of *Homo sapiens* depended on the marine food chain. In *Book of Abstracts*, Dual Congress 1998, eds. M.A. Raath, H. Soodyall, D. Barkham, K.L. Kuykendall & P.V. Tobias. Johannesburg.

Dart, R.A. (1925). *Australopithecus africanus*: the man-ape of South Africa. *Nature*, **115**, 195–199.

Dart, R.A. (1962). The Makapansgat pink breccia australopithecine skull. *American Journal of Physical Anthropology*, **20**, 119–126.

Eiseley, L.C. (1958). *The Immense Journey*. New York: Random House.

Epstein, H.T. (1973). Possible metabolic constraints on human brain weight at birth. *American Journal of Physical Anthropology*, **39**, 135–136.

Falk, D. (1987). Brain lateralization in primates and its evolution in hominids. *Yearbook of Physical Anthropology*, **30**, 107–127.

Falk, D. (1990). Brain evolution in *Homo*: The 'radiator' theory. *Behavioral and Brain Sciences*, **13**, 333–381.

Hemmer, H. (1971). Beitrag zur Erfassung der progressiven Cephalization bei Primaten. In *Proceedings of the 3rd International Congress of Primatology*, eds. J. Biegert & W. Leutenegger, pp. 99–107. Basel: Karger.

Hofman, M.A. (1982). Encephalization in mammals in relation to the size of the cerebral cortex. *Brain, Behavior and Evolution*, **20**, 24–96.

Holloway, R.L. (1972). Australopithecine endocasts, brain evolution in the Hominoidea, and a model of hominid evolution. In *The Functional and Evolutionary Biology of Primates*, ed. R. Tuttle, pp. 175–184. Chicago, New York: Aldine-Atherton.

Holloway, R.L. (1975). Early hominid endocasts: volumes, morphology and significance for hominid evolution. In *Primate Functional Morphology and Evolution*, ed. R.H. Tuttle, pp. 393–416. The Hague: Mouton.

Hounsfield, G.N. (1973). Computerized transverse axial scanning (tomography). *British Journal of Radiology*, **46**, 1016–1022.

Jerison, H.J. (1970). Gross brain indices and the analysis of fossil endocasts. *The Primate Brain*, **1**, 225–244.

Jerison, H.J. (1973). *Evolution of the Brain and Intelligence*. New York, London: Academic Press.

Macchiarelli, R., Galichon, V., Bondioli, L. & Tobias, P.V. (1998). Hip bone trabecular architecture and locomotor behaviour in South African australopithecines. In *Proc. XIII Cong. IUPPS*, pp. 175–184.

Martin, R.D. (1980). Adaptation and body size in primates. *Zeitschrift für Morphologie und Anthropologie*, **71**, 115–124.

Martin, R.D. (1981). Relative brain-size and basal metabolic rate in terrestrial vertebrates. *Nature*, **293**, 57–60.

Puech, P.-F. (1992). Microwear studies of early African hominid teeth. *Scanning Microscopy*, **6**, 1083–1088.

Radinsky, L. (1972). Endocasts and studies of primate brain evolution. In *The Functional and Evolutionary Biology of Primates*, ed. R. Tuttle, pp. 175–184. Chicago, New York: Aldine-Atherton.

Seidler, H., Falk, D., Stringer, C., Wilfing, H., Müller, G., zur Nedden, D., Weber, G., Recheis, W. & Arsuaga, J.L. (1997). A comparative study of stereolithographically modelled skulls of Petralona and Broken Hill: implications for future studies of middle Pleistocene hominid evolution. *Journal of Human Evolution*, **33**, 691–703.

Spoor, F., Wood, B. & Zonneveld, F. (1994). Implications of early hominid labyrinthine morphology for evolution of human bipedal locomotion. *Nature*, **369**, 645–648.

Tobias, P.V. (1968). The age of death among the Australopithecines. *The Anthropologist*, Special Volume, 23–28.

Tobias, P.V. (1971). *The Brain in Hominid Evolution*. New York and London: Columbia University Press.

Tobias, P.V. (1987). The brain of *Homo habilis*: a new level of organization in cerebral evolution. *Journal of Human Evolution*, **16**, 741–761.

Tobias, P.V. (1991). The age at death of the Olduvai *Homo habilis* population and the dependence of demographic patterns on prevailing environmental conditions. In *Studia Archaeologica: Liber Amicorum, Jacques Nenquin*, eds. H. Thoen, J. Bourgeois, F. Vermeulen, P. Crombé & K. Verlaeckt, pp. 57–65. University of Gent.

Tobias, P.V. (1994). The craniocerebral interface in early hominids. In *Integrative Paths to the Past: Paleoanthropological Advances in Honor of F. Clark Howell*, eds. Robert S. Corruccini & Russell L. Ciochon, pp. 185–203. New Jersey: Prentice Hall, Englewood Cliffs.

Tobias, P.V. (1996). Changes in hominid demographic patterns, environment and encephalisation. In *Human Biology – Global Developments*, eds. L.S. Sidhu & S.P. Singh, pp. 261–274. Ludhiana: USG Publishers & Distributors.

Tobias, P.V. (1999). Re-creating ancient hominid brains by CT-Scanning. Paper presented to the XV Congress of the International Federation of Associations of Anatomists, Rome, September 1999.

Vannier, M., Gado, M. & Marsh, J. (1983a). Three-dimensional display of intracranial soft tissue structures. *American Journal of Neuroradiology*, **4**, 520–521.

Vannier, M., Marsh, J., Gado, M., Totty, W., Gilula, L. & Evens R. (1983b). Clinical applications of three-dimensional surface reconstruction from CT scans. *Electromedica*, **51**, 121 132.

Vannier, M., Marsh, J. & Warren, J. (1983c). Three-dimensional computer graphics for craniofacial surgical planning and evaluation. *Computer Graphics*, 17, 263–273.

Vannier, M., Marsh, J., Warren, J. & Barbier, J. (1983d). Three-dimensional CAD for craniofacial surgery. *Electromagnetic Imaging*, 2, 48–54.

Vannier, M., Marsh, J., Warren. J. & Barbier, J. (1983e). Three-dimensional computer aided design of craniofacial surgical procedures. *Diagnostic Imaging*, 5, 36–43.

Vannier, M.W., Marsh, J.L. & Warren, J.O. (1984). Three dimensional reconstruction images for craniofacial surgical planning and evaluation. *Radiology*, 150, 179–184.

Wind, J. (1980). X-ray analysis of fossil hominid temporal bones. *Antropologia Contemporanea*, 2, 299.

Wind, J. (1984). Computerized X-ray tomography of fossil hominid skulls. *American Journal of Physical Anthropology*, 63, 265–282.

Wind, J. & Zonneveld, F. (1985). Radiology of fossil hominid skulls. In *Hominid Evolution: Past, Present and Future*, ed. P.V. Tobias, pp. 437–442. New York: Alan R. Liss.

Zonneveld, F. & Wind, J. (1985). High-resolution computed tomography of fossil hominid skulls: a new method and some results. In *Hominid Evolution: Past, Present and Future*, ed. P.V. Tobias, pp. 427–436. New York: Alan R. Liss.

13

Advances in the study of hominoid brain evolution: magnetic resonance imaging (MRI) and 3-D reconstruction

Original comparative data on the brains of apes are scarce. The study of the evolution of the human brain and the human mind depends largely on the availability of such evidence. Are there certain features or aspects of the organization of various components of the brain that can be identified as uniquely human? What kind of reorganization took place in the neural circuitry of the hominid brain after the split from other hominoids? How can species-specific adaptations in behavior and cognition be recognized in the underlying neural substrates?

Recent advances in non-invasive neuroimaging techniques used for the analysis of brain structures *in vivo* in humans can now also be applied to the comparative study of the extant hominoids. Magnetic resonance imaging (MRI) and 3-D reconstruction allow for the identification and quantification of many neural structures across species. Use of living subjects avoids issues of shrinkage involved in postmortem tissue processing, facilitates the study of larger samples and also permits the study of species chronically underrepresented (e.g. bonobos, gorillas, orangutans). These new techniques allow for the quantification of selected lobes and smaller sectors of the brain as well as for a more accurate analysis of sulcal and gyral patterns.

The anatomy of the human brain has been traditionally studied either on gross postmortem specimens or in processed histological sections under the microscope. Attempts to image the living brain used, until recently, conventional radiography, a technique that relied on the differential absorption of X-rays by different components of the brain and its covers. The oldest form of the technique could only reveal the bones and calcium-accumulating tissues. However, the improved method of computerized axial tomography (CT) allows the additional visualization of gray and white matter in brain tissue (Martin & Brust, 1985).

A revolution in the study of the regional anatomy of the brain and its functional aspects took place with the introduction of two other imaging techniques: magnetic resonance imaging (MRI) and positron emission tomography (PET) respectively. MRI permits the exploration of the neural structures with much better resolution than CT and is based on a set of physical principles that involve the behavior of hydrogen atoms or protons in a magnetic field (Raichle, 1998). This technology, initially used to measure the atomic constituents of chemical samples, became a powerful tool that can distinguish neural structures on the basis of their individual chemical composition. Early applications of the technique on human brains included attempts to improve the resolution needed to visualize the cortex (Damasio *et al.*, 1991) and also investigations of sulcal patterns and asymmetries (Falk *et al.*, 1991; Vannier *et al.*, 1991). The resolution of MRI images of the living human brain now approximates that of fixed and sectioned anatomical material.

PET and functional MRI (fMRI) are used for the study of the function of the living brain. The signal used by PET is based on changes in the cellular activity of the brain that are accompanied by changes in local blood flow. Thus the activity of the brain of normal, awake human subjects is measured. Changes of neuronal activity are accompanied by changes in the amount of oxygen in the tissue. These changes in oxygen, which is carried by hemoglobin, influence the degree to which hemoglobin disturbs a magnetic field. fMRI can detect these *in vivo* changes of blood oxygenation.

A pilot study

The revolution in neuroimaging techniques had not reached the field of comparative neuroanatomy and primate brain evolution until 1993, when such an effort began with a pilot study that Hanna Damasio and I started at the University of Iowa. One postmortem specimen each of a chimpanzee, gorilla, orangutan, gibbon and macaque was available, and we obtained magnetic resonance images from each of them. Each specimen was placed in a plastic container filled with formalin and scanned in a General Electric scanner. Four living human subjects were also scanned. The brains were reconstructed in three dimensions from the MRI sequences using Brainvox, an interactive family of programs designed to reconstruct, segment and measure brains from MR acquired images (Damasio & Frank, 1992; Frank *et al.*, 1997). This program runs on Silicon Graphics computer stations.

In this first study (Semendeferi *et al.*, 1994, 1997a) we concentrated on the frontal lobes, because they are associated with aspects of cognition, such as decision making, planning of future actions, language, and artistic expression, many of which are thought to be uniquely human. There is also the widespread notion that the frontal lobes are enlarged out of proportion in humans (Deacon, 1988; Finger, 1994), but few comparative studies have tried to test this notion on original, primary data. Are the frontal lobes really disproportionately larger in our species than in the rest of the hominoids? Did the frontal lobes undergo a particular enlargement during human evolution after the split of the hominid line from the African apes? Use of MR imaging in combination with software designed to reconstruct the brain in three dimensions and calculate the size of segmented subvolumes (Damasio & Frank, 1992) made such a study possible. In this first study we outlined the hemispheres and the frontal lobe in each species and obtained volumetric estimates. The cortex of the frontal lobes was further subdivided into three sectors known to have distinct functional attributes: dorsal (manipulation of space, numbers and language), mesial (attention mechanisms), and orbital (social behavior). A clear separation between gray and white matter was not consistently visible in the postmortem specimens. Therefore the regions of interest included the immediately underlying white matter (white matter core of each gyrus).

As expected, the frontal lobes of the human brain were found to be the largest in absolute terms followed by those of the great apes, then the gibbon and last the macaque. Contrary to expectation, we found that in relative terms human values did not stand out among the hominoids. As a percentage of the total hemisphere the chimpanzee frontal lobe value fell within the range of the human values and the other apes followed closely. Furthermore, when regressed against total hemispheric size, the frontal lobe of humans did not prove to be larger than expected for an ape brain of human size.

The three sectors of the frontal cortex (dorsal, mesial, orbital) also formed three plateaus with the same general distribution of their absolute values as seen in the case of the hemispheres and the frontal lobes. The macaque and gibbon had the smallest values, followed by the great apes and then the human brain. The only noticeable exception was the small size of the orangutan orbital sector, whose value lay between that of the gibbon and the other great apes. In all species the orbital sector is the smallest followed by the mesial and the dorsal sectors. The relative values of the three sectors (calculated as a ratio of the volume of the cortex of the frontal lobe and immediately underlying white matter) were quite similar across all hominoids and the only value that stood out was that of the orangutan orbital sector. When the volumes of the dorsal, mesial and orbital sectors of the frontal lobe were regressed against the volume of the hemisphere and a best fit line was determined on the basis of the nonhuman primate data, the human values were, in all three cases, as large as expected for a primate brain of human size.

The new, larger data set of living hominoid brains

The study involving postmortem specimens included only one subject per species, and we were concerned with the possibility of differential shrinkage in the different sectors of the ape brains which might possibly have influenced the results. Our provocative results on the frontal lobe would remain controversial unless these concerns could be addressed. Images of living subjects were needed for all the ape species in a larger number of individuals. Late in 1994 we approached the new director of the Yerkes Regional Primate Research Center, Tom Insel, who agreed to undertake the scanning of the apes. After numerous trials and a large scale collaboration between the staff of the Department of Neurology at the University of Iowa and the staff and students of Emory University we managed to obtain the first acceptable scans of a chimpanzee. The scanning of several more apes and other anthropoids from both Yerkes and the Atlanta Zoo followed.

The 3-D reconstruction of the specimens, the volumetric estimates and the analysis began in Iowa using Brainvox. Figure 13.1 includes the 3-D reconstruction from MR images of selected subjects representing all hominoid taxa. The subjects are all adult individuals of both sexes (ten humans, three bonobos, six chimpanzees, two gorillas, four orangutans and four gibbons). A human subject was scanned both in Iowa and Emory (the author) in order to ensure consistency across measurements obtained from brains scanned at these two different sites (apes scanned at Emory and humans scanned in Iowa).

The results of this new study (Semendeferi et al., 1996, 1997a,b; Semendeferi & Damasio, 2000) in fact demonstrates that humans have the largest frontal lobes *only* in absolute terms, and are followed by the great apes and then the gibbons. Any relative measure of the size of the human frontal lobe points to the fact that human frontal lobes are *not* larger than expected for an ape brain of human size. Figure 13.2*a* shows this allometric relationship where the human data are clearly aligned along the regression line that is estimated on the basis of the nonhuman hominoids. The size of the frontal lobes as a percentage of the total size of the two hemispheres does not stand out either and the ranges of these values in individual human and ape subjects overlap. The mean relative values for these taxa lie between 35–37%.

However, not all sectors of the brain exhibit such a pattern. The temporal lobe, heavily involved in recognition and memory, is well developed in the human brain and a qualitative inspection of the allometric relationship (Fig. 13.2*b*) shows human values to be larger than expected on the basis of the nonhuman hominoids. The same applies to another sector of the brain, the insula (Fig. 13.2*c*), an area involved in autonomic function, taste and processing of internal stimuli. It was also recently shown that the left precentral gyrus of the insula seems to be involved in the coordination of speech articulation (Dronkers, 1996). Nevertheless, statistical significance is not reached in either case and use of a larger sample would be necessary to investigate possible quantitative differences. In contrast, the large parieto-occipital sector, like the frontal lobe, does not stand out in the human brain, but is as large as expected for an ape brain of the human size. The parietal and occipital cortices integrate sensory and visual information, and are involved in functions such as visuospatial coordination and attention mechanisms.

Of interest is the finding on the cerebellum, a structure involved in fine motor tuning, balance and, more recently, also aspects of cognition. The human cerebellum proved to be smaller than expected for an ape brain of human size (Semendeferi & Damasio, 2000), and the difference does reach statistical significance (Fig. 13.2*d*). What can such a finding mean especially in light of recent evidence that this structure is not only involved in motor related functions as previously thought, but also in cognitive aspects of behavior (Fiez, 1996; Muller *et al.*, 1998)? It is most likely that different components of this structure evolved at different rates during primate evolution. The studies of Matano *et al.* (1985) and Matano & Hirasaki (1997), who studied the cerebellar system and its components on histological sections in several mammals, support the idea of differential enlargement of certain parts of the system. The lateral

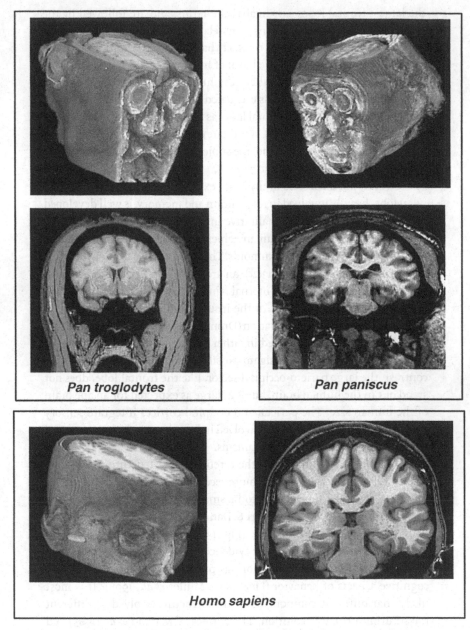

Fig. 13.1. Three-dimensional reconstruction of magnetic resonance images obtained from living ape and human subjects.

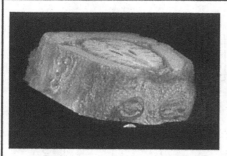
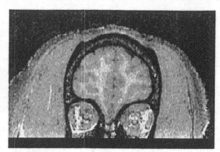

Pongo pygmaeus

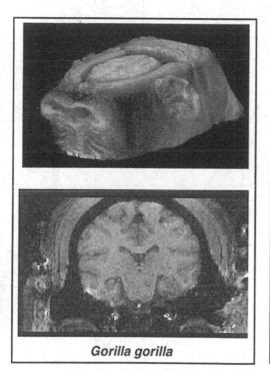

Gorilla gorilla

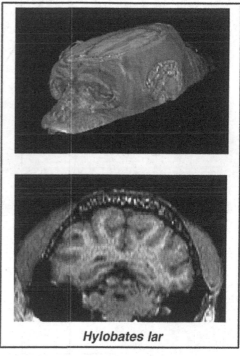

Hylobates lar

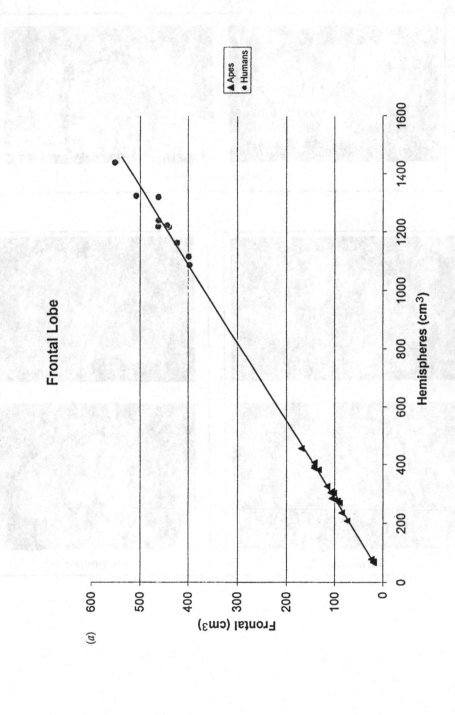

(a)

Frontal Lobe

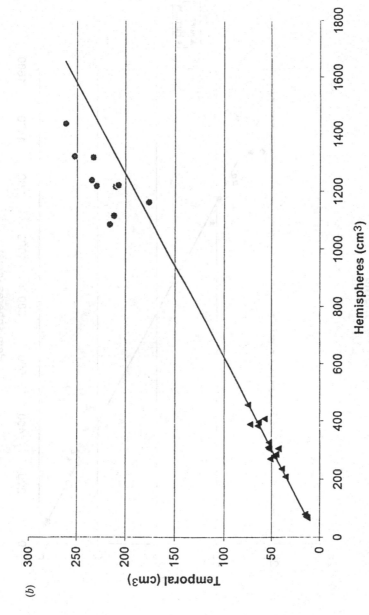

Temporal Lobe

Fig. 13.2. Allometric relationships between the hemispheres and large sectors of the brain. The best fit line is based on the nonhuman subjects (great and lesser apes).

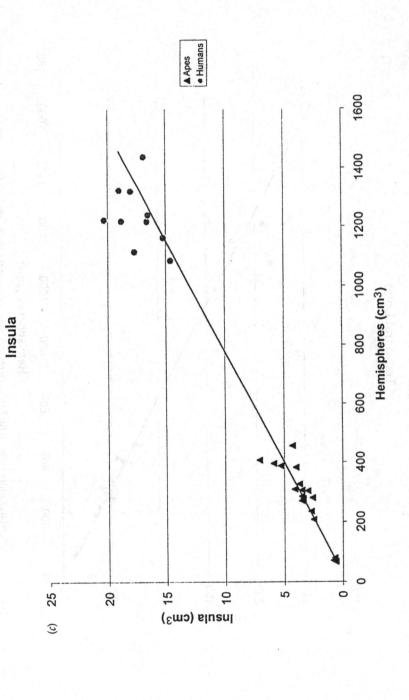

Insula

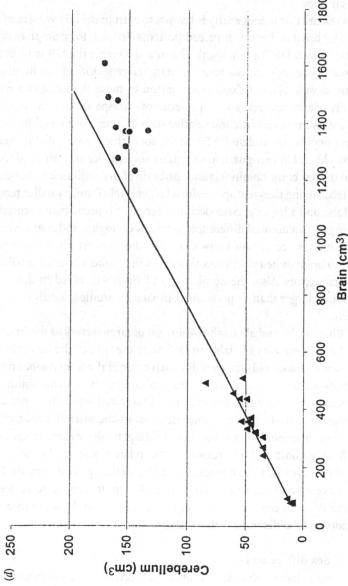

Fig. 13.2. (cont.)

cerebellar system, including the ventral pons, is relatively larger in primates such as gibbons and chimpanzees, and the dentate nucleus, which is connected with the lateral cortex of the cerebellum, is larger in humans than in apes.

A remarkable homogeneity is known to exist in the relative size of the primate brain and many of its components (Jerison, 1973; Stephan *et al.*, 1981; Finlay & Darlington, 1995). The new data from the MR studies discussed above support this idea for many large sectors of the hominoid brain as well. Nevertheless, examination of more than one subject in closely related taxa reveals the presence of intraspecific and interspecific variability in the absolute and relative sizes of certain sectors of the brains of hominoids (Semendeferi & Damasio, 2000) that are identifiable even at a gross level. The orangutan has a remarkably smaller orbitofrontal sector than the rest of the hominoids and the brain of the gorilla seems to be specialized among the great apes, with a larger cerebellum, a smaller temporal lobe, and a larger parieto-occipital sector. It is premature to correlate these gross anatomical differences with any ecological and cognitive specialization, since we now know that even the simplest functions involve coordination of neural circuits that cross the borders of traditional anatomical sectors. Also, the number of individuals involved in the study, although larger than in previous comparative studies, is still relatively small.

What can be said about the evolution of large sectors of the brain on the basis of the data available so far? After the split of the hominid line from other hominoids the overall relative size of the frontal lobe and the parieto-occipital region does not seem to have increased in hominids. It is possible that the frontal lobes increased in size well before the appearance of the first Plio-Pleistocene hominids, sometime after the split of the Miocene hominoids from the line leading to the extant lesser apes. Following those early increases in the relative size of the hominoid frontal lobe, no further changes seem to have taken place during the Plio-Pleistocene with regard to relative overall size. It remains to be seen if subdivisions of the frontal lobe and other regions of the brain into subsectors reveal differences in their relative size.

Sex differences

The above data on the various lobes and sectors of the hominoid brain have recently been analyzed in terms of possible sex differences and right–left asymmetries (unpublished observations). The hominoids scanned included five male and five female humans, two male and one female bonobo, three male and three female chimpanzees, one male and one female gorilla, three male and one female orangutan and two male and two female gibbons. The mean raw values (in cm³) of the brain (hemispheres plus cerebellum), cerebellum, hemispheres, frontal, parieto-occipital, and temporal lobes, and insula are larger in males than females across the great apes and humans (Fig. 13.3). Some exceptions are present, as in the case of the chimpanzee cerebellum and parieto-occipital sectors and the human insula where values, although very close, favor the females. The values for the gibbons are also close, but in most sectors females have a larger mean value than males. The gorillas and orangutans exhibit the largest degree of sexual dimorphism and the two chimpanzees the smallest. Nevertheless, the above observations of sex differences were not statistically significant for the two groups, humans and apes, in any of the sectors. Individual ape species, like the gorilla and the orangutan, present large differences between males and females, but the size of the sample (two and four individuals respectively) does not allow for statistical testing.

Right–left asymmetries are not detectable in either males or females in the mean raw values of the hemispheres or the frontal lobes (Fig. 13.3). In the case of the temporal and the parieto-occipital lobes a qualitative inspection of the graphs reveals small asymmetries across species that vary depending on the lobe examined. The insula presents a consistently asymmetrical pattern in favor of a larger size in the left hemisphere in both males and females across all species examined with the exception of the male gibbons. This asymmetry of the insula reaches statistical significance in the case of the apes, when a paired t-test is performed on right versus left insula (Fig. 13.4). Similarly, humans appear to have a larger left insula, but the difference is not significant. It should be noted nevertheless that even in the case of the apes, none of the differences are significant once Bonferroni's correction for multiple comparisons is used, although the p-values are borderline significant.

The mean *relative* values of the sectors were also analyzed (Fig. 13.5). The mean relative size of the cerebellum and the hemispheres (as a percentage of the brain), and the temporal and parieto-occipital lobes (as a percentage of the hemispheres) varies between males and females up to one or two percent, but the range of variation in individual subjects overlaps. A visual inspection of the graphs reveals that the right frontal lobe is larger than the left in both males and females across all hominoids

(a)

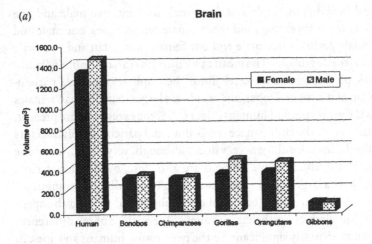

(b)

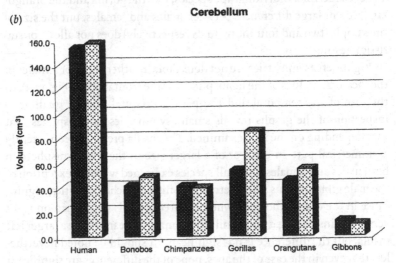

Fig. 13.3. Graphs illustrating raw values of major brain sectors according to sex and right-left hemispheres.

(except for male gibbons) (Fig. 13.5c). In contrast, the left insula is larger than the right insula in both males and females across species with the exception of the male gibbon (Fig. 13.5f).

The larger relative size of the right frontal lobe in the apes, but not in humans, reaches statistical significance (Fig. 13.6a,b), although significance is lost when Bonferroni's correction is applied. In contrast, the

(c)

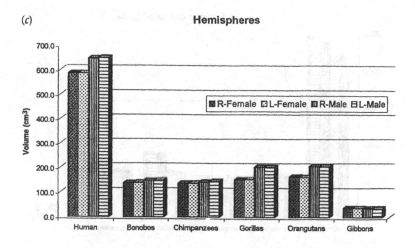

(d)

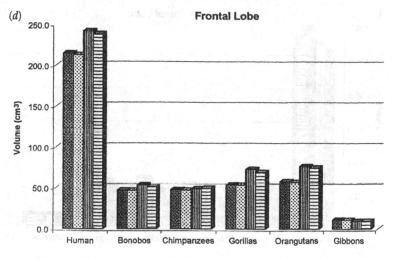

Fig. 13.3. *(cont.)*

larger relative size of the left insula in humans, but not in apes, has a significant *p*-value (Fig. 13.6*c*, *d*). Neither survives Bonferroni's correction for multiple comparisons, although these asymmetries are observable visually in both apes and humans and are consistent with the asymmetries observed with raw values.

Is the insula, a region primarily involved in autonomic functions, processing of internal stimuli, taste, and coordination of speech articulation,

(e)

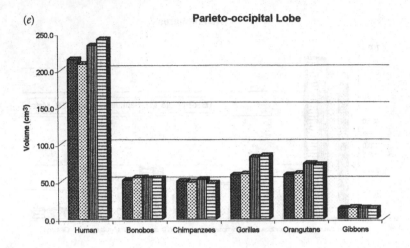

(f)

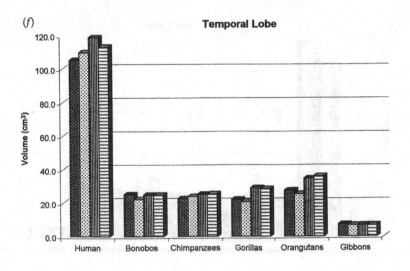

Fig. 13.3. (cont.)

organized differently in the left and right hemispheres of humans and
apes? Will the relative size of the right frontal lobe prove to be larger than
the left in apes and humans when a larger sample becomes available?
More hominoids need to be examined in order to test these preliminary
findings.

(g)

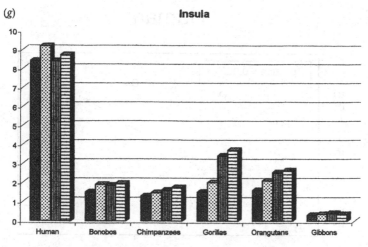

Fig. 13.3. (cont.)

Sulci

The great apes have complex sulcal patterns that exhibit interspecific and intraspecific variation similar to that of the human brain. Major sulci and their configurations have been described in the past on the surface of postmortem specimens of apes (Connolly, 1950). Use of three-dimensionally reconstructed images of the external views of the scanned brains in combination with two-dimensional slices throughout each brain now allow for the investigation of the sulci below the surface. It is thus possible to follow the branching patterns and connections otherwise not visible. In a pilot study addressing such variation (Semendeferi & Damasio, 1997) we investigated some of the major sulci and their distribution. The central, precentral, postcentral, cingulate, and superior temporal sulci and the Sylvian fissure were examined in terms of continuity, branching patterns, connections with other sulci and overall distribution in six chimpanzee, two bonobo, one gorilla and three orangutan brains. Figure 13.7 illustrates a common chimpanzee brain with marked sulci on various views. This specimen has some of the most representative sulcal patterns found in most of the great ape brains examined.

The most stable sulcus in terms of continuity among the 12 brains examined is the Sylvian fissure, the course of which is uninterrupted in all hemispheres examined. The central sulcus and the superior temporal sulcus are also continuous in most cases (with the exception of one

(a)

Human

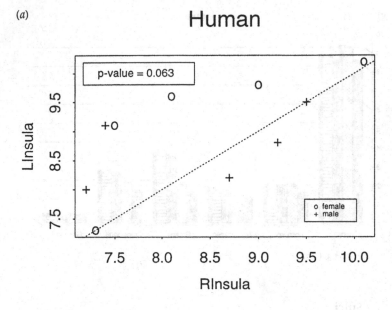

(b)

Ape

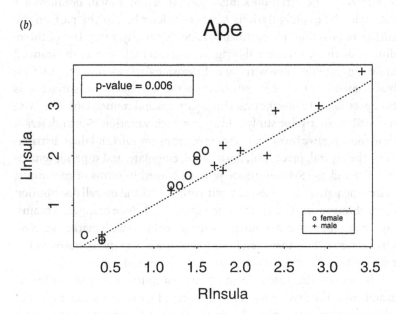

Fig. 13.4. Regressions of individual raw values of the left and right insula for males and females in humans and apes.

(a)

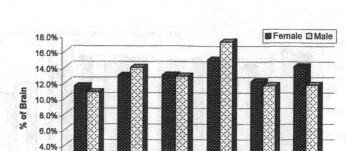

(b)

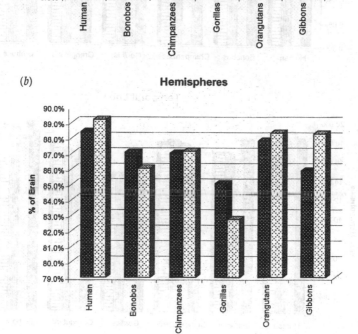

Fig. 13.5. Graphs illustrating relative values of major brain sectors according to sex and right-left hemispheres.

(c)   **Frontal Lobe**

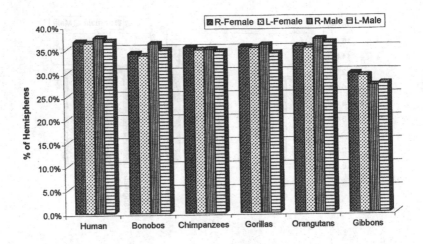

(d)   **Temporal Lobe**

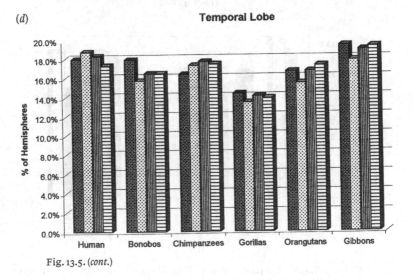

Fig. 13.5. (cont.)

chimpanzee and one orangutan hemisphere respectively). A comparison
in terms of continuity between the precentral and postcentral sulci
reveals that the precentral sulcus is mostly discontinuous, being composed of two or more segments. The postcentral sulcus is continuous in
almost half the hemispheres examined across species and the cingulate
sulcus is continuous in two-thirds of the hemispheres.

(e)

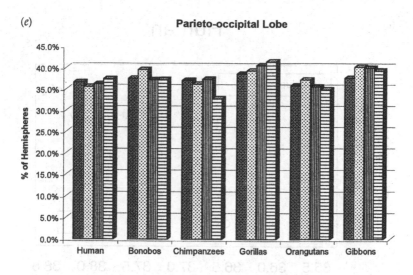

(f)

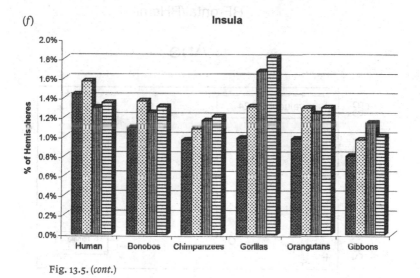

Fig. 13.5. (cont.)

The central sulcus extends onto the mesial surface of most of the great ape hemispheres, as it does in most human brains but not in the brain of the macaque. Also unlike the case for the macaque, the superior temporal sulcus does not merge with the Sylvian fissure in any of the hemispheres, except for that of one bonobo.

Most of these major sulci are connected with neighboring sulci to

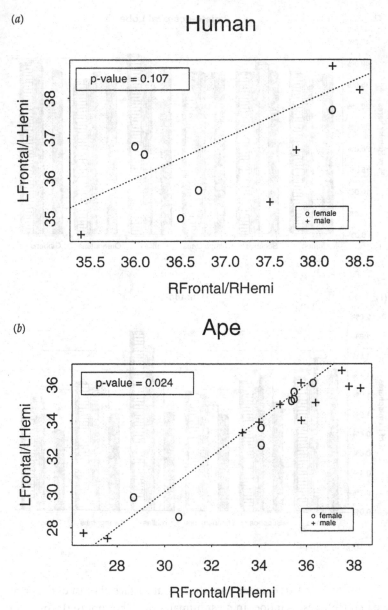

Fig. 13.6. (a, b) Regression of individual relative values of the right and left frontal lobes as a percentage of the right and left hemisphere for males and females in humans and apes. (c, d) Regression of individual relative values of the right and left insula as a percentage of the right and left hemisphere for males and females in humans and apes.

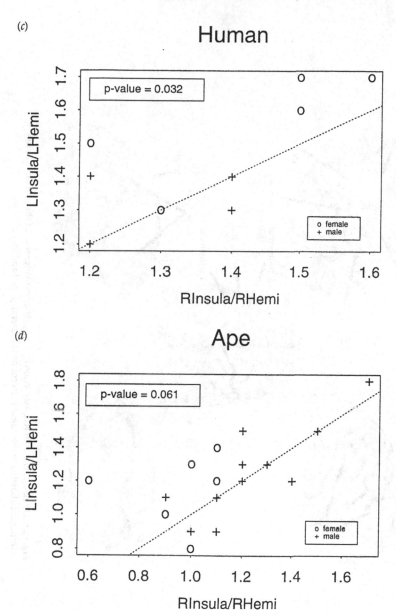

(c)

Human

(d)

Ape

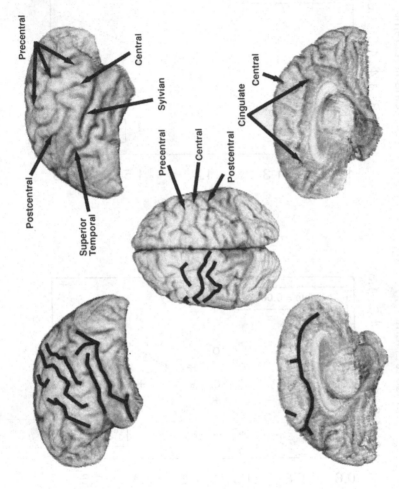

Fig. 13.7. Three-dimensional reconstruction of a magnetic resonance scan of the brain of a living chimpanzee showing major sulcal patterns on the lateral, dorsal and mesial views.

Precentral

Central

Postcentral

Sylvian

Superior Temporal

Precentral

Central

Postcentral

Cingulate

Central

some degree either at the surface or in their convoluted course below the surface. Although the central sulcus and the Sylvian fissure have connections with other sulci in less than half of the cases, the rest of the sulci are interconnected in the majority of the hemispheres across species. The complex sulcal patterns are also expressed in the large number of branching in all of these sulci. Only a few of the hemispheres examined exhibit no branching in the precentral (six hemispheres), postcentral (two) and superior temporal (two) sulci, while the others have various patterns of ramification in the frontal, parietal and temporal lobes. Sulci do not necessarily mark the borders of neighboring cortical areas in primates (Bailey *et al.*, 1950; Welker, 1990) and the significance of the variation in their complex configurations is not yet completely understood. A combination of histological studies of the underlying cortical structure and a larger number of scanned individuals per species will allow for a better appreciation of species-specific sulcal patterns and their importance.

A valuable database for a variety of studies

The newly acquired MR scans provide the opportunity for a variety of insights into the organization and evolution of the primate brain. Using the same data set, Rilling & Insel (1998) found that the cerebellum in selected New and Old world monkeys is smaller than that of apes in relative terms and that apes have a larger cerebellum than expected for a non-hominoid primate of their brain size. They suggest that a grade shift occurred through natural selection in favor of an enlarged cerebellum in the apes. This finding reinforces the idea proposed here that the relationship between the cerebellum and the cerebrum changed in favor of a larger cerebrum and a smaller cerebellum during hominid evolution.

Another idea that has been entertained for a while is that changes in the size of the cortex during primate evolution do not keep up with changes in the size of the white matter and that larger primate brains include larger amounts of white matter (Hofman, 1989, Chapter 6 this volume; Semendeferi *et al.*, 1994). The MR scans were used to measure cross-sectional areas of the corpus callosum, brain size, neocortical surface and white matter (Rilling & Insel, 1999). Intraconnectivity within each cerebral hemisphere, as expressed by the amount of white matter, was found to be larger in larger brains and to exceed in pace neocortical surface area. In contrast, interhemispheric connectivity as expressed by surface area measurements of the corpus callosum was smaller in larger brains, like humans, than in smaller primate brains and seems not to keep pace with increasing brain size.

A controversial issue regarding the presence or absence of the planum temporale (PT) in primates other than humans was recently resolved, when Gannon *et al.* (1998) reported their findings based on postmortem specimens of chimpanzees. They found that PT, a structure implicated in the lateralization of language function in humans, is also present in these apes and is asymmetrical. PT is larger in the left hemisphere than in the right, a condition similar to that which characterizes the human brain (Geschwind & Galaburda, 1984). Whether an asymmetrical PT is a shared derived chimpanzee/human feature that is not present in other hominoids was resolved using the newly acquired MR data set. Hopkins *et al.* (1998) investigated the presence/absence of PT in the great apes, lesser apes and selected Old World and New World monkey species. The presence of PT was identified in the great apes, but not in the lesser apes or the other anthropoids. PT was found to be larger in the left hemisphere than in the right, and the number of individuals with a left asymmetry was shown to be significantly larger than those with a right asymmetry. Some of the great ape brains presented no left–right bias in the size of PT.

In a separate effort to apply Magnetic resonance imaging techniques to issues regarding the evolution of the primate brain, Gilissen *et al.* (1996) and Zilles *et al.* (1996) reported findings on cortical shape of humans and chimpanzees. Right-handed humans were known to exhibit a right frontal/left occipital petalia, which means that the posterior portion of the left hemisphere is wider and protrudes further than the right, while the anterior portion of the right hemisphere is wider and protrudes further than the left. Petalias are also known to be present in the brains of the great apes, but occur to a lesser extent (LeMay, 1976; LeMay *et al.*, 1982; Holloway & De La Coste-Lareymondie, 1982). The studies by Zilles *et al.* and Gilissen *et al.* included 32 living human subjects and nine postmortem chimpanzee brains and did not reveal any statistically significant asymmetry in the right frontal/left occipital petalia in the chimpanzees. (See also Gilissen, Chapter 10, this volume.) In contrast, statistically significant asymmetries were found to be present in humans in favor of the left visual cortex (striate and extra-striate areas) and the right frontal lobe (areas 46, 10, and 44). The authors comment that the above structural difference in the shape of human and chimpanzee brains might not reflect a principal difference between humans and all great apes, but rather a species-specific pattern of the chimpanzee brain. They note that unpublished observations on gorilla and orangutan brains argue for the presence of petalias in these species.

On the basis of the above data set, Gilissen *et al.* (1997) and Gilissen (Chapter 10, this volume) also addressed the variability in cortical shape in humans and chimpanzees. Human cortical shape is regionally inhomogeneous and the pattern in the chimpanzee brains was found to be similar to that of humans. Highest variability in both hemispheres exists in regions processing higher sensory and associative functions and motor programming. More specifically in the chimpanzee brains these regions include areas of the occipital lobe (areas OC, OB according to Bailey *et al.*, 1950), frontal lobe (FE, FDp, FCBm), temporal and parietal lobes (TA + PG + PF, TG, TE1 + TE2) and mesial FA (supplementary motor cortex). Variability in the human brain was identified in similar locations with the exception of the occipital lobe where it is restricted only to the polar region and the supplementary motor cortex.

Pilot studies using functional imaging

Positron emission tomography (PET) and functional magnetic resonance imaging (fMRI) is now being used extensively on human subjects to localize activity-dependent signals that take place during motor, sensory and cognitive tasks (Posner *et al.*, 1988). The signal reflects changes in local cerebral blood flow and oxygenation. Some attempts have recently been made to apply these imaging techniques to the brains of nonhuman primates. It should be noted that many technical challenges are involved in successfully using functional imaging in nonhuman subjects, especially when alert (non-anesthetized) subjects have to be immobilized in a confined space.

Stefanacci *et al.* (1998) used an awake adult female rhesus monkey (*Macaca mulatta*) that was previously habituated to sit with her body restrained and head immobilized in the MR scanner. The fMR experiment aimed at demonstrating activity-dependent signals in the visual cortex during the passive viewing of a visual stimulus. Although slight motion of the subject during the experiment created some artifact, strong activations were detected in primary and extrastriate visual cortices as was expected. Strong activation was present in the banks and fundus of the superior temporal gyrus (areas STP and FST), while no activation was observed in other, non-visual sectors of the brain, such as the somatosensory and auditory cortices or the hippocampus. Such findings are in agreement with previous data from single-cell recording studies showing activity in striate and extrastriate visual areas. As the authors point out, problems involving motion contamination, rewarding the animal during the experiment, tracking eye movements and resolution of the fMRI signal need to be addressed in future studies.

Dubowitz *et al.* (1998) have used fMRI to demonstrate cerebral activation in the cortex of the macaque. Their study included an awake 4-year-old male rhesus macaque that was presented with a variety of visual stimuli. Activation was again observed in the primary visual cortex and extrastriate visual cortex, but the left primary visual cortex showed more activation than the right (possibly due to artifact).

Vanduffel *et al.* (1998) also reported the application of fMRI on an awake rhesus monkey during the presentation of an animated video. Differential activity was noted in V1, V2 and V3 that reflected changes in the signal during the presence versus absence of visual stimulation.

Positron emission tomography (PET) was used with baboons (*Papio anubis*) in a recent study by Kaufman *et al.* (1999). Using ^{15}O-labeled water they measured regional cerebral blood flow on twenty anesthetized subjects and found significant left–right asymmetries in the motor cortex and subcortical regions. The authors suggest that these findings, which are similar to results from human studies, may relate to issues of handedness and laterality in primates.

The future

The contributions of new imaging techniques to the study of brain evolution are already significant and the future looks promising. Long standing questions in our field, pertaining to the size of the frontal lobes and the cerebellum in apes and humans or the asymmetry of the planum temporale have now been answered thanks to the non-invasive tools that are now available. If we are to talk about what is uniquely human and what took place in the organization of the brain during hominid evolution, we cannot rely exclusively on comparisons coming from more distant taxa like other mammals or even other anthropoids to the exclusion of the great and lesser apes. A comparison between the human and gibbon data only, would certainly lead to different conclusions regarding the evolution of the human frontal lobe if other hominoids were not present (gibbons have smaller frontal lobes). The ethical dilemmas involved in the experimental use of the apes and the scarcity of postmortem specimens resulting from natural deaths make current imaging techniques very attractive. These non-invasive tools allow for the study of our closest relatives, the apes, who have been excluded in most neuroscientific investigations of the last several decades.

The paleoneurological study of extinct hominids can largely benefit from studies using imaging techniques on living ape and human subjects. If human and great ape frontal lobes have similar relative sizes, as was shown to be the case, then it is not likely that the frontal lobes of any hominid will show considerable relative differences. If individual endocasts show small differences in the relative size of the frontal lobe, it is very likely that intraspecific variation, clearly present in all hominoids, is responsible for the finding. In contrast, identification of the presence of differences in the relative size of the cerebellum among Plio-Pleistocene hominid species would be very revealing and would assist in timing the onset of the differential increase between the cerebellum and the cerebrum during human evolution.

Is the application of imaging techniques adequate for understanding the organization of the hominoid brain? Are we at the point where the microscope and the histology can be abandoned and replaced by these new tools? Improvements of these new techniques are taking place at a very fast pace and it is likely that in the near future we will be able to see finer details of the neural tissue in living subjects, but the answer to the above questions is clearly no, not yet at least. Studies using imaging techniques can at this point address a specific set of questions that involve the gross structure and, in the case of functional imaging, the *approximate* location of increased neural activation. Imaging tools can successfully address unresolved issues in the field, such as the size of various macroscopic segments of the brain, and may be able to point to specific cortical or subcortical areas that need detailed investigation with a combination of more techniques. But the new imaging techniques cannot give the cellular and connectional information gathered under the microscope. There is an obvious need and place for both.

MR images can serve as a valuable link between future functional imaging studies and the evaluation of histological sections. Functional imaging does not provide the detail needed to evaluate the organization of the structure activated. On the other hand, the microscopic study of the brain based on histological sections, if used alone, cannot provide many insights into the larger picture of the evolution of the human brain due to its own limitations (availability of tissue, small samples and pure logistics of large scale investigations). As I said before, we need both.

Efforts to map the human and macaque brain by combining MR, PET and histology studies have already started (Roland *et al.*, 1994; Zilles *et al.*, 1995; Mazziota *et al.*, 1995; Sereno, 1998). Histological sections are aligned with MR images of postmortem specimens. Such images are aligned with MR images of living subjects that can also be co-registered with results from PET experiments. This is the kind of approach that can take our field, the study of the evolution of the primate brain, beyond simplistic interpretations, such as the old idea that human cognition evolved largely due to a disproportionate enlargement of the frontal lobe in the hominid line. A variety of techniques involving structural and functional imaging along with histological methods can now be used to map the brain of closely related primate taxa on larger samples than has hitherto been possible.

Acknowledgments

I thank Dean Falk, Kathleen Gibson and Hanna Damasio for their comments.

References

Bailey, P., Bonin, G. & McCulloch, W.S. (1950). *The Isocortex of the Chimpanzee*. Urbana, Illinois: The University of Illinois Press.

Connolly, C.J. (1950). *External Morphology of the Primate Brain*. Springfield, Illinois: C.C. Thomas Publisher.

Damasio, H. & Frank, R. (1992). Three dimensional *in vivo* mapping of brain lesions in humans. *Archives of Neurology*, **49**, 137–143.

Damasio, H., Kuljis, R.O., Yuh, W., Van Hoesen, G.W. & Ehrhardt, J. (1991). Magnetic resonance imaging of human intracortical structure *in vivo*. *Cerebral Cortex*, **1**, 374–379.

Deacon, T. W. (1988). Human brain evolution: II. Embryology and brain allometry. In *Intelligence and Evolutionary Biology*, eds. H. J. Jerison & I. Jerison, pp. 383–415. Springer-Verlag Publishers.

Dronkers, N.F. (1996). A new brain region for coordinating speech articulation. *Nature*, **384**, 159–161.

Dubowitz, D.J., Chen, D., Atkinson, D.J., Grieve, K.L., Gillikin, B., Bradley, W.G. & Anderson, R.A. (1998). Functional magnetic resonance imaging in macaque cortex. *Neuroreport*, **9**(10), 2213–2218.

Falk, D., Hildebolt, C., Cheverud, J., Kohn, L. A.P., Gigiel, G. & Vannier, M. (1991). Human cortical asymmetries determined with 3-D MR technology. *Journal of Neuroscience Methods*, **39**, 185–191.

Fiez, J.A. (1996). Cerebellar contributions to cognition. *Neuron* **16**(1), 13–15.

Finger, S. (1994). *Origins of Neuroscience: A History of Explorations into Brain Function*. Oxford: Oxford University Press.

Finlay, B. L. & Darlington, R. B. (1995). Linked regularities in the development and evolution of mammalian brains. *Science*, **268**, 1578–1583.

Frank, R. J., Damasio, H. & Grabowski, T. J. (1997). Brainvox: An interactive, multimodal, visualization and analysis system for neuroanatomical imaging. *Neuroimage*, **5**, 13–30.

Gannon, P. J., Holloway, R. L., Broadfield, D. C. & Braun, A. R. (1998). Asymmetry of chimpanzee planum temporale: humanlike pattern of Wernicke's brain language area homolog. *Science*, **279**, 220–222.

Geschwind, N. & Galaburda, A. M. (eds.) (1984). *Cerebral Dominance: The Biological Foundations*. Cambridge, Mass: Harvard University Press.

Gilissen, E., Dabringhaus, A., Schlaug, G., Schormann, T., Steinmetz, H. & Zilles, K. (1996). Structural asymmetries in the cortical shape of humans and common chimpanzees: a comparative study with Magnetic Resonance Tomography. In *Proceedings of the 3rd Joint Symposium On Neural Computation*, **6**, 89–102.

Gilissen, E., Dabringhaus, A., Schlaugh, G., Steinmetz, H., Schromann, T. & Zilles, K. (1997). Structural asymmetries in the cortical shape of humans and common chimpanzees: a comparative study with magnetic resonance tomography. *American Journal of Physical Anthropology*, (Supplement) **24**, 117–118.

Hofman, M. A. (1989). On the evolution and geometry of the brain in mammals. *Progress in Neurobiology*, **32**, 137–158.

Holloway, R. L. & De La Coste-Lareymondie, M. C. (1982). Brain endocast asymmetry in pongids and hominids: some preliminary findings on the paleontology of cerebral dominance. *American Journal of Physical Anthropology*, **58**, 101–110.

Hopkins, W. H., Marino, L., Rilling, J. K. & MacGregor, L. (1998). Planum temporale asymmetries in great apes but not in lesser apes. *Neuroreport*, **9**, 2913–2918.

Jerison, H. J. (1973). *Evolution of the Brain and Intelligence*. New York: Academic Press.

Kaufman, J. A., Phillips-Conroy, J., Black, K. J. & Perlmutter, J. S. (1999). Regional cerebral blood flow in anaesthetized baboons (Papio anubis): the use of Positron Emission Tomography in anthropology. *American Journal of Physical Anthropology*, (Supplement) **28**, 166.

LeMay, M. (1976). Morphological cerebral asymmetries of modern man, fossil man, and nonhuman primates. *Annals of New York Academy of Science*, **280**, 349–366.

LeMay, M., Billig, M. S. & Geshwind, N. (1982). Asymmetries of the brains and skulls of nonhuman primates. In *Primate Brain Evolution: Methods and Concepts*, eds. E. Armstrong & D. Falk, pp. 263–277. New York: Plenum Press.

Martin, J. H. & Brust, J. C. M. (1985). Imaging the living brain. In *Principles of Neural Science*, eds. E. R. Kandel & J. H. Schwartz, pp. 259–283. New York: Elsevier Science Publishing Co.

Matano, S. & Hirasaki, E. (1997). Volumetric comparisons in the cerebellar complex of anthropoids, with special reference to locomotor types. *American Journal of Physical Anthropology*, **103**, 173–183.

Matano, S., Baron, G., Stephan, H. & Frahm, H. (1985). Volume comparisons in the cerebellar complex of primates II. Cerebellar Nuclei. *Folia Primatologica*, **44**, 182–203.

Mazziotta, J. C., Toga, A. W., Evans, A., Fox P. & Lancaster, J. (1995). A probabilistic atlas of the human brain: theory and rationale for its development. The International Consortium for Brain Mapping (ICBM). *Neuroimage*, 2(2), 89–101.

Muller, R. A., Courchesne, E. & Allen, G. (1998). The cerebellum: so much more. *Science*, 282, 879–880.

Posner, M. I., Petersen, S. E., Fox, P. T. & Raichle, M. E. (1988). Localization of cognitive operations in the human brain. *Science*, 240, 1627–1631.

Raichle, M. E. (1998). Behind the scenes of functional brain imaging: a historical and physiological perspective. *Proceedings of the National Academy of Science USA*, 95, 765–772.

Rilling, J. K. & Insel, T. R. (1998). Evolution of the primate cerebellum: differences in relative volume among monkeys, apes and humans. *Brain, Behavior and Evolution*, 52, 308–314.

Rilling, J. K. & Insel, T. R. (1999). Differential expansion of neural projection systems in primate brain evolution. *Neuroreport*, 10, 1453–1459.

Roland, P. E., Graufelds, C. J., Wahlin, J., Ingelman, L., Andersson, M., Ledberg, A., Pedersen, J., Akerman, S., Dabringhaus, A. & Zilles, K. (1994). Human brain atlas: for high-resolution functional and anatomical mapping. *Human Brain Mapping*, 1, 173–184.

Semendeferi, K. & Damasio, H. (1997). Comparison of sulcal patterns in the living brain of the great apes. *Society for Neuroscience Abstracts*, 23 (1–2), 1308.

Semendeferi, K. & Damasio, H. (2000). The brain and its main anatomical subdivisions in living hominoids using magnetic resonance imaging. *Journal of Human Evolution*, 38(2), 317–332.

Semendeferi, K. Damasio, H. & Van Hoesen, G. W. (1994). Evolution of frontal lobes: An MRI study on apes and humans. *Society for Neurosciences Abstracts*, 20(1–2), 1415.

Semendeferi, K, Rilling, J., Insel, T. R. & Damasio, H. (1996). Brain volume and its components in living apes and humans. *Society for Neuroscience Abstracts*, 22 (1–3), 675.

Semendeferi, K., Damasio, H., Frank, R. & Van Hoesen, G. W. (1997a). The evolution of the frontal lobes: a volumetric analysis based on three-dimensional reconstructions of magnetic resonance scans of human and ape brains. *Journal of Human Evolution*, 32(4), 375–388.

Semendeferi, K., Damasio, H., Rilling, J. & Insel, T. (1997b). The volume of the cerebral hemispheres, frontal lobes and cerebellum in living humans and apes using *in vivo* magnetic resonance morphometry. *American Journal of Physical Anthropology*, (Supplement) 24, 208–209.

Sereno, M. I. (1998). Brain mapping in animals and humans. *Current Opinion in Neurobiology*, 8(2), 188–194.

Stefanacci, L., Reber, P., Costanza, J., Wong, E., Buxton, R., Zola, S., Squire, L. & Albright, T. (1998). fMRI of monkey visual cortex. *Neuron*, 20, 1051–1057.

Stephan, H., Frahm, H. & Baron, G. (1981). New and revised data on volumes of brain structures in insectivores and primates. *Folia Primatologia*, 35, 1–29.

Vanduffel, W., Beatse, E., Sunaert, S., Van Hecke, P., Tootell, R. B. H. & Orban, G. A. (1998). Functional magnetic resonance imaging in an awake rhesus monkey. *Society for Neuroscience Abstracts*, 24(1–2), 11.

Vannier, M. W., Brunsden, B. S., Hildebolt, C. F., Falk, D., Cheverud, J. M., Figiel, G. S., Perman, W. H., Kohn, L. A., Robb, R. A., Yoffie, R. L. & Bresina, S. J. (1991). Brain surface cortical sulcal lengths: quantification with three-dimensional MR imaging. *Radiology*, **180**, 479–484.

Welker, W. (1990). Why does the cerebral cortex fissure and fold? In *Cerebral Cortex*, eds. E.G. Jones & A. Peters, pp. 3–136. Plenum Publishing Company.

Zilles, K., Schlaug, G., Matelli, M., Luppino, G., Schleicher, A., Qu, M., Dabringhaus, A., Seitz, R. & Roland, P.E. (1995). Mapping of human and macaque sensorimotor areas by integrating architectonic, transmitter receptor, MRI and PET data. *Journal of Anatomy*, **187**, 515–537.

Zilles, K., Dabringhaus, A., Geyer, S., Amunts, K., Qu, M., Schleicher, A., Gilissen, E., Schlaug, G. & Steinmetz, H. (1996). Structural asymmetries in the human forebrain and the forebrain of nonhuman primates and rats. *Neuroscience and Biobehavioral Reviews*, **20**(4), 593–605.

KATRIN SCHÄFER, HORST SEIDLER, FRED L. BOOKSTEIN,
HERMANN PROSSINGER, DEAN FALK & GLENN CONROY

14

Exo- and endocranial morphometrics in mid-Pleistocene and modern humans

In hominid evolution, the shape of the inner frontal bone in the median sagittal plane has, in contrast to the outer vault, not changed since at least the Plio-Pleistocene (Bookstein et al., 1999). Nonetheless, inner vault size increased significantly (by ~11%) while the size of the outer frontal profile did not. Thus, two of the more interesting questions to pose are: 'At which other positions of the skull have major shape and size changes taken place?' and 'Could it be that the exocranium is involved in shape changes while the endocranium is involved in size changes?'. We approach these questions by analyzing general shape and size of both the exo- and endocranium in the median sagittal plane. Importantly, because the inner surface of the braincase provides information concerning brain evolution (Jerison, 1973) and because of the syn-evolution of cerebellar and frontal lobes (Seidler et al., 1997), our investigation also includes the occipital bone.

Geometric relations in the median-sagittal plane

Our sample includes 21 crania of modern humans of both sexes (10 females, 11 males): 15 from Central Europe, two San and two Bantu, and two Papuans. To these we added the stereolithographs of three mid-Pleistocene fossil hominid crania (Seidler et al., 1997): Kabwe (Broken Hill 1; Woodward, 1921), Petralona (Kokkoros & Kanellis, 1960), both of uncertain age – but probably in excess of 200 000 years old; and Atapuerca SH5 cranium (Arsuaga et al., 1993), about 300 000 years old.

We measured the 3D coordinates of nine important endo- and exocranial landmarks in the mid-sagittal plane and points along a perimeter of the posterior cranial fossa (defined below). These 3D coordinates were

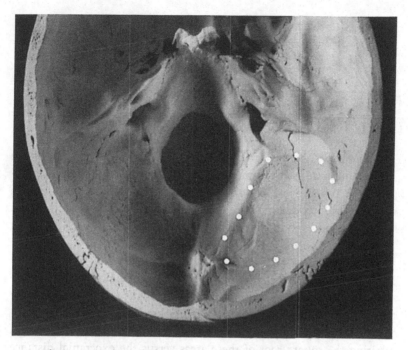

Fig. 14.1. Posterior-inferior part of the cranium (superior view, calotte removed). White dots indicate the points that were placed along the boundaries of the posterior cranial fossae in order to estimate the surface area.

measured with the 3D Polhemus 3Space FASTRAK® tracking system which uses the interference of electromagnetic fields to determine the position of the probe's tip in space.

Because, at present, there is no straightforward, established methodology to determine the volume of the cerebellum from cranial shape, we used as a surrogate the area of an almost planar surface whose perimeter runs along the inferior transverse sulcus, along the internal occipital crest, parallel to the elevated margin of the foramen magnum, then completing the contour along the occipital–temporal suture. Owing to the highly variable morphology of the boundaries of these fossae, 12–15 points were placed on the perimeter (Fig. 14.1) and the surface area calculated by triangulation. For every individual cranium the average of both sides was used, except for Kabwe (whose right side is missing).

For the analysis of the exocranium, we used the following landmarks: nasion (n), bregma (b), lambda (l), inion (i), basion (ba) and a median sagittal landmark at the anterior rim of the spheno-occipital synchondrosis

Table 14.1. *Cerebellum surface area S (mm²)*

Homo sapiens						
min.	mean	max.	SD	Atapuerca	Kabwe	Petralona
375	432	473	27	349	415	385

(Aiello & Dean, 1990) referred to in this paper as exo-clivus (cl). For the endocranium we used: foramen caecum (fc), bregma (b), lambda (l), endo-inion (ei; Tobias, 1991), basion (ba) and a median-sagittal point on the clivus at the interior rim of the spheno-occipital synchondrosis (referred to in this paper as endo-clivus; ecl).

Results

We found (Table 14.1) that the mean aforementioned cerebellum plani-metric area in *H. sapiens* exceeds that of the fossils by 5–20%, similar to the size of the inner frontal cranial profiles (Bookstein *et al.*, 1999).

We compared the posterior fossae areas with linear chord distances, plotting the square root of these areas versus the exocranial distance ('exocranial surface ratio') and versus endocranial distance ('endocranial surface ratio'), respectively. As a representative exocranial distance we used the nasion–inion chord, and endocranially, the foramen caecum–endoinion chord. There is a clear separation (Fig. 14.2) of the mid-Pleistocene from the modern sample in the exocranial surface ratio but not in the endocranial one.

Relative to the mid-Pleistocene specimens, the inion of the moderns has an inferior, anterior displacement which decreases the mean angle bregma–lambda–inion and increases the mean angle lambda–inion–basion (Table 14.2). On the other hand, because the endoinion is displaced posteriorly, perhaps because of reduced occipital thickness, the 'inner' angle bregma–lambda–endoinion increases in the moderns relative to fossils while the mean angle lambda–endoinion–basion is smaller in the moderns.

The angles inion–basion–nasion and basion–nasion–bregma are also smaller than the mean angles of the moderns in the mid-Pleistocenes, while the angle basion–foramen caecum–bregma does not separate the two groups. Furthermore, the distance lambda–inion is greater in the moderns, resulting in a shortening of the distance inion–basion, irrespec-

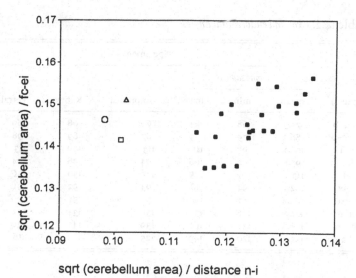

Fig. 14.2. Square root of cerebellar surface relative to an exo- and an endocranial distance. The abscissa values (i.e. ratio to exocranial surface) are much larger for the moderns – and thus indicate a clear separation from the mid-Pleistocenes; the ordinate values show no such separation. Solid symbols: *H. sapiens*; open symbols: fossil crania (circle: Petralona, triangle: Kabwe, square: Atapuerca).

tive of cranial height. The landmark distances clarify some of the angle variations: the inion in modern humans is closer to the endoinion and the nasion is closer to the foramen caecum (Fig. 14.3). Interestingly, Andrews (1986) postulated this shift of endoinion relative to inion as typical of *H. erectus*.

The decreasing pneumatization in moderns led to a caudal, posterior displacement of nasion, resulting in a small decrease of the angle nasion–bregma–inion (Fig. 14.4); however, both groups overlap in the angle foramen caecum–bregma–endoinion.

This separation/overlap mechanism is associated with a lack of change in the distance foramen caecum–endoinion since the mid-Pleistocene (Fig. 14.5) in conjunction with a decrease in the exocranial distance nasion–inion, most markedly relative to Petralona and Kabwe.

Consistent with the other results, the angles fc–b–ei and fc–l–ei do not change from the mid-Pleistocene to the present. Likewise, Fig. 14.6 shows the corresponding exo- and endocranial linear distances from inion (Fig. 14.6*a*) and endoinion (Fig. 14.6*b*) to lambda and basion. Figure 14.6*a*

Table 14.2. *Exo- and endocranial angles*

angle (°)	Homo sapiens mean	Homo sapiens min.	Homo sapiens max.	Atapuerca	Kabwe	Petralona
ba–n–b	75.3	68	83	69	68	69
ba–fc–b	86.3	79	93	87	89	98
n–b–l	102.1	97	111	113	109	113
n–fc–l	97.8	92	106	104	98	104
b–l–i	113.4	107	125	122	130	126
b–l–ei	102.1	94	118	93	92	91
l–i–ba	102.4	87	111	97	91	90
l–ei–ba	122.3	106	132	131	134	132
i–ba–n	146.5	132	162	139	142	140
ei–ba–fc	132.4	120	149	125	127	116

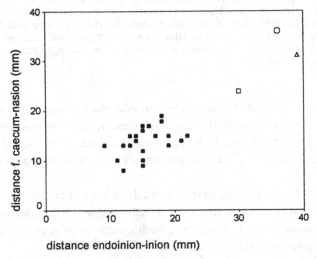

Fig. 14.3. Distances from foramen caecum to nasion, and from endoinion to inion. The graph shows that both distances are markedly larger in the mid-Pleistocene crania. Solid symbols: *H. sapiens*; open symbols: fossil crania (circle: Petralona, triangle: Kabwe, square: Atapuerca).

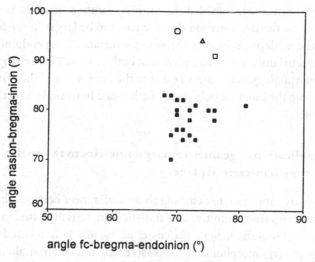

Fig. 14.4. The relation between two specific exo- and endocranial angles. The angle of exocranial landmarks separates the fossil and the modern samples completely, whereas the endocranial landmark angle shows complete overlap between the two samples. Solid symbols: *H. sapiens*; open symbols: fossil crania (circle: Petralona, triangle: Kabwe, square: Atapuerca).

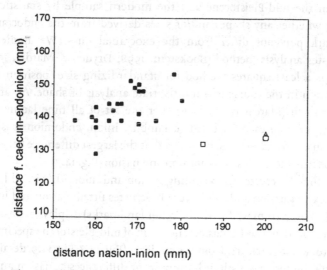

Fig. 14.5. The relation between two specific exo-and endocranial distances. The distance from nasion to inion is much greater in the mid-Pleistocene than in the modern sample (except for Atapuerca, which is nearer to the *H. sapiens* range). In contrast, the endocranial distances (fc-ei) overlap for all specimens. Solid symbols: *H. sapiens*; open symbols: fossil crania (circle: Petralona, triangle: Kabwe, square: Atapuerca).

indicates that the exocranial distance inion–lambda overlaps in both groups, while the inion–basion distance tends to be larger in the fossils than in the moderns. Figure 14.6b shows the distance from endoinion to basion and to lambda to be comparable in both groups. These changes in cranial morphology may simply be due to the outer table of the cranium approaching the inner table, because of a decrease in frontal and occipital thickness.

Application of geometric morphometrics to the analysis of the median-sagittal plane

An alternative approach to detecting shape differences between the two samples derives from a multivariate statistical analysis of Cartesian coordinate data (Bookstein, 1991; Marcus et al., 1996). This methodology, called geometric morphometrics, preserves all information about the spatial relations of the points and permits the visualization of between-group and within-group differences, sample variation, and other results in the space of the raw point mesh (Slice et al., 1998).

We used geometric morphometrics to find possible distinctions between the mid-Pleistocene and the modern sample by statistically testing whether any shapes and/or sizes derived from the endocranial landmark polygons differ from the exocranial ones. We applied a Procrustes analysis method (Bookstein, 1998; Dryden & Mardia, 1998) which is a least squares method for standardizing size, position and orientation in the course of a multivariate analysis of shape. An affine Procrustes fit (Marcus et al., 1996) over the set of all nine landmarks (nasion, foramen caecum, bregma, lambda, inion, endoinion, basion, exo-clivus, and endo-clivus) indicates that the largest difference between the moderns and the fossils is at inion and nasion (Fig. 14.7).

An affine Procrustes fit excluding nasion and inion (that is, all landmarks except nasion and inion were Procrustes fitted; nasion and inion were, however, co-moved with the other landmarks) displays an overlap of both groups; in this fit, nasion and inion of mid-Pleistocene specimens separate even more clearly from the moderns (Fig. 14.8; Fig. 14.9: detail). A permutation test reveals highly significant differences at nasion and at inion between the two groups, and no such differences in the other seven landmarks (Fig. 14.9).

We conclude that the shape of the endocranium remained remarkably stable since the mid-Pleistocene whereas the shape of the exocranium

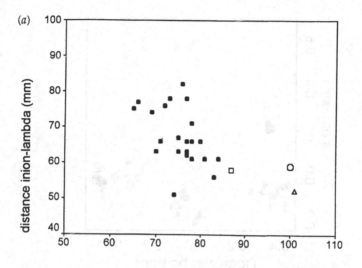

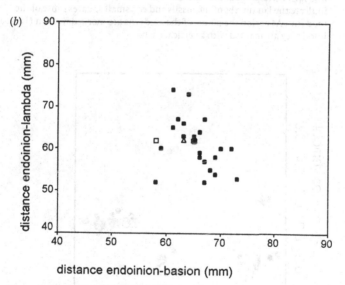

distance endoinion-basion (mm)

Fig. 14.6. (a) Linear exocranial chord distances relating to inion. In the inion–basion distance the mid-Pleistocenes fall above the modern specimens; Atapuerca is nearer to the *H. sapiens* than to Kabwe and Petralona. Solid symbols: *H. sapiens*; open symbols: fossil crania (circle: Petralona, triangle: Kabwe, square: Atapuerca). (b) Endocranial chord distances relating to endoinion. For both distances, the mid-Pleistocenes are completely within the modern range. Solid symbols: *H. sapiens*; open symbols: fossil crania (circle: Petralona, triangle: Kabwe, square: Atapuerca).

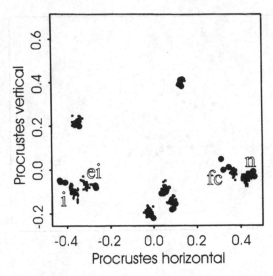

Fig. 14.7. Nine-point affine Procrustes fit (right lateral view). The large dots indicate the landmarks of the fossils and the small squares those of the moderns. At nasion the points of the moderns are marked with an N and at inion they are marked with a vertical dash.

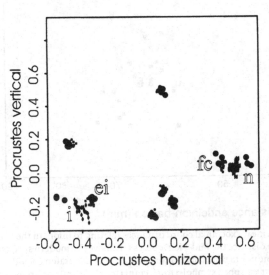

Fig. 14.8: Seven-point affine Procrustes fit (right lateral view). The large dots indicate the landmarks of the fossils and the small squares those of the moderns. At nasion the points of the moderns are marked with an N and at inion they are marked with a vertical dash. Note how clearly both groups separate at these two landmarks.

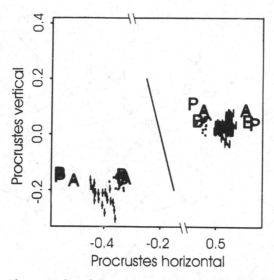

Fig. 14.9. Enlarged view of the seven-point affine Procrustes fit of Fig. 8 (right lateral view). Foramen caecum and nasion are plotted on the right and inion and endoinion on the left. At both endo-landmarks mid-Pleistocene and modern specimens overlap, whereas at the corresponding exo-landmarks no overlap can be detected. Key: A, Atapuerca; B, Broken Hill; P, Petralona; small squares: foramen caecum and endoinion of *H. sapiens*, N nasion and vertical dashes inion of *H. sapiens*.

changed considerably (Fig. 14.10). In particular, major shape changes took place at the anterior and posterior ends of the exocranium.

One can also carry out principal component analysis of the coordinates of the N landmarks as a set of 2N variables using the method of relative warps (Bookstein, 1998). Relative warp analyses of the exocranial (N = 6) and the endocranial (N = 5) data sets separately (Fig. 14.11) corroborate the findings from Procrustes fit (Fig. 14.8). For the outer table analysis (Fig. 14.11a) the first relative warp scores separate the two samples spectacularly, while for the inner table (Fig. 14.11b) there is substantial overlap.

An adequate surrogate for the intuitive perception of size is the so-called Centroid Size (SC; Dryden & Mardia, 1998), which is the square root of the sum of squared distances of the landmarks from the centroid (x-coordinate: average of all landmarks' x-coordinates; y-coordinate: average of all landmarks' y-coordinates). Centroid Size analysis also corroborates the insights gained from affine Procrustes fit and from relative warp analysis. There is a significant change in exocranial but not in the endocranial size from mid-Pleistocene to moderns. The size of the

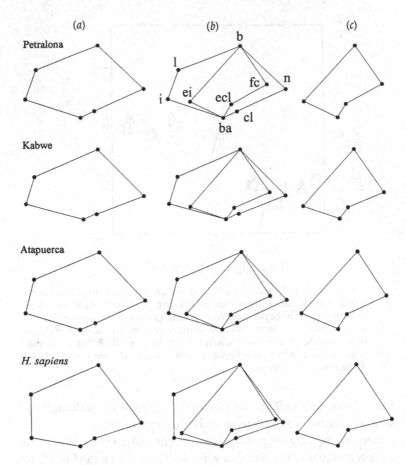

Fig. 14.10. Procrustes fits of the three fossils and of one modern specimen (right lateral view). In the middle column all landmarks are plotted, in the left column only the exocranial ones (plus b and ba) and in the right column only the endocranial ones (plus b and ba). Notice how exocranial shapes differ more than endocranial shapes between mid-Pleistocene specimens and modern humans. (Key: ba, basion; b, bregma; cl, clivus; ecl, endoclivus; ei, endoinion; fc, foramen caecum; i, inion; l, lambda; n, nasion.)

exo-polygon (n–b–l–i–ba–cl) of the mid-Pleistocenes (CS = 7.90) is significantly (P ~ 0.002, t-test) larger than that of the moderns (CS = 7.35). When comparing the endo-polygons (fc–b–l–ei–ba–ecl) of the mid-Pleistocenes with those of the moderns, we find no significant size difference (mid-Pleistocenes: CS = 6.57; moderns: CS = 6.74; P > 0.20, t-test).

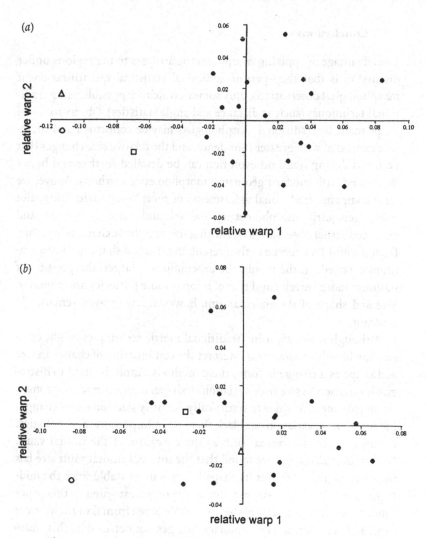

Fig. 14.11. (*a*) Relative warp scores (principal component scores for Procrustes-registered shape co-ordinates) of the exocranial landmarks. Solid symbols: *H. sapiens*; open symbols: mid-Pleistocenes (square: Atapuerca; circle: Petralona; triangle: Kabwe). Axes are in units of Procrustes length. The two samples are widely separated in the first relative warp, but not in the second relative warp. (*b*) Relative warp scores (principal component scores for Procrustes-registered shape co-ordinates) of the endocranial landmarks. Solid symbols: *H. sapiens*; open symbols: mid-Pleistocenes (square: Atapuerca; circle: Petralona; triangle: Kabwe). Axes are in units of Procrustes length. First and second relative warp scores show overlap between the two samples.

Conclusions

The advantage of applying morphometric analyses to the regions under discussion is that they permit additional statistical quantification of morphological observations, only some of which are possible using traditional techniques (such as distance and angle statistics). Observations of shape made by traditional morphologists may be confirmed and therefore expressed with greater confidence, and the relative size changes that occurred during hominid evolution can be detailed further and better quantified with modern geometric morphometric methods. Above, we have compared traditional assessments of morphology with outcomes using geometric morphometric analyses and have confirmed and extended earlier observations regarding size and shape changes in crania: from the mid-Pleistocene to the present, the size and shape of the exocranium changed. In the fossils, the exocranium is larger, the position of nasion is more anterior and that of inion is more posterior and superior. Size and shape of the endocranium, however, have stayed remarkably constant.

Although scientists using traditional metric techniques might occasionally be able to assess and interpret the combination of change in size and shape as a change in form, these methods cannot be used to distinguish variation in size from variation in shape. Because modern geometric morphometrics is able to statistically quantify size and shape changes independently, variation (and lack thereof) in important morphological features can be discovered, such as the curvature of the frontal vault. Bookstein *et al.* (1999) have found that the internal frontal vault size has increased significantly, yet its shape has remained stable since the mid-Pleistocene. As the mid-sagittal endopolygon investigated in this paper cannot probe the geometry of the inner table of the frontal vault, we must conclude that there are evolutionary changes not detected by this endopolygon. Furthermore, Bookstein *et al.* (1999) found that the outer table did change in shape but not in size, while we show here that the overall mid-sagittal exocranial polygon changed in both size and shape. Straightforward interpretation, it seems, is not yet possible: different regions of the cranium must be analyzed with a much finer mesh, which will invariably include sliding landmarks. The discovery of invariance in internal vault curvature and its increase in size, and the stability in the overall size and shape of the endocranium in the mid-sagittal plane since the mid-Pleistocene encourages further analyses using these modern methods. Furthermore, these findings raise new questions, among them, 'Are there other invariants in the endocranium and, if so, where?'. The endocranial surface reproduces the external gross morphology of the cerebral and cerebellar cortices (Jerison, 1973), so this question is of paramount interest to researchers who are investigating hominid brain evolution.

The changes and invariances detected with geometric morphometrics also raise questions about equating change in size and shape of the skull with evolution of cognitive abilities. Hopefully, future analyses of the shape variations in different parts of the endocranium will help to clarify the trends that constrained the evolution of the brain and intelligence in our ancestors (Jerison, 1973).

Acknowledgements

This work was supported by ÖNB grant Jubiläumsfonds 8050 to H.S., and NSF grant SBR-9729796 to D. F.

References

Aiello, L. & Dean, C. (1990). *An Introduction to Human Evolutionary Anatomy*. San Diego: Academic Press.

Arsuaga, J. L., Martinez I., Gracia, A., Carretero, J. M. & Carbonell, E. (1993). Three new human skulls from the Sima de los Huesos. *Nature*, **362**, 534–537.

Andrews, P. J. (1986). On the characters that define *Homo erectus*. *Courier Forschungsinstitut Senckenberg*, **69**, 167–178.

Bookstein, F., Schäfer, K., Prossinger, H., Fieder, M., Seidler, H., Stringer, C., Weber, G.W., Arsuaga, J.L., Slice, D., Rohlf, F.J., Recheis, W., Mariam, A.J. & Marcus, L.F. (1999). Comparing frontal cranial profiles in archaic and modern *Homo* by morphometric analysis. *The Anatomical Record (New Anatomist)*, **257**, 217–224.

Bookstein, F.L. (1991). *Morphometric Tools for Landmark Data: Geometry and Biology*. Cambridge: Cambridge University Press.

Bookstein, F.L. (1998). A hundred years of morphometrics. *Acta Zool. Hung.*, **44**, 7–59.

Dryden, I.L. & Mardia, K.V. (1998). *Statistical Shape Analysis*. Chichester, UK: Wiley.

Jerison, H.J. (1973). *Evolution of the Brain and Intelligence*. New York: Academic Press.

Kokkoros, P. & Kanellis, A. (1960). Découverte d'un crâne d'homme paléolithique dans péninsule Chalcidique. *Anthropologie*, **64**, 132–147.

Marcus, L.F., Corti, M., Loy, A., Naylor, G.J.P. & Slice, D.E. (1996). *Advances in Morphometrics*. New York: Plenum Press.

Seidler, H., Falk, D., Stringer, C., Wilfing, H., Müller, G., zur Nedden, D., Weber, G.W., Recheis, W. & Arsuaga, J.L. (1997). A comparative study of stereolithographically modelled skulls of Petralona and Broken Hill: Implications for future studies of middle Pleistocene hominid evolution. *Journal of Human Evolution*, **33**, 691–703.

Slice, D. E., Bookstein, F. L., Marcus, L. F. & Rohlf, F. J. (1998). A Glossary for *Geometric Morphometrics*. http://life.bio.sunysb.edu/morph/ Bibliographies and glossary.

Tobias, P. V. (1991). *Olduvai Gorge Volume IV*. Cambridge: Cambridge University Press.

White, T. D. & Folkens, P. A. (1991). *Human Osteology*. San Diego: Academic Press.

Woodward, A. S. (1921). A new cave man from Rhodesia, South Africa. *Nature*, **108**, 371–372.

Epilogue

The study of primate brain evolution: where do we go from here?

I am pleased to accept the title that Dean Falk and Kathleen Gibson assigned me for this concluding essay. And of course I thank them for arranging the meeting of the American Association of Physical Anthropologists in my honor. Most of all I must thank the contributors at that meeting and the others who have taken time to prepare the chapters in this book, which commemorates that meeting. In my judgment it would be inappropriate for me to comment on those excellent chapters, to argue with some of them or to agree with others. The chapters speak well for themselves, I will leave commentary to the journals, such as *Current Anthropology* or *Brain and Behavior Sciences*, that specialize in it. It has been a great pleasure to be involved with these activities.

I will depart from my assignment in three ways. First I must write about where I would go from here rather than prescribe for others. The chapters in this book present better prescriptions than I am competent to offer for the route our field as a whole can take. Second, I would like to write about where we have been, because my particular route is so much one involving the fossil evidence that I think it takes some explaining. Finally, I have to write about more than only primates, because my emphasis has been and continues to be on the evolution of the vertebrate brain, including the primates among the mammals.

Although I avoided specific citations of the chapters of this book, I was thinking about dolphin brains and the strange problems they pose for quantifiers and behaviorists when writing this essay. I had to discuss Preuss's chapter when reviewing my concerns with the whale brain and its evolution and the quantification of cortical thickness functions. I was able to maintain my resolve for the other contributors although some, of course, are mentioned by name.

I will emphasize themes that I have developed before, which I think need more work or correction, and indicate the way I would work on them now. I will be less ambitious about the details of mammalian and primate brain evolution than these deserve, covering mainly the quantitative analyses that come easiest for me and that I can handle. And I will discuss my current interest in the technology of computer graphics, which will improve the answers to old questions and, perhaps, suggest some new ones.

Personal and other history

I call my discipline paleoneurology, following my mentor, Tilly Edinger. Tilly died when I began writing my 'big book' (Jerison, 1973), which I dedicated to her. I have recently written a preface to Edinger's biography (Kohring & Kreft, in press) which I have added as an appendix to this chapter, as a footnote to the history of my discipline. In that preface I describe the circumstances of my meeting Tilly and my introduction to what she described as fossil brains (Edinger, 1929, 1975).

Almost from the beginning of my scientific life I sought to incorporate the fossil data into evolutionary schemes. I was especially impressed by Karl Lashley's famous presidential lecture to the American Society of Naturalists on the evolution of mind in which he mentioned brain–body analysis. Lashley, in turn, had probably discovered that analysis in informal meetings of a group of distinguished neurobiologists in Chicago in 1920s and 1930s. The group included Warren McCulloch (McCulloch, 1965) and Gerhard von Bonin (von Bonin, 1963), and I heard about these meetings from another of the participants, the pioneer neuropsychologist Ward Halstead (Halstead, 1947).

I reconstruct this relatively modern history as beginning with von Bonin's long-time interest as a neuroanatomist in brain evolution, and his penchant for quantitative analysis. He may have been inspired by early work published by Eugene Dubois (see Theunissen, 1989, especially chapter 5), but perhaps learning from Halstead, von Bonin performed an elementary statistical analysis to determine the regression of log brain weight on log body weight in mammals (von Bonin, 1937). He reported that 2/3 was the allometric exponent, the slope of the regression line for log–log data. In this way von Bonin introduced objective mathematical and statistical methods to studies of brain evolution.

Halstead told me years later that von Bonin had presented his results to the Chicago club, which may have been where Lashley first heard of them, and this led to their being cited in Lashley's presidential lecture. I read the lecture's published version (Lashley, 1949), and discovered von Bonin's work, eventually verifying von Bonin's result in my first publication on brain evolution (Jerison, 1955). With that I began my commitment to my first 'error' which I discuss later under the heading 'The allometric exponent.'

In verifying von Bonin I did some scientific filtering of data, because I recognized that cetaceans, evolving in a gravitationally odd environment, had different constraints on the size of their bodies than land mammals, and that there must have been something equally odd about primates as a mammalian order of brain-size specialists. I did my regression analysis of what I thought of as typical mammal species, excluding cetaceans and primates from the sample that I used to calculate the slope of a 'mammalian' line, the value of the allometric exponent. This filtering was of course a no-no for statistical purists who want to let all the data do the talking, but it strengthened my commitment to 2/3 rather than other candidates for the role of a 'true' value.

Whatever the right thing to do is, the impressive results of allometric analysis of brain–body data, and of the role of encephalization that Lashley described as providing the only anatomical correlate of mind, led me to look at brain size as a kind of a statistic and to look for neural and behavioral parameters that it estimated. I wanted to learn why the simple measures of the size of the whole brain and of the body could be used in this way. After I began to work on the problem, I met Roland Bauchot who gave me a copy of his PhD thesis (Bauchot, 1963) on the volumes of thalamic nuclei. Tilly Edinger told me that she had published on fossil camel brains in a book edited by Bauchot's collaborator, Heinz Stephan (Hassler & Stephan, 1966). (I had been invited to the meeting that led to Stephan's book, but could not afford the flight to Germany.) Eventually I found the several compendia published by Stephan and his collaborators (e.g. Stephan, Frahm & Baron, 1981; cf. Stephan, Baron & Frahm, 1991) on the laboriously acquired data on the volumes of various components of the brains of insectivores, prosimians, and other primates. It was only later that I realized that Stephan was working in Tilly Edinger's father's laboratory at the brain research institute in Frankfurt, Germany, a laboratory that I mention in the appendix to this epilogue.

Using Stephan's and Bauchot's data and those of their students, I was able to verify that the simple measure of brain size was worth studying and analyzing. These contribute to the quantification of brain size as a statistic with respect to the neural and informational parameters that it estimates. I was fascinated by the idea of developing the fossil evidence, which consist of an image of the external surface of the brain in mammals and birds. Accepting criticisms from anatomists such as von Bonin, I was suspicious of the use of gyral and sulcal patterns as correlates of behavior. Brain size was the most reliable measurement that was available, and it became my basic handle to interpret the data on fossil brains.

Numerology?

I can be correctly accused of enjoying numbers of a mindless way. I cannot describe my pleasure when I can attach numbers to a phenomenon, even when I know it is a pretty stupid way to spend one's time. After publishing my 'big book' I actually tallied the dates of publication of my citations to check on my biases. I have the graph I drew somewhere, I hope lost, because otherwise I might inflict it on you. But it was nevertheless interesting as a study of the sociology of science. As I recall, like most authors I tended to be up-to-date, citing recent publications more often than older ones. I had more than 500 references, and since my book is now a standard source, I must apologize for being so conventional. In my defense I should note that I did try to cite the earliest rather than the latest publication that I found for a particular idea. I tried to honor the creator of a concept if I identified the author, rather than someone who had cited the publication as part of a review.

Later in this epilogue I present some of my updated quantifications on the brain, graphs that I intend to illustrate what I think of as the most interesting results that I have run into. These graphs are my personal excuse for exercising my compulsion. It is not only fun, but the results are important.

My 'big book' is now nearly thirty years old. It should be extinct as a scientific monograph, which would usually be given a half-life of about five years. But my book lives on, and as the first example of my compulsion being acted out, let me illustrate the history of its rate of citation as determined from Citation Index. The citation rate has remained steady throughout the book's history, which surprised me. I like to think that people found my scientific results interesting (Figure 1).

The book may have also had special value as a useful target for attack by correcting its 'mistakes'. Let me discuss these first, because their

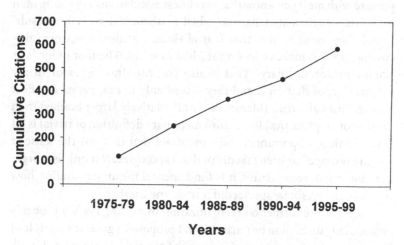

Evolution of the Brain and Intelligence

Fig. 1. Cumulative rate of citation for Jerison (1973).

correction, rejection, or recognition as not mistaken at all are the first element in my describing where I would go from here.

There are, of course, real mistakes in the book, such as discussing the brainlessness of marsupials as a group in a paragraph intended to hoist only the didelphids on that petard. I was personally most offended by a mistake that I still cannot understand. Some of the graphs in the book were drawn by professional artists, but I made a half-log unit error in misplacing convex polygons in two graphs that I drew myself (Jerison, 1973, Figs. 7.4 and 8.4), exaggerating the difference between mammals and their ancestors. Advances in computer graphics make such errors rare. When I present graphs nowadays my numbers are on data sheets and my graphs are drawn automatically by a graphics program that never makes mistakes. (Well, hardly ever!) The graphs for this epilogue were all drawn by my graphics program, not by me. The only possible mistakes are with the numbers, I think most of mine are now gone from my data sheets.

Mistake 1. Brain reorganization and other linguistic mistakes

My biggest mistake was probably in describing differences among species in the organization of the brain as trivial. I do not apologize. My mistake was semantic. I wasn't thinking as a writer, alert to avoid misunderstandings. Look up 'trivial' in your dictionary. You may sympathize with me if you know that my closest associations as a young man were with mathematicians, and when mathematicians call a 'result' trivial they mean merely that it is obvious, a truism not worth discussing. That is more or less what I had in mind. The first usage is as 'commonplace, ordinary.' That is also OK. My drawing error in my graphs were of that type, and they served only to exaggerate an effect that was basically true. (Mammals are all relatively larger brained than reptiles or amphibians.) But a third dictionary definition of trivial is 'of little worth or importance', and I am afraid that this was the sense at which my usage has been taken. For that I apologize. Not only is reorganization worth recognizing, it is fundamental for understanding how brains of all vertebrate species differ from one another.

When I wrote further on reorganization in my 'big book' I probably obscured my discussion by renaming it. I proposed a general principle of brain structure–function relations, which I termed 'proper mass.' I think of it as a principle applicable to all verebrate brains, not limited to human evolution. The idea was that the mass of brain tissue devoted to a specialized function in a species was related to the importance of the activity supported by that brain tissue in the life of a member of that species. I was being semantically stupid in my choice of words, because even colleagues sympathetic to my general views mistook my usage as supporting Lashley discredited idea of mass action.

The idea that the size of a neural system is usually related to its importance is obviously right, and I thought that it must have been named. I consulted with my old friend, Wally Welker, on the matter. Wally had published the clearest research result exemplifying proper mass (Welker, 1990; Welker & Campos, 1963) in the diverse adaptations of living procyonids. He described and illustrated the enlargement of sensorimotor neocortical representation of the paws of the raccoon as compared with the enlarged representation of the rhinarium in the neocortex of the coati mundi. Raccoons use their paws as hands, whereas coatis nose about to explore their environment. Wally could think of no word or phrase for the idea, which was as obvious to him as it was to me. Hence, 'proper mass.' The only textbook in which I have seen the designation accepted is Butler & Hodos (1996), but it is a valid organizing principle for understanding the diversity of brains as they evolved in vertebrates.

The unfortunate side of the unnecessary controversy, to which I may have contributed by my misuse of 'reorganization', has been the emphasis on the specialized evolution of the human brain compared to other primates and other mammals, as if the structural reorganization of the human brain was unique in vertebrate history (Deacon, 1997). Of course the human brain is unique, perhaps because of the evolution of our language sense. But all species are unique, and the organization of their brains is unique. It is uniqueness that identifies a species. Reorganization as a phenomenon is a feature of evolution, which is part of what establishes the uniqueness of a species. It reflects changes that became fixed in the genetic material of various species as they evolved to enter their adaptive niches, and although we remain ignorant about the details of the genetic control of the diversity in brain structure, we can recognize it as one of the things to explain as we improve our understanding of the genetics of brain development.

Mistake 2. The allometric exponent

In my first publication on brain–body relations (Jerison, 1955) I reported an allometric exponent of 0.73 for the entire mammalian sample on which I calculated the regression of log brain size on log body size. This value, or the commonly recognized one of 0.75 that we accept now (Martin, 1990), made no sense to me, whereas the value of 2/3 first proposed by Brandt (1867) and later rationalized by Snell (1891) made good sense. It reflected the brain's work in mapping information between surfaces and volumes, and it was easy to incorporate into a theory of encephalization (Jerison, 1977). Dubois's empirical value of 5/9 (see Jerison, 1973; Theunissen, 1989) made no sense either, and von Bonin's 0.66 found by regression analysis provided relief from the nonsense results with other values. I am distressed by the easy acceptance of 3/4 in the present literature, and am not optimistic that this brief statement will fix things, but I will try.

There are two problems. First, does it make sense to seek some correct value for the exponent in the genetic instructions that tell mammalian bodies and brains how to grow to their mature size? Second, if there is a theoretical true value of the exponent, how should we expect empirical estimates of that value to deviate from the true value. There is a third problem, which I am not competent to discuss, but which may be one of the paths to prescribe for the future of our field. This is to rethink the general issue of allometry in relation to recent developments in fractal geometry (West, Brown & Enquist, 1997). Although exponents calculated by regression analysis may be interpretable in terms of fractal dimensions, I find only those in Bridgman's dimensional analysis of 1931 easy to understand.

Allometry as theoretical biometrics was a theory of growth (Huxley, 1932). The idea was that if you knew the rates of growth of different body systems, their correlated changes should be related to one another in some specifiable way. The biometric problem is well described by Harvey & Pagel (1991). The aspect that intrigues me is that the growth pattern during development of an individual animal generates an equation that is equally useful for describing relationships among adults of different species. There is no question that the equation works, and it does describe brain–body relations. I am concerned with what this suggests about how the genetic system works and what it implies about how the brain works in mammals.

My prejudices will show. Although I have reported statistics as often as most people in our field, and I think I use them sensibly, my view has never been very respectful of statistical niceties. If a regression coefficient is reported, my first reaction is to ask about its referent: what does it describe? My second reaction is to ask whether there is any fundamental significance to its actual value.

In the case of brain–body allometry I have assumed that the fundamental referent for the exponent was some genetic constraint on overall growth of the body and brain in an animal. In mammals I assume that the constraint is related to the role of the brain in mapping information from sensory to neural surfaces, and that a rule evolved that prescribed the number of neural elements in different parts of the system. For brain–body allometry, I have assumed that the rule was related to the fact that sensory systems are distributed across what are approximately two dimensional bodily surfaces, such as the skin, the retina, the basilar membrane of the ear, and the olfactory epithelia, but that the size of the analytic systems (neocortex, etc.) involves volumes as well as surfaces, since their mass involves layers of nerve cell bodies distributed about white matter. The surface–volume relationship has always appealed to me intuitively, and for this reason a 2/3 exponent has seemed to me *a priori* correct exponent to reflect the fundamental constraint on neural growth in a mammalian brain.

Empirically, however, one finds a 3/4 exponent. This strikes me as a problem for theoretical analysis, not an issue about 'true' exponents. It is especially valuable for guiding the tactics of theory building. The theoretical problem is, why are brains as big as they are, and why is their size related as it is to body size in vertebrates. I have published a bit of my answer for mammals in several places, and it is not inappropriate to repeat the argument now.

We must first differentiate between an empirical and theoretical exponent. The theoretical exponent can reflect fundamental relationships among information processing elements with respect to the transformation of information. The empirical value of the exponent should reflect structural relationships involved in the packing of the information-processing elements within organ systems such as brains and bodies. I presented the fundamental analysis in my generally ignored theory of encephalization (Jerison, 1977). To simplify the analysis I treated cortical thickness in mammals as a constant length (depth), although I knew that its measure was related approximately to the 1/6 power of brain size or the 1/9 power of body size. I had determined those from illustrations in Kappers, Huber & Crosby (1936). Here are a few more facts.

I took cortical thickness as constant because it very nearly is. Mouse neocortex averages about 0.5 mm in thickness, whereas human neocortex averages about 2 or 3 mm in thickness. Not much of an increase. I have never published data on the issue, since I could find none and would have to collect them myself. Schüz and I are currently working on the problem, relying on digitized brain data that are available. Taking some measurements from charts published by Rockel, Hiorns & Powel (1980) and trying to be statistically correct by avoiding anything to bias the measures, I assembled the data for Figure 2. It is clear that neocortical thickness is not constant among species. Its relationship to brain size across species appears to be relatively orderly.

Since there is a substantive issue about the value of an empirical allometric exponent, let me free-associate about the correction required for my 1977 theory of encephalization. The theory was based on the idea that an equation relating brain size (a three-dimensional volume) to body size (another three-dimensional volume) had to be dimensionally balanced in Bridgman's sense. After a bit of analysis I presented my concluding theoretical statement:

$$E = 0.1 \, mP^{2/3} + A \tag{1}$$

The units are in the centimeter–gram–second system. E and P are brain and body size (grams or milliliters), m is a dimensionless constant, and to balance the equation, I pointed out that the multiplier 0.1 was a depth in centimeters, i.e. 1 mm. The two sides of the equation are then balanced.

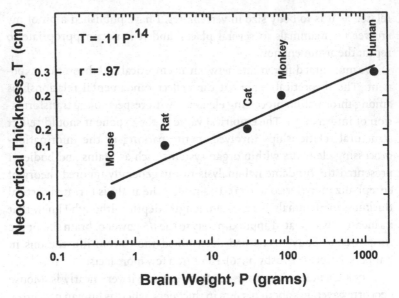

Fig. 2. Neocortical thickness as a function of brain size in five species of mammals. Measured from graph on motor cortex in Rockel *et al.*, 1980.

One point, of course, is that the exponent 2/3 reduces the dimensionality of the body to that of a two-dimensional sheet of 0-thickness. I wrote that the depth of 0.1 cm could represent the depth of neocortex, which is of that order of magnitude in living mammals. *A* was an added amount of brain tissue, a three-dimensional term in grams or millileters, and represented the amount of encephalization in a species.

The 'mistake' in Eq. (1) is in having neocortical depth as constant. To be represented by the actual depth of the neocortex, we need the kind of information presented in Figure 2, and we have to remember that the right-hand side of the equation has to be exactly three-dimensional for the equation to be balanced.

You can do the numbers yourselves. The data of Figure 2 are needed only to clarify the dimensionality of the multiplier, and we should also remember that Figure 2 is only an *ad hoc* representation of a 'true' relationship. To make things a bit easier, we can begin by replacing the 0.14 exponent with 1/6 (=0.167), implying a relationship to the depth dimension (the square root of the depth as the dimension that is the cube root of the volume, whatever that suggests). The physical source of the right-hand side of the equation is body size, hence the suggestion from Figure 2 has to be converted into something that affects the dimensionality of the measure of body size. A reasonable way to handle that is to consider brain size as a theoretical function of the 2/3 power of body size, i.e. that it is proportional to the area of a map of the information spread over a kind of body surface. The multiplier would then have a dimension of $(P2/3)(P1/6)$, or $(P1/9)$. (Dimensional analysis would replace P with $L3$, to indicate that the operations are on the dimensions.) The expected empirical exponent if one measured body size in a regression analysis of brain-body relations is therefore $(2/3) + (1/9)$, or 0.78. In other words, if the dimensional approach is correct we should expect a regression analysis to show brain size as approximately a function of the 0.78, or 3/4 power of body size whereas the fundamental allometric relationship for the system would still be given by terms involving the 2/3 exponent to convert volumes to surfaces.

$$E = m\ (P1/9)P2/3 + A \tag{2}$$

The term $(P1/9)$ represents a dimensional transformation of the depth term, m is no longer dimensionless; its dimension would bring the dimensionality of the right side of the equation to 3. The term A remains a three-dimensional term, the residual encephalization. For the 'average' mammal it has a value of 0 and disappears in the regression equation.

I am doing no more than pointing out the direction I would take to try to resolve this problem, and mine is not a pretty solution. To require a fractional dimension for the multiplier is the sort of thing that fractal geometry might handle but not the Bridgman physics that I prefer. The approach reported by West and colleagues (1997) may be relevant.

Although it is incomplete, my statement supports theorizing about brain size with the idea that the brain works as a mapping machine. For the theory, the map is two-dimensional. However, the empirical map to which the theory refers is a sheet of cells (neurons) with some thickness. When the extent of the mapping is determined from a measure of body size, as it is in allometric analysis, one of the issues is to understand departures from theoretical expectations about a mapping system. From this cursory review it seems to me that the appearance of a 3/4 exponent in empirical regression studies is pretty much what one would anticipate if the fundamental activity is a mapping but that the physical map that is generated by the brain, though thin, does have a thickness, and that thickness is related to brain size. The thickness relationship must be determined empirically, as in the analysis I offer in Figure 2. It is this that

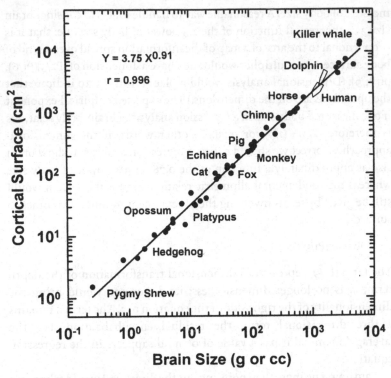

Fig. 3. Cortical surface area as a function of brain size in fifty species of mammals, including orders Monotremata, Marsupialia, Artiodactyla, Carnivora (including pinnipeds), Cetacea, Perissodactyla, Primates, and Xenarthra. Minimum convex polygons enclose individual human (N = 20) and dolphin (*Tursiops truncatus*, N = 13) data and indicate within-species variability. (From Jerison, 1991b, by permission.)

affects the dimensional relationships that can be inferred from regression equations and allometric exponents.

Uniformities and diversity

In recent years, my favorite graph has been Figure 3, which is based on data from Brodmann (1913), Elias & Schwartz (1971), Ridgway (1981) and Ridgway & Brownson (1984). I use it to argue that brain size is a statistic that estimates the total neural information processing capacity in a mammalian species. The argument can be developed in several ways, but the simplest is based on the Rockel *et al.* (1980) report that excepting the visual cortex of anthropoid primates, the number of neurons under a measured area of cortical surface is constant among species. The report was based on only five species. A more relevant datum is from Schüz & Demianenko (1995) who counted the number of synapses in neocortex of hedgehog and squirrel monkey. Consistent with an old speculation of mine (Jerison, 1973, p. 70), they found that the number of synapses per unit neocortical volume was constant in the two brains. As a first approximation, cortical volume is estimated from brain size independent of species (Jerison, 1991b), from which one can infer that the number of neocortical synapses in a mammalian brain is estimated by brain size. All of these measurements are worth reexamination and refinement, and given my enjoyment of Figure 3, I especially appreciated the critical review of the anatomical issues in Preuss's chapter, which can temper my enthusiasm. On the other hand I would hope that anatomists concerned with these issues show more concern with the uniformities in their data when they compare species. One expects them to emphasize the diversities.

We are unlikely to find a more diverse sample of species than in Figure 3, but the measurement of cortical surface area has been chancy in the past. With the advent of computer graphics applied to imaging the brain, the measurements can be redone, and the data for these are presently available in computerized databases (e.g., at http://www.neurophys.wisc.edu/brain/, on the internet as this volume goes to press). The uncertainty about Figure 3 is the apparent irrelevance of gyrencephaly. Smooth and convoluted brains are included, and a single equation fits all of the species.

It is helpful to debate problems of uniformity versus diversity as Preuss raised them in his chapter, but I think that it is really a matter of style and emphasis. There is no real conflict. There are uniform features in neural organization and important differences as well. The danger in overemphasizing one or the other is that we can miss important issues. My impression has been that anatomists tend to emphasize diversity whereas evolutionists look for uniformities. The uniformities serve as benchmarks of a sort, to which diversity is referred.

As a historical aside, I think that Karl Lashley's reputation as a neurobiologist suffered from his report with George Clark (Lashley & Clark, 1946) in which he challenged the ability of anatomists to use cytoarchitectonic data as available then for the parcellization of cortical functional areas. It challenged the validity of classical cytoarchitectonic studies. I think that there was almost universal disapproval of the conclusion of Lashley & Clark among anatomists and fairly general approval among physiologists and psychologists working with the same material. But I also think that some of the rejection of Lashley's concept of mass action was related to the sense that he and Clark had gone too far in their criticisms, and that, in fct, cytoarchitectonics provide valid criteria.

On dolphin cytoarchitectonics, it is hard to imagine a mammal operating without a layer 4 in its neocortex, but to my knowledge there is no debate that this layer is effectively absent in the cetacean brain, as Preuss reports. But there must be thalamic relays in the dolphin neocortex that are involved with neurons in layer 4 in land mammals, so the question may simply be to discover where the neurons are hiding in the dolphin's brain.

To complete this aside, I would add that Lashley's mass action, which was thought of as opposed to a strict localization-of-function view of the brain, may be more correct than the views of localizationists, at least as the problem is presently understood. It is very likely a question of which functions are being looked at. More than a half century ago Lashley himself provided some of the foundation for our understanding of localized visual function, although we now understand the issues much more adequately (Zeki, 1993). But broad cognitive functions may indeed be controlled by so broadly distributed a system that a kind of mass action would be the best description, and the functions would be difficult to localize. This may have been true for Lashley's rats running in their mazes, in which the performance deficit following brain lesions was correlated with the size of the lesion rather than its locus in the brain. One thinks of the brain's cognitive control systems as working as distributed systems in which the activity may be spread through broad regions (Goldman-Rakic, 1988). There is, nevertheless, a continuing search for foci of activity, which is a localization of a sort.

The issue is not dead. It arose in a paper by Duncan and his associates (Duncan *et al.*, 2000), which I saw as I began work on this essay. They reported the localization of intelligence (at least the *g* factor) in the human brain as focal frontal lobe activation in human subjects when performing high-*g* tasks. Controversy is not dead either as one can read in the critique in an unusual review of the paper by Sternberg (2000), one of the leading students of studies of human intelligence.

I should present an additional caveat. The work by Duncan and his colleagues involved the measurements of PET (Positron Emission Tomography) scans in people during mental work and looking at the pattern of activation. They found 'localization' in the frontal lobes. The issue can be, what does one mean by localization? The size of the activated areas was of the order of several square centimeters, which would include perhaps 100 million neurons in the activated region of each frontal lobe. That is hardly a precisely localized control. Their point was that the control was not scattered throughout the brain. But who would expect scattered activation in this kind of study? It is quite comparable to recognizing visual system activation focused in visual cortex, or activity in motor cortex associated with voluntary movement. We should not think it necessary to contrast a localization view with a distributed-system view. Both are probably correct, depending on what one is looking for.

Perhaps even more important for the analysis of the evolution of the brain, in particular for an understanding of unique features in human brain evolution, is that one can make PET scans and fMRI (functional magnetic resonance imagery) scans in animals as well as humans. Such research is new and not easy to do. Animals have to be well trained to sit through the restraints required for scanning while performing appropriate mental work. The University of Georgia Language Research Center (represented here by Professor Gibson and Professor Rumbaugh), famous for their work on language-like behavior in bonobos (*Pan paniscus*), has reported preliminary results of such work (Rilling *et al.*, 1999) in which they mapped PET (positron emission tomography) scan data onto pictured brains of chimpanzees and humans working on experimental language-related problems. Although the areas lit up in the two species were somewhat different, the total amount of activity appeared to be similar in the two species and it clearly reflected the brain's role in conscious experience in the subjects of the study. The tentative conclusions reported thus far suggests that the language of the chimpanzee is organized neurally in different ways from human language.

To return to the manifest diversity of neural organization and the anomalous histology of the cetacean brain, I recognize that this remains an unresolved puzzle. There was no dolphin brain in the Rockel *et al.* report on which Figure 2 is based, and there is no question that had a datum been available it would have been an unusual outlier. But in a large enough sample of species it would have had little effect on the overall analysis of the utility of brain size as a statistic that estimated mammalian neural information processing capacity. When appropriate, I have cited Garey & Leuba (1986) on dolphins, since they reported that dolphins had about 60 percent as many neurons per unit cortical surface area compared to the land mammal species in Rockel *et al.*

Just as we can be surprised but not overwhelmed by how much more extensive the surface area of the dolphin brain is than that of the human brain, we are equally surprised by its thin population of neurons. One can note from Figure 3 that although dolphins have much thinner cortices, their cortex is half again as extensive as the human cerebral cortex. (We can also learn how to think about log-units from the graph, since the dolphin polygon is only slightly displaced from the regression line.) These opposite trends, which are examples of the diversity in quantitative measures of mammalian brains, pretty much balance one another. When these are combined they support the simple measure of brain size to characterize the overall information-processing capacity of both the human and the dolphin brain as being about the same.

Does this mean that dolphins are as smart as we are? I suppose that depends on what one means by smart. But it is a nonsense question. It should be obvious that all species use their processing capacity in species-typical ways. The analytic problem is to determine what it is that dolphins do that encumbers so much processing capacity. The approach points one to selecting species for behavioral studies, and for seeking examples of behavior that are likely to require a lot of neural information-processing capacity. It was the unusual encephalization of dolphins that led me to speculations about the ways the very large amounts of processing capacity might be used to support unusual cognitive processes (Jerison, 1986). We continue to receive reports about the unusual capacities of cetaceans, and their use of auditory information, sometimes in more complex ways than we humans can (Janik, 2000; Tyack, 2000).

The uniformities that we find, such as that represented by Figure 3, tell us what we can expect, but the diversities point us to exceptions. A major diversity within the mammals, for example, is with respect to encephalization. Anthropoid primates as a group are about twice as encephalized as other mammals, that is, they have about two or three times as much brain for a given body size. A 50 kg wolf (*Canis lupus*) has about a 150 g brain; a chimpanzee weighing about the same may have a 400 g brain. A kangaroo with the same body weight may have a 60 g brain.

Fossil brains

Having taken so much space to discuss dolphin brains, it is time to introduce the fossil record of the brain for an unusual speculation that I would like to offer. We know that dolphins have big brains, and in my 'big book' I was able to report that the cetacean brain has always been big as mammal brains go (Jerison, 1973, chapter 15). There is a problem with their watery environment and the lack of selection pressures to keep their bodies small, hence we are not surprised by the body size of very large whales. That was my original reason for excluding them from my first search for a 'true' allometric equation. There is a singular fact about the evolutionary history of cetaceans that may be related to their having evolved very large brains. I want to present that, as a teaser about how clues may appear in the fossil record. It is not convincing, just suggestive. There is a lot more from the record of fossil brains, which I will not trouble you with here.

The present consensus is that cetaceans are most closely related to living artiodactyls, and that their ancestors were early Eocene archaic ungulates. We have data on a member of the ancestral group, the middle Eocene Mesonyx obtucidens, which lived about 50 million years ago and was a contemporary and close relative of the earliest whales. We have illustrations of its brain (Radinsky, 1976), which was surprisingly modern in appearance. In body configuration it was not at all like any living ungulate or any marine mammals for that matter; it might have passed for a small bear or wolf (see Savage & Long, 1986). Most unusual was the extent to which it was neocorticalized, more than any of its contemporaries except, perhaps, the early primates.

Figure 4 is one of the graphs that I have published before on the fossil evidence of the evolution of the neocortex (Jerison, 1991a), modified for this epilogue by identifying data contributed by Mesonyx and by a creodont Pterodon dasyuroides, a late Eocene species of about 40 million years ago. The mesonychids, though technically ungulates, may have filled a niche for carnivorous mammals, prior to the appearance of large carnivores (Carroll, 1987), and the first carnivores in that niche were the creodonts, such as Pterodon. Neither was a 'true' carnivore of the mammalian order Carnivora. Radinsky (1978) considered the Mesonyx and Pterodon as approximately equally encephalized (EQ = 0.5, approximately), which is about half as much as living true carnivores of the order Carnivora. With the exception of the primates, middle Eocene mammals were less encephalized than Mesonyx; typical values of EQ were about 0.3.

Figure 4 graphs data derived from two-dimensional lateral projections of the brains of 35 fossil and 24 living species of carnivores and ungulates. The sample covers the last 60 million years of mammalian

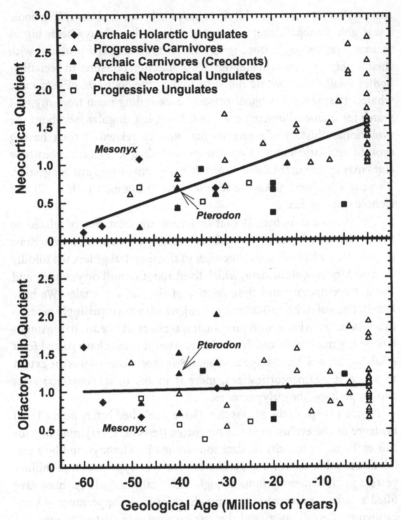

Fig. 4. Top: change in relative neocortical surface area (neocortical quotient) as a function of geological age. 'Progressive' change noted here (positive slope of regression line) indicates increased neocorticalization over time. Each point is a species. Bottom: absence of change in relative surface area of the olfactory bulbs as a function of geological age. (From Jerison, 1991b, by permission.)

history. A lateral projection of the brain of a species in this sample shows a clear rhinal fissure, and neocortex is forebrain dorsal to that fissure. In the same projection one has a view of the olfactory bulbs, and I could analyze the evolution of the peripheral olfactory apparatus in the same way as that of neocortex.

The analysis was comparable to that of encephalization, determining an expected size of either the neocortex or the olfactory bulbs from the regression of these measures against body size, estimated from the height of the foramen magnum. These enabled me to calculate the neocortical and olfactory bulb quotients graphed in Figure 4. Additional details on the procedure are in Jerison (1990).

The main inferences from Figure 4 are about neocorticalization. Secondary inferences are methodological, that the method was good enough to distinguish between the neocortical system, which was evolving progressively during the Cenozoic era, and the peripheral olfactory system, which was at a steady state during those 60 million years. Presenting data on the evolution of the olfactory bulbs, based on the same data set, is essentially evidence on the adequacy of the method, namely that it could distinguish between evolutionary progress and evolutionary stasis. This graph is presently the only quantitative evidence from the fossil record that neocortex increased in relative size when the mammals evolved, i.e. that neocorticalization was a fact of mammalian evolution.

A less certain, though statistically significant, conclusion from the graph is that progressive species as defined by extinction data may have enjoyed their selective advantage because of the enlarged neocortex. The regression line has more progressive species above the regression line and fewer archaic species above the line than would be expected by chance.

I am accustomed to data on brain morphometrics that are as orderly as the surface–volume relationship shown in Figure 3. Typical correlations are greater than 0.98. The product–moment correlation coefficient for the neocortex vs. age relationship in Figure 4 is 0.69, significantly different from 0 ($N = 59$), but there seemed to me to be quite a bit of scatter about the regression line. This may reflect a true diversity within this sample, but I suspect that some of the scatter is simply a failure of the two-dimensional projection to assess an effect that is, in fact, three-dimensional. In the next section I describe my current work on three-dimensional (3-D) imagery, which includes the reanalysis of the same endocasts, the same fossil brains. It should be possible then to measure the actual exposed surface area of the neocortex.

There is more to be inferred from Figure 4. As an early Eocene mammal, Mesonyx was obviously unusual in brain development. This is evident in the appearance of the brain (see Radinsky, 1976). A measurable criterion is its size, and this fossil brain was significantly larger than that of its contemporaries, with significantly more neocortex.

As major groups of animals competing for the available niches of their time, the mesonychids (Mesonyx and its relatives) were ungulates within a carnivore's niche. As a group they were probably replaced by a carnivorous order, the Creodonta, and the earliest true carnivores (order Carnivora) which were smaller in body size at that time. Did the brain have a role in the replacement? Figure 4 says no, at least for the mesonychid-to-creodont transition. The representatives of the two orders in Figure 4 were similar both in brain size and body size. The Mesonyx brain was about 80 ml and that of Pterodon about 60 ml. They weighed about 38 and 27 kg, respectively (Radinsky, 1978).

Interestingly, Figure 4 is affirmative on the transition that eventually occurred between the creodonts and true carnivores, the transition indicated as from archaic to progressive carnivores. The second transition is difficult to ascertain from inspection of the endocast, and as experienced a student as Len Radinsky argued against the suggestion that brain size could have been an element in the success of the true carnivores. The quantitative data of Figure 4, however, favor a role for encephalization. In the graph the progressive species are distinguished from the archaic species. Although the numbers are low, by conventional statistical criteria the probability that it was a random thing for the archaic species to fall below the regression line while the progressive carnivores were above it, is less than 5 per cent. In short, statisticians might say that the difference was significant beyond the 0.05 level. (If a species is a member of an order that is entirely extinct it is defined as archaic, whereas members of surviving orders are progressive. It is a matter of survival not modernity.)

Now for the conjecture. It is a bit of a stretch, but if the determinants of brain size in the mesonychids were similar to those of the earliest whales, then they may have been operative in both groups. Cetacean encephalization may have a history as ancient as that of the primates. The earliest true primates, relatives of living tarsiers, were the most encephalized mammals of their time (Jerison, 1979), and there may be some genetic features that evolved in the earliest anthropoids, retained through the rest of anthropoid evolution, that support instructions for relative brain enlargement. The Eocene primates, the Eocene mesonychids and the earliest

whales, were contemporaries. Although it is not presently possible to gen-
eralize in the same way about cetaceans, or about the mesonychids, the
extent of their encephalization relative to other mammals of their time is
relatively easy to establish and it would provide an additional element for
our knowledge of the history of encephalization.

Measurement and high and low technology

I don't want to outstay my welcome, but I have two more items to present
about where we go from here. Some are based on my own research and
others on my ability to speculate. You can appreciate the first, my plans
for 3-D imaging, by inspecting Figure 4. I was surprised when I made the
measurements that two-dimensional projections of the extent of neocortex compared to other parts of the brain would yield as clear a picture as
they do. The projection, after all, is a profile of the brain. It cannot show
curvature. The analysis worked adequately for neocortex, because in the
species in which I made the measurements none of the neocortex was
hidden except that buried in the folds of the convolutions. And those
hidden ones will never be seen in fossils, because we are dealing with
rocks not with brains. Fossil brains are endocasts, not brains, and they
merely mirror what is molded by the cranial cavity.

If we can make 3-D images, however, the data would not be distorted
by the fact that brains that differ in overall size may also differ in the
extent to which the external surface is visible in a lateral view. When I first
analyzed the data I tried to include measurements on 'paleocortex' or 'old
brain', that is, cortex below the rhinal fissure. It was immediately evident
that much of this part of the brain is not visible in a 2-D projection; it is on
the ventral surface of the endocast, and it curves around differently in different brains. From the time that I recognized that data on surface area
measures would be useful I sought a way to make the measurements.
With the advent of computer imaging methodology the problem has
been solved and has become simple if one can scan the endocast.

Figure 5 is one of the first scans that I made, of Pterodon, the creodont
mentioned earlier. The particular endocast with which I worked had
olfactory bulbs missing, but you will see the information that is available
from one of these 'virtual' fossil brains. I leave it to you to identify
significant fissures, and I have resisted the temptation to point to the
rhinal fissure, which is clearly visible in the skeleton frame at the bottom
of the illustration, though it is less obvious in the rendered version at the

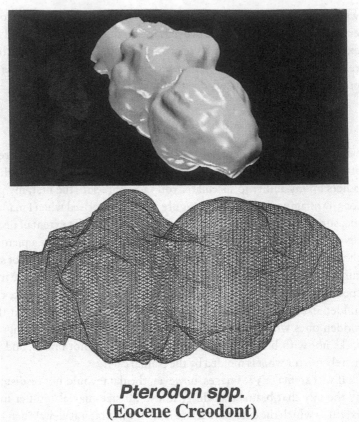

Pterodon spp.
(Eocene Creodont)

Fig. 5. A 3-D scan of the fossil 'brain' (endocranial cast) of *Pterodon dasyuroides*. 'Wire diagram' generated by the scanning device below, rendered illlustration (filling the gaps and smoothing the wire diagram) above.

top. In scans like these one can mark a region for measurement and determine surface and volume measures almost instantaneously. My present plan is to generate a graph like Figure 4 but with data based on virtual endocasts. The procedure could also eliminate much of the uncertainty with respect to body size.

A major benefit of the computerized procedure is that one will be able to make the measurements on more species, in particular on primate brains. We have excellent endocasts for the earliest of these, the lower Eocene *Tetonius*. The fossil brain was relatively large, almost as encephalized as average living mammals and about half as encephalized as living tarsier-like prosimians. Until the advent of computer imaging, it has been impossible to include it or any other primate in the analysis presented in Figure 4, because the rhinal fissure is obscured by the curvature of the temporal lobe. With a virtual endocast one can 'paint' the entire neocortical surface that can be read from the endocast in three-dimensions, and in that way perform the analysis in a wider range of species. Carnivores and ungulates were selected for the sample, because only in these species could I gather enough data to answer the questions about neocortical evolution.

If there is enough information to reconstruct a 'virtual' body, then its volume is equally easy to measure. This would be an improvement over the procedure based on the size of the foramen magnum as a surrogate for body size. (I should add that the size of the medulla is an excellent surrogate; the difficulty with the foramen magnum is that it includes the great cistern, the size of which is proportional to brain size and is correlated with encephalization. I have guessed that this enlargement of the foramen magnum reflects the utility of providing sacks of blood that can cushion the medulla from shocks incurred by the movement of larger brains within the cranial cavity as an animal runs or leaps.) The procedure of creating virtual equivalents of the body and its parts using 3-D imagery and computer graphics is an enormous contribution to the study of vertebrate morphology and biomechanics. Within a few years procedures for working in this way should be routine.

The low technology is the familiar technology: weighing whole brains, measuring the area of sections through the brain and so forth. It continues to be the way much of our gross data are generated. For comparative studies of brain size that included the analysis of the parts of the brain, we have all been indebted to Heinz Stephan and his research group at the Max Planck Institute for Brain Research. These laborious methods can be replaced or supplemented by computerized approaches to measuring area and volume, including the measures taken from histological sections of brains from living species. For many of these it will be sufficient to use digitized images of histological slides prepared classically. The main outstanding problem with these is uncertainty about shrinkage and distortion introduced by the histological procedures.

The great contributions of analyses of brain–body relations may be in the way outliers can be identified. I have recently reviewed my data on these, updating old graphs and adding data and correcting errors.

The graph of the present situation in living vertebrates in Figure 6 includes all presently available data (Jerison, 2001). I don't think a contribution from me would be complete without such a summary. It is less neat

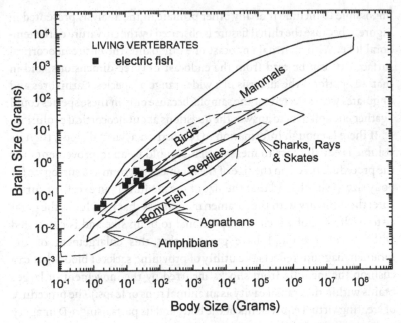

Fig. 6. Brain–body relations in 2018 living vertebrate species enclosed in minimum
   convex polygons. The samples are 647 mammals, 180 birds, 1027 bony fish, 41
   amphibians, 59 reptiles, 59 cartilaginous fish (sharks, rays, and skates), and 5
   agnathans, or jawless fish. Electric fish are Mormyriformes, unpublished data,
   courtesy of Professor Andy Bass of Cornell University. Most of the other bony
   fish data are unpublished except as in this graph, data courtesy of Professor
   Roland Bauchot of the University of Paris VII. Note that birds and mammals
   overlap one another as 'higher vertebrates,' and reptiles, amphibians and fish
   overlap one another as 'lower vertebrates.' Electric fish, however, are in the
   'higher vertebrate' range of encephalization, and chondrichthyans (sharks,
   rays and skates) overlap the lower and higher vertebrate ranges.

than some I have published before, mainly because I have added more
groups than I usually show: electric fish, cartilaginous fish, and jawless
fish. Usually one summarizes such data with regression lines, but in my
view the polygons are more valid devices. The method is to draw convex
polygons about the points belonging to a group of interest. To the extent
that the polygons are distinct one distinguishes the groups from one
another, and from Figure 6 we can see the extent to which one is justified in
discussing 'lower' versus 'higher' vertebrates. The sharks and electric fish
confound the picture, but the distinction is generally easy to maintain.

The role of graphs like Figure 6 is to provide a map of brain–body space,
of brain-size opportunities that are presently realized by vertebrates. One

can add fossils to the graph, and doing that indicates that the present situation remains representative of the diversity of brain size within the vertebrates. A graph made before the Mesozoic era would have shown no birds or mammals and the range of body sizes would have been smaller, but all species would have fallen within appropriate polygons. There would have been no outliers. The most unusual specimen may have been a Carboniferous era shark, about 300 million years old, which would have been graphed in the chondrichthyan polygon, in the mammalian region. It was the first 'experiment' with encephalization in the vertebrates.

Graphs made during the Mesozoic, after the appearance of birds and mammals would have contributed points to the avian and mammalian polygons, although all would have been near the lower borders but above the other polygons. There is an exception. Some of the late Mesozoic dinosaurs, in particular the ostrich-dinosaurs (struthiomimids) were more encephalized than any living reptiles and fell in the lower part of the avian polygon. The main effect of adding dinosaurs to the data set is to expand the reptilian polygon to be more similar in body-size range to that of the living mammals. The 'mammal-like reptiles' (amniotes ancestral to the mammals, including synapsids and therapsids) were reptilian in encephalization. Their data fall within the reptilian polygon.

Finally most living electric fish (Mormyriformes) are large brained, falling within the living mammal polygon. Their brains are enlarged because of an expanded cerebellum rather than forebrain. Cenozoic graphs would show the mammals gradually filling the polygons by expanding upward with more encephalized species appearing. By about 20 million years ago it probably would look much as it does today, because the cetaceans would have been diverse enough, and encephalized enough to provide species for the upper border of the mammalian polygon. Early hominids would be with living pongids, upper class, as it were, but not the largest brained animals of their time. Only within the past million years did hominids expand to approximately their present grade of encephalization and they definitely achieved it only with the advent of *Homo sapiens* and the neandertals, less than a half-million years ago.

Figure 6 is a chart for future research. It points to species about which we need to know more, in particular about their activities in which there could have been selection for increased information-processing capacity. We can guess that this might explain the expanded brain in electric fish, though we might be hard put to explain why handling information from electric organs should be more greedy a task relative to brain control than, say, the handling of visual information by frogs or any of the many unusual adaptations in fish revealed by ethological research.

We should be impressed by the data on cartilaginous fish. It is one of the benefits of the analysis that it points one to comparisons that might not otherwise be considered. One does not know how to measure or define animal intelligence behaviorally, but from their encephalization, it is clear that sharks and their relatives deserve much closer scrutiny by ethologists and comparative psychologists than they have received. There are additional comparisons that should be made. The approach would single out parrots as birds to study, because they are among the most encephalized of living birds, justifying Pepperberge's (1994) efforts. The only other living avian group that is in their range are the corvids, and the common crow is surely worth a close look. Among the cartilaginous fish, the most encephalized appears to be the manta ray (*Manta birostris*), and we know almost nothing about the normal behavior of this gentle giant, but other shark species are also unusually encephalized (Northcutt, 1989). My approach does not, and, as I indicate elsewhere, (Jerison, in press) cannot in principle explain the details of the behavior of a species, but it is clearly useful in helping us choose the species to study. It is a challenge to ethologists and comparative psychologists to analyze the utility of the extra neural processing performed by that system. The analogy might be to the enlarged inferior colliculi in bats specialized for echolocation, since these structures are especially implicated in the analysis. Of course, the forebrain in these bats is not unusually enlarged, but it is specialized for auditory analysis (Grinnell, 1995).

Neurogenetics?

The ignorance that I can bring to molecular biology and neurogenetics is great enough that I can speculate with ease. A major issue, which my laboratory work has never addressed though my speculations have, is what kind of genetic programs will effect the kinds of brain evolution that is evident from the fossil record. I have, of course, been impressed as we all must be by the discovery of common genetic systems in humans and fruitflies for differentiating the head region of an embryo (see Deacon, 1997, for a review). It is one of the finest biological uniformities that one can cite. An equally difficult problem that I can only state, but to the solution of which I have nothing to suggest, is the translation of genetic programs into phenotypic structures and functions. I can imagine part of a neural network to be prescribed in the genetic code, but I cannot imagine that enough code can be squeezed on to the chromosomes to prescribe a full network. Here is one example that I gave, to show how to convert a chimpanzee into a person.

It may be helpful to consider the way the genetic information might be encoded. A possible genetic blueprint of a species might include code for the following instruction to regulate growth in a primordial nerve cell: 'perform 32 cell divisions and then stop.' If that instruction were followed and no cells died, 4 294 967 296 nerve cells would be produced. Imagine now a major (but small) mutation, which changed '32' to '34'. This small change would yield 17 179 869 184 nerve cells. Were these fated to be neo-cortical neurons the mutation would be about right to distinguish the number of neurons in the brain of a chimpanzee from that in a human (Pakkenberg & Gundersen, 1997). In this example, the code may seem overly simple, but it is that kind of code that can be written, and it is a code that would have a very great morphometric effect. Instructions that are significantly more complex may be beyond the capacity of genes to encode information. (Jerison, 2000, p. 218)

In this example there is nothing about localized functions, or the creation of specialized systems such as the language system of the brain. I have shared the example with a few geneticists, and I have one testimonial that it is not a crazy way to ask the questions. I sent the paragraph as an e-mail to M. V. Olson (cf. Olson, 1999) who replied that he had not published a complete statement of his analysis to describe how the necessary counting of the sort that I asked about could be done. He added the following: 'I agree entirely that it is likely that "simple" genetic changes of the type hypothesized will account for the really major differences between chimps and humans. My molecular point has been that such changes are likely to involve loss of regulation rather more subtle genetic innovations. We know that the regulatory systems that govern development are full of nearly redundant and nearly dispensable features. Hence, one could get the effect envisioned just by dropping one of the regulatory subsystems that limits the number of cell divisions in a particular chimp cell lineage' (Olson, personal communication).

Conclusions

Scattered through this essay I have made a number of suggestions about ways for the future. One obvious requirement is for more and better data, suitably prepared for analysis. We need data on species currently under-represented in our broad analysis of vertebrate brain evolution. We are too reliant on Stephan's work and those of his colleagues for background on the diversity of mammalian brains, and the new data are insufficiently quantifies to be added to his set. One of the delightful features of Barbara Finlay's contributions has been the way the set has been expanded.

It is a fairly obvious prescription to announce that 'more research is needed' even if we slip into the passive voice to make this banal statement seem more profound. Yet that is clearly what we need. The substantive chapters in this book have pointed the way, and we need only follow.

References

Bauchot, R. (1963). L'architechtonique comparée qualitative et quantitative du diencéphale des insectivores. *Mammalia*, 27(Suppl. 1), 1–400.

Brandt, A. (1867). Sur le rapport du poids du cerveau à celui du corps chez différents animaux. *Bulletin du Société impériale Naturalistes Moscou*, 40(III–IV), 525–543.

Bridgman, P.W. (1959). *Dimensional Analysis*. New Haven, Conn: Yale University Press.

Brodmann, K. (1913). Neue Forschungsergebnisse der Grosshirnrindenanatomie mit besonderer Berucksichtung anthropologischer Fragen. *Verhandlungen des 85ste Versammlung Deutscher Naturforscher und Aerzte in Wien*, pp. 200–240.

Butler, A.B. & Hodos, W. (1996). *Comparative Vertebrate Neuroanatomy*. New York: Wiley Liss.

Carroll, R.L. (1987). *Vertebrate Paleontology and Evolution*. New York: Freeman.

Deacon, T.W. (1997). *The Symbolic Species: The Co-evolution of Language and the Brain*. New York: W. W. Norton.

Duncan, J., Seitz, R.J. Kolodny, J., Bor, D., Herzog, H., Ahmed, A., Newell, F.N. & Emslie, H. (2000). A neural basis for general intelligence. *Science*, 289, 457–460.

Edinger, T. (1929). Die fossilen Gehirne. *Ergeb. Anat. Entwicklungsgesch*, 28, 249.

Edinger, T. (1962). Anthropocentric misconceptions in paleoneurology. *Proceedings of the Rudolf Virchow Medical Society of the City of New York*, 19 56–107.

Edinger, T. (1975). Paleoneurology, 1804–1966: An annotated bibliography. *Advances in Anatomy, Embryology and Cell Biology*, 49, 12–258.

Elias, H. & Schwartz, D. (1971). Cerebro-cortical surface areas, volumes, lengths of gyri and their interdependence in mammals, including man. *Zeitschrift für Saugetierkunde*, 36, 147–163.

Garey, L.J. & Leuba, G. (1986). A quantitative study of neuronal and glial numerical density in the visual cortex of the bottlenose dolphin: evidence for a specialized subarea and changes with age. *Journal of Comparative Neurology*, 247, 491–496.

Goldman-Rakic, P.S. (1988). Topography of cognition: parallel distributed networks in primate association cortex. *Annual Review of Neurosciences*, 11, 137–166.

Grinnell, A.D. (1995). Hearing in bats: an overview. In Fay, R.R. & Popper, A.M. (eds.) *Hearing by Bats*, pp. 1–36. Heidelberg: Springer Verlag.

Halstead, W.C. (1947). *Brain and Intelligence: A Quantitative Study of the Frontal Lobes*. Chicago: University of Chicago Press.

Harvey, P.H. & Pagel, M.D. (1991). *The Comparative Method in Evolutionary Biology*. Oxford, New York, Tokyo: Oxford University Press.

Hassler, R., & Stephan, H. (eds.) (1966). *Evolution of the Forebrain*. Stuttgart: Thieme.

Huxley, J.S. (1932). *Problems of Relative Growth*. London: Allen & Unwin.

Janik, V.M. (2000). Whistle matching in wild bottlenose dolphins (*Tursiops truncatus*). *Science*, **289**, 1355–1357.

Jerison, H.J. (1955). Brain to body ratios and the evolution of intelligence. *Science*, **121**, 447–449.

Jerison, H.J. (1973). *Evolution of the Brain and Intelligence*. New York: Academic Press.

Jerison, H.J. (1977). The theory of encephalization. *Annals of the New York Academy of Sciences*, **299**, 146–160.

Jerison, H.J. (1979). Brain, body, and encephalization in early primates. *Journal of Human Evolution*, **8**, 615–635.

Jerison, H.J. (1986). The perceptual worlds of dolphins. In Schusterman, R.J., Thomas, J., & Wood, F.G. (eds.) *Dolphin Cognition and Behavior: a Comparative Approach*, pp. 141–166. Hillsdale, N.J.: Erlbaum.

Jerison, H.J. (1990). Fossil evidence on the evolution of the neocortex. In Jones, E.G. & Peters, A. (eds.) *Cerebral Cortex*, Vol. 8A, 285–309. New York: Plenum.

Jerison, H.J. (1991a). Fossil brains and the evolution of the neocortex. In Finlay, B., Innocenti, G. & Scheich, H. (eds.) *The Neocortex: Ontogeny and Phylogeny*, pp. 5–42. New York: Plenum Press.

Jerison, H.J. (1991b). *Brain Size and the Evolution of Mind: 59th James Arthur Lecture on the Evolution of the Human Brain*. New York: American Museum of Natural History.

Jerison, H.J. (2000). Evolution of intelligence. In Sternberg, R.J. (ed.) *Handbook of Human Intelligence*, 2nd edn, pp. 216–244. Cambridge: Cambridge University Press.

Jerison, H.J. (2001). The evolution of neural and behavioral complexity. In Roth, G. & Wulliman, M.F. (eds.) *Cognitive Neuroscience*. New York: Wiley.

Jerison, H.J. (in press). On theory in comparative psychology. In Sternberg, R.J. & Kaufman, J. (eds.) *The Evolution of Intelligence*, Mahwah, NJ: Lawrence Erlbaum Associates.

Kohring, R. & Kreft, G. (eds.) (in press). *Tilly Edinger: Leben einer juedischen Wissenschaftlerin*. [Tilly Edinger: The life of a female Jewish Scientist.] Senckenberg-Buch No. 73. Frankfurt/Main.

Lashley, K.S. (1949). Persistent problems in the evolution of mind. *Quarterly Review of Biology*, **24**, 28–42.

Lashley, K.S. & Clark, G. (1946). The cytoarchitecture of the cerebral cortex of Ateles: a critical examination of architectonic studies. *Journal of Comparative Neurology*, **85**, 223–306.

Martin, R.D. (1990). *Primate Origins and Evolution: A Phylogenetic Reconstruction*. London: Chapman & Hall.

McCulloch, W.S. (1965). *Embodiments of Mind*. Cambridge, MA: MIT Press.

Northcutt, R.G. (1989). Brain variation and phylogenetic trends in elasmobranch fishes. *Journal of Experimental Zoology Supplement*, **2**, 83–100.

Olson, M.V. (1999). When less is more: gene loss as an engine of evolutionary change. *American Journal of Human Genetics*, **64**, 18–23.

Pakkenberg, B. & Gundersen, H.J.G. (1997). Neocortical neuron number in humans: effect of sex and age. *Journal of Comparative Neurology*, **385**, 312–320.

Pepperberg, I.M. (1994). Vocal learning in African Grey parrots: effects of social interaction. *Auk*, **111**, 300–313

Radinsky, L. (1976). The brain of Mesonyx, a Middle Eocene mesonychid condylarth. *Fieldiana Geology*, **33**, 323–337.

Radinsky, L. (1978). Evolution of brain size in carnivores and ungulates. *American Naturalist*, **112**, 815–831.

Ridgway, S.H. (1981). Some brain morphometrics of the Bowhead whale. In Albert, T.F. (ed.) *Tissues, Structural Studies, and Other Investigations on the Biology of Endangered Whales in the Beaufort Sea. Final Report to the Bureau of Land Management, U.S. Dept. of Interior*, vol. 2, pp. 837–844, from University of Maryland, College Park, Maryland.

Ridgway, S.H. & Brownson, R.H. (1984). Relative brain sizes and cortical surfaces of odontocetes. *Acta Zoologica Fennica*, **172**, 149–152.

Rilling, J.K., Kilts, C., Williams, S., Kelley, J. Beran, M., Giroux, M., Hoffman, J.M., Savage-Rumbaugh, S. & Rumbaugh, D. (1999). Functional neuroimaging of linguistic processing in chimpanzees. *Society for Neuroscience Abstracts*, **25**(2), 2170.

Rockel, A.J., Hiorns, R.W. & Powell, T.P.S. (1980). The basic uniformity in structure of the neocortex. *Brain*, **103**, 221–244.

Savage, R.J.G. & Long, M.R. (1986). *Mammal Evolution: An Illustrated Guide*. London: British Museum (Natural History).

Schüz, A. & Demianenko, G.P. (1995). Constancy and variability in cortical structure: a study on synapses and dendritic spines in hedgehog and monkey. *Journal für Hirnforschung*, **36**, 113–122.

Snell, O. (1891). Die Abhängigkeitangigkeit des Hirngewichtes von dem Körpergewicht und den geistigen Fähigkeiten. *Arch. Psychiat. Nervenkr.* **23**, 436–446.

Stephan, H., Baron, G. & Frahm, H.D. (1991). *Insectivora: With a Stereotaxic Atlas of the Hedgehog Brain. Comparative Brain Research in Mammals*, Vol. 1. New York: Springer Verlag.

Stephan, H., Frahm, H. & Baron, G. (1981). New and revised data on volumes of brain structures in insectivores and primates. *Folio Primatologica*, **35**, 1–29.

Sternberg, R.J. (2000). The holey grail of general intelligence. *Science*, **289**, 399–401.

Theunissen, B. (1989). *Eugene Dubois and the Apeman from Java*. Dordecht, Holland: Kluwer.

Tyack, P.L. (2000). Dolphins whistle a signature tune. *Science*, **289**, 1310–1311.

von Bonin, G. (1937). Brain weight and body weight in mammals. *Journal of General Psychology*, **16**, 379–389.

von Bonin, G. (1963). *The Evolution of the Human Brain*. Chicago: University of Chicago Press.

Welker, W.I. (1990). Why does cerebral cortex fissure and fold? A review of determinants of gyri and sulci. In Jones, E.G. & Peters, A. (eds.) *Cerebral Cortex*, Vol. 8B, pp. 1–132. New York: Plenum Press.

Welker, W.I. & Campos, G.B. (1963). Physiological significance of sulci in somatic sensory cerebral cortex in mammals of the family Procyonidae. *Journal of Comparative Neurology*, **120**, 19–36.

West, G.B., Brown, J.H. & Enquist, B.J. (1997). A general model for the origin of allometric scaling laws in biology. *Science*, **276**, 122–126.

Zeki, S. (1993). *A Vision of the Brain*. London: Blackwell.

Appendix

Tilly Edinger (1897–1967) was affiliated with the Senckenberg Museum of Natural History in Frankfurt, Germany, until 1938. She had published her PhD thesis, in which she named endocranial casts of fossils as 'fossil brains' (Edinger, 1929) during her tenure at the Senckenberg. Her father, Ludwig Edinger (1855–1918) founded what is now the Max Planck Institute for Brain Research in Frankfurt. Tilly fled to the United States at about the time of Kristalnacht when Nazi hoodlums smashed windows of Jewish shops and vandalized Jewish property as part of an organized anti-Semitic campaign by Hitler's Germany. Through the efforts of leading American paleontologists, Alfred Romer and George Gaylord Simpson, she was appointed a research associate at Harvard's Museum of Comparative Zoology. I was asked to prepare this preface for her biography, which will be published in 2001: Kohring, R. & Kreft, G. (eds.) *Tilly Edinger – Leben einer juedischen Wissenschaftlerin* [*Tilly Edinger – The Life of a Jewish Woman Scientist*], Senckenberg-Buch No. 73. Frankfurt/Main.

Preface

When I dedicated my book on brain evolution (Jerison, 1973) to Tilly Edinger, I tried to convey my special intellectual debt to her in the following words:

"Among the individuals whose help and support I would like to acknowledge, I must name, first, Tilly Edinger, to whom this book is dedicated. Her frequent letters, sharing with me, an experimental psychologist, the advances and retreats of vertebrate paleontology as it was concerned with the evolution of the brain, were major contributions to my education and important introductions to the data of this book. When she died shortly before I began writing, my anticipated pleasure in the work diminished because I could no longer look forward to her reactions. These, I am sure, would have combined pleasure in having data about endocasts used in unusual ways with bewilderment at some of the details of that use – as she put it to me, she never could understand logarithms and other magic." (Jerison, 1973, p. xiii)

It is a great pleasure to be able to discuss our friendship in a more personal way in this introduction to her biography.

I first met Tilly in the red-bound Memoir 25 of the "Publications of the Geological Society of America," her first major English publication, which has the unusual title, Evolution of the Horse Brain. That was in 1953 when I found the book on the shelves of the library of Antioch College, in Yellow Springs, Ohio, in the USA. The book was a revelation. I was amazed to learn that the evolutionary evidence that she presented could be read directly from the fossil record. Can I be blamed for seeking to learn more and to get to know her? I wrote her, and a few years later we met in person at the Museum of Comparative Zoology at Harvard.

Although she has been described as the daughter of a rich German Jewish family, there was no evidence of that background in the small flat in Cambridge, Massachusetts where I brought a bottle of inexpensive white wine for the light dinner that we shared at our first meeting. She often remarked on that gift later, a successful beginning for our friendship. Tilly was a gentle and kind friend, who tried very hard to appreciate the quantitative arguments that I developed to analyze the fossil brains.

To appreciate her kindness to me, one should keep in mind her deep hatred for Othniel Marsh, which I never fully understood. In many publications (e.g. Edinger, 1961) Tilly took great pains to expose what she considered the fraudulence of Marsh's claims. She was convinced that he invented the images of bird brains (Hesperornis and Ichthyornis) that he published, and that he had never prepared the specimens. I could vouch for two criticisms of Marsh, which Tilly enjoyed. First was his fantastic picture of the cerebellum of Coryphodon and second, his enlarged olfactory bulbs in one uintathere endocast that made the cast look like an enlarged rodent brain. Both of these were preparation errors. Whoever made the preparations had removed "matrix" from the cranial cavity that was, in fact, fossilized bone. Another of Marsh's "errors," as Tilly saw it, was his advocacy for an evolutionary teleology that saw brain-enlargement as one of the imperatives of vertebrate evolution. It was, therefore, certainly wrenching and difficult for her to accept my own demonstrations of something close to substantiation for some of those views in my quantitative analyses, in particular of mammalian and avian brain evolution.

What I showed was that there were many instances of measurable encephalization within the lineages of birds and mammals, although I hope I successfully avoided the teleology and aristogenesis often offered then as explanations. My explanations, which Tilly could accept, was that there was some selective benefit for encephalization in some environmental niches, and that species evolving in such niches would have responded by selection for encephalization. She could appreciate this qualitative statement, though its quantitative justification puzzled her. On one occasion I remember looking at data on rodent evolution with her, in which she questioned my statements, showing me measurements of squirrel brains and bodies that seemed to be outlandish outliers compared to brain/body data in rodents and other mammals. I "taught" her by taking out a piece of log-log graph paper on which I plotted the points. These fell very close to a general mammalian regression line. It was then that she commented to me on logarithms and other magic.

Although like Tilly I am Jewish, and my wife, Irene, is a survivor of the Nazi holocaust, I remember no reference to Judaism in conversations with Tilly. It would hardly have been appropriate. Our relationship was entirely as scientists, and mine was as an admirer of her dedicated work on the fossil evidence for the evolution of the brain. When I learned more of her personal history, her major scientific and economic losses upon her exile to the United States, and when I realized that she was the daughter of the great neurologist, Ludwig

Edinger, it only added to the deep respect and love that I felt for her. Her tragic death was evidently directly related to her deafness. I was told that because she could not hear a truck's approach, she had walked into its path near the steps of the Museum of Comparative Zoology.

Index

Page numbers in *italics* refer to figures and tables